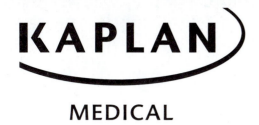

USMLE® STEP 1 Lecture Notes 2017

Biochemistry and Medical Genetics

USMLE® is a joint program of the Federation of State Medical Boards (FSMB) and the National Board of Medical Examiners (NBME), neither of which sponsors or endorses this product.

This publication is designed to provide accurate information in regard to the subject matter covered as of its publication date, with the understanding that knowledge and best practice constantly evolve. The publisher is not engaged in rendering medical, legal, accounting, or other professional service. If medical or legal advice or other expert assistance is required, the services of a competent professional should be sought. This publication is not intended for use in clinical practice or the delivery of medical care. To the fullest extent of the law, neither the Publisher nor the Editors assume any liability for any injury and/or damage to persons or property arising out of or related to any use of the material contained in this book.

© 2017 by Kaplan, Inc.

Published by Kaplan Medical, a division of Kaplan, Inc.
750 Third Avenue
New York, NY 10017

10 9 8 7 6 5 4 3 2 1

Course ISBN: 978-1-5062-0872-5

All rights reserved. The text of this publication, or any part thereof, may not be reproduced in any manner whatsoever without written permission from the publisher. This book may not be duplicated or resold, pursuant to the terms of your Kaplan Enrollment Agreement.

Retail ISBN: 978-1-5062-0835-0

Kaplan Publishing print books are available at special quantity discounts to use for sales promotions, employee premiums, or educational purposes. For more information or to purchase books, please call the Simon & Schuster special sales department at 866-506-1949.

BIOCHEMISTRY

Editor
Sam Turco, Ph.D.
Professor, Department of Biochemistry
University of Kentucky College of Medicine
Lexington, KY

MEDICAL GENETICS

Editor
Vernon Reichenbecher, Ph.D.
Professor Emeritus, Department of
Biochemistry & Molecular Biology
Marshall University School of Medicine
Huntington, WV

Contributors
Roger Lane, Ph.D.
Professor, Department of Biochemistry
University of South Alabama College of Medicine
Mobile, AL

Ryan M. Harden, M.D., M.S.
Physician, Family Medicine
Gateway Family Health Clinic, Ltd
Sandstone, MN

Assistant Professor, Department of Family Medicine and Community Health
University of Minnesota Medical School, Duluth Campus
Duluth, MN

We want to hear what you think. What do you like or not like about the Notes? Please email us at **medfeedback@kaplan.com**.

Contents

Section I: Biochemistry

Chapter 1: Nucleic Acid Structure and Organization 3

Chapter 2: DNA Replication and Repair. 17

Chapter 3: Transcription and RNA Processing. 33

Chapter 4: The Genetic Code, Mutations, and Translation. 49

Chapter 5: Regulation of Eukaryotic Gene Expression 73

Chapter 6: Genetic Strategies in Therapeutics. 83

Chapter 7: Techniques of Genetic Analysis 99

Chapter 8: Amino Acids, Proteins, and Enzymes 115

Chapter 9: Hormones 131

Chapter 10: Vitamins 145

Chapter 11: Overview of Energy Metabolism 159

Chapter 12: Glycolysis and Pyruvate Dehydrogenase 169

Chapter 13: Citric Acid Cycle and Oxidative Phosphorylation 187

Chapter 14: Glycogen, Gluconeogenesis, and the Hexose Monophosphate Shunt. 199

Chapter 15: Lipid Synthesis and Storage 217

Chapter 16: Lipid Mobilization and Catabolism 239

Chapter 17: Amino Acid Metabolism 261

Chapter 18: Purine and Pyrimidine Metabolism 287

Section II: Medical Genetics

Chapter 1: Single-Gene Disorders 303

Chapter 2: Population Genetics 333

Chapter 3: Cytogenetics 347

Chapter 4: Genetics of Common Diseases 371

Chapter 5: Recombination Frequency 379

Chapter 6: Genetic Diagnosis 389

Index 405

SECTION I

Biochemistry

Nucleic Acid Structure and Organization

Learning Objectives

❏ Explain information related to nucleotide structure and nomenclature
❏ Answer questions about nucleic acids
❏ Use knowledge of organization of DNA

CENTRAL DOGMA OF MOLECULAR BIOLOGY

An organism must be able to store and preserve its genetic information, pass that information along to future generations, and express that information as it carries out all the processes of life. The major steps involved in handling genetic information are illustrated by the central dogma of molecular biology (Figure I-1-1). Genetic information is stored in the base sequence of DNA molecules. Ultimately, during the process of gene expression, this information is used to synthesize all the proteins made by an organism. Classically, a gene is a unit of the DNA that encodes a particular protein or RNA molecule. Although this definition is now complicated by our increased appreciation of the ways in which genes may be expressed, it is still useful as a general, working definition.

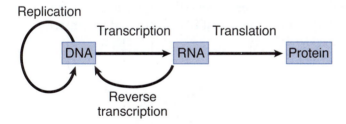

Figure I-1-1. Central Dogma of Molecular Biology

Gene Expression and DNA Replication

Gene expression and DNA replication are compared in Table I-1-1. Transcription, the first stage in gene expression, involves transfer of information found in a double-stranded DNA molecule to the base sequence of a single-stranded RNA molecule. If the RNA molecule is a messenger RNA, then the process known as translation converts the information in the RNA base sequence to the amino acid sequence of a protein.

When cells divide, each daughter cell must receive an accurate copy of the genetic information. DNA replication is the process in which each chromosome is duplicated before cell division.

Section I • Biochemistry

Table I-1-1. Comparison of Gene Expression and DNA Replication

Gene Expression	DNA Replication
Produces all the proteins an organism requires	Duplicates the chromosomes before cell division
Transcription of DNA: RNA copy of a small section of a chromosome (average size of human gene, 10^4–10^5 nucleotide pairs)	DNA copy of entire chromosome (average size of human chromosome, 10^8 nucleotide pairs)
Transcription occurs in the nucleus throughout interphase	Occurs during S phase
Translation of RNA (protein synthesis) occurs in the cytoplasm throughout the cell cycle.	Replication in nucleus

The concept of the cell cycle (Figure I-1-2) can be used to describe the timing of some of these events in a eukaryotic cell. The M phase (mitosis) is the time in which the cell divides to form two daughter cells. Interphase is the term used to describe the time between two cell divisions or mitoses. Gene expression occurs throughout all stages of interphase. Interphase is subdivided as follows:

- G_1 phase (gap 1) is a period of cellular growth preceding DNA synthesis. Cells that have stopped cycling, such as muscle and nerve cells, are said to be in a special state called G_0.

- S phase (DNA synthesis) is the period of time during which DNA replication occurs. At the end of S phase, each chromosome has doubled its DNA content and is composed of two identical sister chromatids linked at the centromere.

- G_2 phase (gap 2) is a period of cellular growth after DNA synthesis but preceding mitosis. Replicated DNA is checked for any errors before cell division.

Note

Many chemotherapeutic agents function by targeting specific phases of the cell cycle. This is a frequently tested area on the exam. Below are some of the commonly tested agents with the appropriate phase of the cell cycle they target:

- S-phase: methotrexate, 5-fluorouracil, hydroxyurea
- G2 phase: bleomycin
- M phase: paclitaxel, vincristine, vinblastine
- Non cell-cycle specific: cyclophosphamide, cisplatin

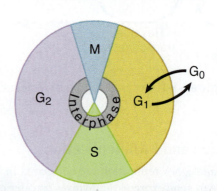

Figure I-1-2. The Eukaryotic Cell Cycle

Control of the cell cycle is accomplished at checkpoints between the various phases by strategic proteins such as cyclins and cyclin-dependent kinases. These checkpoints ensure that cells will not enter the next phase of the cycle until the molecular events in the previous cell cycle phase are concluded.

Reverse transcription, which produces DNA copies of an RNA, is more commonly associated with life cycles of retroviruses, which replicate and express their genome through a DNA intermediate (an integrated provirus). Reverse transcription also occurs to a limited extent in human cells, where it plays a role in amplifying certain highly repetitive sequences in the DNA (Chapter 7).

NUCLEOTIDE STRUCTURE AND NOMENCLATURE

Nucleic acids (DNA and RNA) are assembled from nucleotides, which consist of three components: a nitrogenous base, a five-carbon sugar (pentose), and phosphate.

Five-Carbon Sugars

Nucleic acids (as well as nucleosides and nucleotides) are classified according to the pentose they contain. If the pentose is ribose, the nucleic acid is RNA (ribonucleic acid); if the pentose is deoxyribose, the nucleic acid is DNA (deoxyribonucleic acid).

Bases

There are two types of nitrogen-containing bases commonly found in nucleotides: purines and pyrimidines (Figure I-1-3):

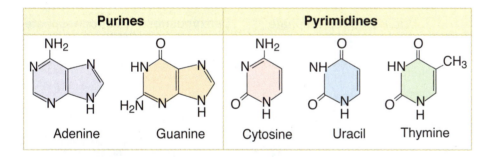

Figure I-1-3. Bases Commonly Found in Nucleic Acids

- Purines contain two rings in their structure. The two purines commonly found in nucleic acids are adenine (A) and guanine (G); both are found in DNA and RNA. Other purine metabolites, not usually found in nucleic acids, include xanthine, hypoxanthine, and uric acid.

- Pyrimidines have only one ring. Cytosine (C) is present in both DNA and RNA. Thymine (T) is usually found only in DNA, whereas uracil (U) is found only in RNA.

Nucleosides and Nucleotides

Nucleosides are formed by covalently linking a base to the number 1 carbon of a sugar (Figure I-1-4). The numbers identifying the carbons of the sugar are labeled with "primes" in nucleosides and nucleotides to distinguish them from the carbons of the purine or pyrimidine base.

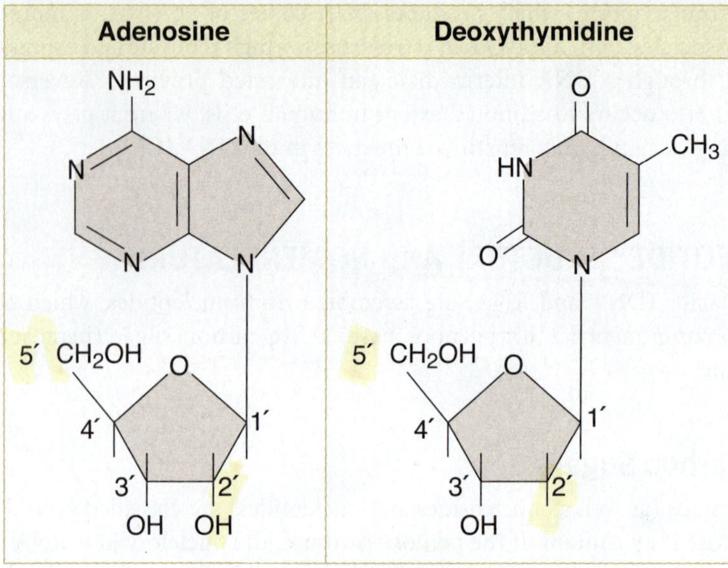

Section I • Biochemistry

Figure I-1-4. Examples of Nucleosides

Nucleotides are formed when one or more phosphate groups is attached to the 5′ carbon of a nucleoside (Figure I-1-5). Nucleoside di- and triphosphates are high-energy compounds because of the hydrolytic energy associated with the acid anhydride bonds (Figure I-1-6).

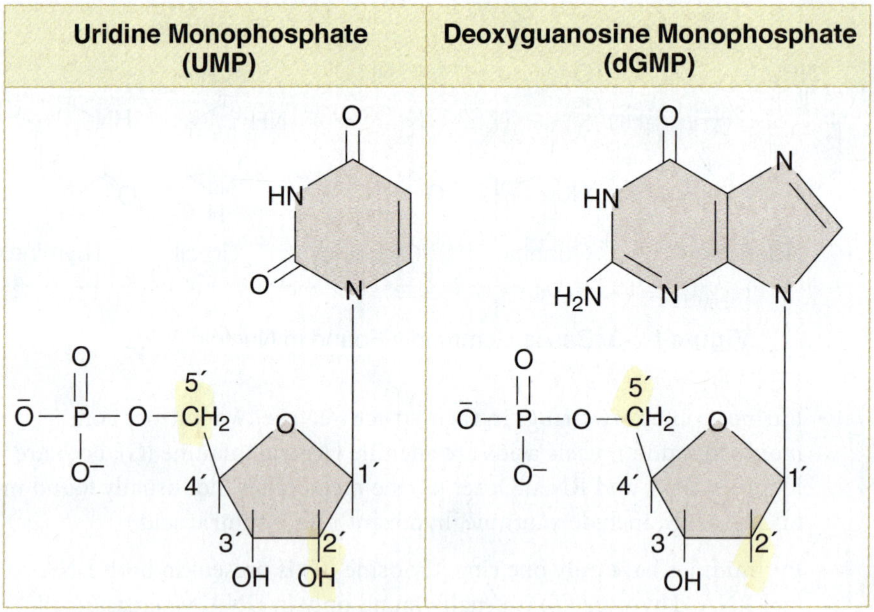

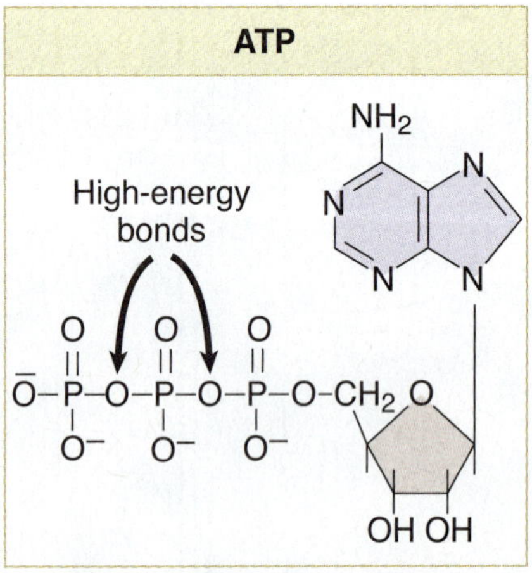

Figure I-1-6. High-Energy Bonds in a Nucleoside Triphosphate

Figure I-1-5. Examples of Nucleotides

The nomenclature for the commonly found bases, nucleosides, and nucleotides is shown in Table I-1-2. Note that the "deoxy" part of the names deoxythymidine, dTMP, etc., is sometimes understood, and not expressly stated, because thymine is almost always found attached to deoxyribose.

Table I-1-2. Nomenclature of Important Bases, Nucleosides, and Nucleotides

Base	Nucleoside	Nucleotides		
Adenine	Adenosine (Deoxyadenosine)	AMP (dAMP)	ADP (dADP)	ATP (dATP)
Guanine	Guanosine (Deoxyguanosine)	GMP (dGMP)	GDP (dGDP)	GTP (dGTP)
Cytosine	Cytidine (Deoxycytidine)	CMP (dCMP)	CDP (dCDP)	CTP (dCTP)
Uracil	Uridine (Deoxyuridine)	UMP (dUMP)	UDP (dUDP)	UTP (dUTP)
Thymine	(Deoxythymidine)	(dTMP)	(dTDP)	(dTTP)

Names of nucleosides and nucleotides attached to deoxyribose are shown in parentheses.

NUCLEIC ACIDS

Nucleic acids are polymers of nucleotides joined by 3′, 5′-phosphodiester bonds; that is, a phosphate group links the 3′ carbon of a sugar to the 5′ carbon of the next sugar in the chain. Each strand has a distinct 5′ end and 3′ end, and thus has polarity. A phosphate group is often found at the 5′ end, and a hydroxyl group is often found at the 3′ end.

The base sequence of a nucleic acid strand is written by convention, in the 5′→3′ direction (left to right). According to this convention, the sequence of the strand on the left in Figure I-1-7 must be written

5′-TCAG-3′ or TCAG:

- If written backward, the ends must be labeled: 3′-GACT-5′
- The positions of phosphates may be shown: pTpCpApG
- In DNA, a "d" (deoxy) may be included: dTdCdAdG

In eukaryotes, DNA is generally double-stranded (dsDNA) and RNA is generally single-stranded (ssRNA). Exceptions occur in certain viruses, some of which have ssDNA genomes and some of which have dsRNA genomes.

In a Nutshell

Nucleic Acids

- Nucleotides linked by 3′, 5′ phosphodiester bonds
- Have distinct 3′ and 5′ ends, thus polarity
- Sequence is always specified as 5′→3′

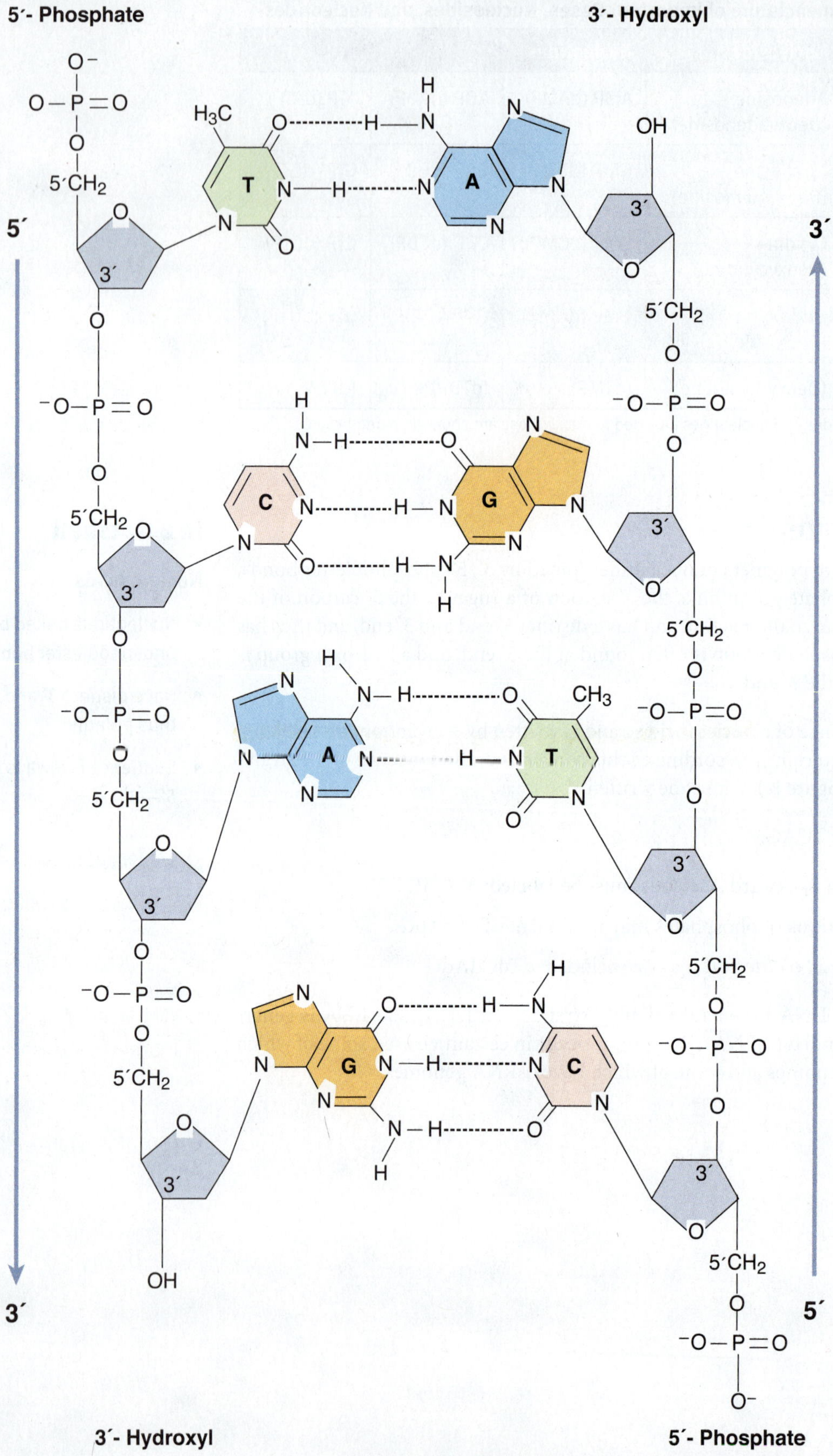

Section I • Biochemistry

Figure I-1-7. Hydrogen-Bonded Base Pairs in DNA

DNA Structure

Figure I-1-8 shows an example of a double-stranded DNA molecule. Some of the features of double-stranded DNA include:

- The two strands are antiparallel (opposite in direction).
- The two strands are complementary. A always pairs with T (two hydrogen bonds), and G always pairs with C (three hydrogen bonds). Thus, the base sequence on one strand defines the base sequence on the other strand.
- Because of the specific base pairing, the amount of A equals the amount of T, and the amount of G equals the amount of C. Thus, total purines equals total pyrimidines. These properties are known as Chargaff's rules.

With minor modification (substitution of U for T) these rules also apply to dsRNA.

Most DNA occurs in nature as a right-handed double-helical molecule known as Watson-Crick DNA or B-DNA (Figure I-1-8). The hydrophilic sugar-phosphate backbone of each strand is on the outside of the double helix. The hydrogen-bonded base pairs are stacked in the center of the molecule. There are about 10 base pairs per complete turn of the helix. A rare left-handed double-helical form of DNA that occurs in G-C-rich sequences is known as Z-DNA. The biologic function of Z-DNA is unknown, but may be related to gene regulation.

Note

Using Chargaff's Rules

In dsDNA (or dsRNA)
(ds = double-stranded)

% A = % T (% U)

% G = % C

% purines = % pyrimidines

A sample of DNA has 10% G; what is the % T?

10% G + 10% C = 20%

therefore, % A + % T must total 80%

40% A and 40% T

Ans: 40% T

Bridge to Pharmacology

Daunorubicin and doxorubicin are antitumor drugs that are used in the treatment of leukemias. They exert their effects by intercalating between the bases of DNA, thereby interfering with the activity of topoisomerase II and preventing proper replication of the DNA.

Other drugs, such as cisplatin, which is used in the treatment of bladder and lung tumors, bind tightly to the DNA, causing structural distortion and malfunction.

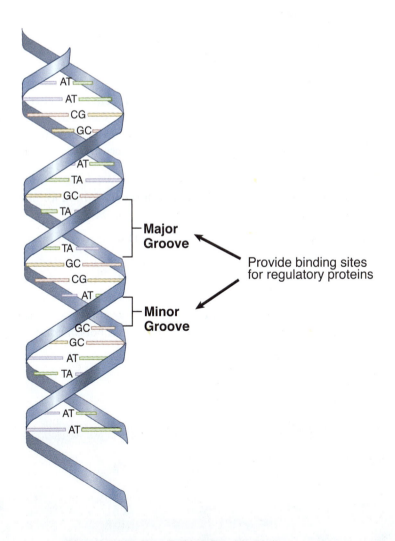

Figure I-1-8. The B-DNA Double Helix

Denaturation and Renaturation of DNA

Double-helical DNA can be denatured by conditions that disrupt hydrogen bonding and base stacking, resulting in the "melting" of the double helix into two single strands that separate from each other. No covalent bonds are broken in this process. Heat, alkaline pH, and chemicals such as formamide and urea are commonly used to denature DNA.

Denatured single-stranded DNA can be renatured (annealed) if the denaturing condition is slowly removed. For example, if a solution containing heat-denatured DNA is slowly cooled, the two complementary strands can become base-paired again (Figure I-1-9).

Such renaturation or annealing of complementary DNA strands is an important step in probing a Southern blot and in performing the polymerase chain reaction (reviewed in Chapter 7). In these techniques, a well-characterized probe DNA is added to a mixture of target DNA molecules. The mixed sample is denatured and then renatured. When probe DNA binds to target DNA sequences of sufficient complementarity, the process is called hybridization.

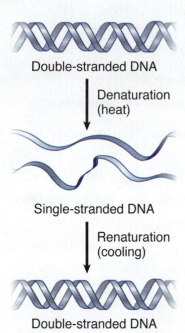

Figure I-1-9. Denaturation and Renaturation of DNA

ORGANIZATION OF DNA

Large DNA molecules must be packaged in such a way that they can fit inside the cell and still be functional.

Supercoiling

Mitochondrial DNA and the DNA of most prokaryotes are closed circular structures. These molecules may exist as relaxed circles or as supercoiled structures in which the helix is twisted around itself in three-dimensional space. Supercoiling results from strain on the molecule caused by under- or overwinding the double helix:

- Negatively supercoiled DNA is formed if the DNA is wound more loosely than in Watson-Crick DNA. This form is required for most biologic reactions.

- Positively supercoiled DNA is formed if the DNA is wound more tightly than in Watson-Crick DNA.

- Topoisomerases are enzymes that can change the amount of supercoiling in DNA molecules. They make transient breaks in DNA strands by alternately breaking and resealing the sugar-phosphate backbone. For example, in *Escherichia coli*, DNA gyrase (DNA topoisomerase II) can introduce negative supercoiling into DNA.

Nucleosomes and Chromatin

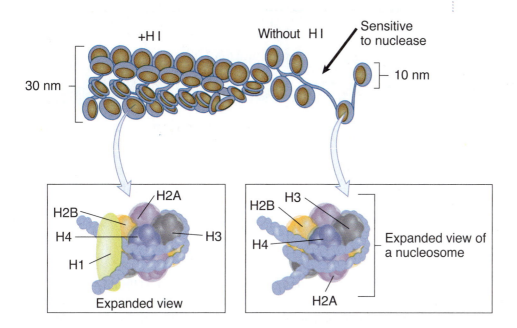

Figure I-1-10. Nucleosome and Nucleofilament Structure in Eukaryotic DNA

Nuclear DNA in eukaryotes is found in chromatin associated with histones and nonhistone proteins. The basic packaging unit of chromatin is the nucleosome (Figure I-1-10):

- Histones are rich in lysine and arginine, which confer a positive charge on the proteins.

- Two copies each of histones H2A, H2B, H3, and H4 aggregate to form the histone octamer.

- DNA is wound around the outside of this octamer to form a nucleosome (a series of nucleosomes is sometimes called "beads on a string", but is more properly referred to as a 10nm chromatin fiber).

- Histone H1 is associated with the linker DNA found between nucleosomes to help package them into a solenoid-like structure, which is a thick 30-nm fiber.

- Further condensation occurs to eventually form the chromosome. Each eukaryotic chromosome in G0 or G1 contains one linear molecule of double-stranded DNA.

Cells in interphase contain two types of chromatin: euchromatin (more opened and available for gene expression) and heterochromatin (much more highly condensed and associated with areas of the chromosomes that are not expressed.) (Figure I-1-11).

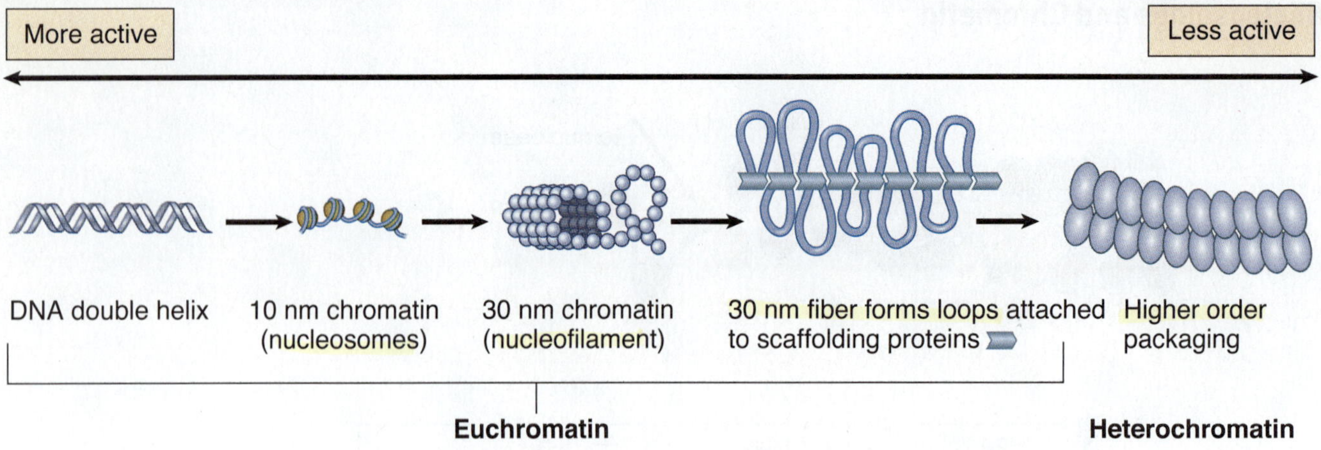

More active
Less active
DNA double helix
10 nm chromatin (nucleosomes)
30 nm chromatin (nucleofilament)
30 nm fiber forms loops attached to scaffolding proteins
Higher order packaging
Euchromatin
Heterochromatin

Figure I-1-11. DNA Packaging in Eukaryotic Cell

Euchromatin generally corresponds to the nucleosomes (10-nm fibers) loosely associated with each other (looped 30-nm fibers). Heterochromatin is more highly condensed, producing interphase heterochromatin as well as chromatin characteristic of mitotic chromosomes. Figure I-1-12 shows an electron micrograph of an interphase nucleus containing euchromatin, heterochromatin, and a nucleolus. The nucleolus is a nuclear region specialized for ribosome assembly (discussed in Chapter 3).

Euchromatin
Heterochromatin
Nucleolus

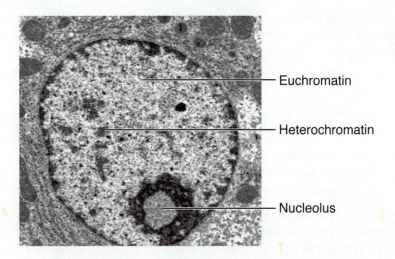

Figure I-1-12. An Interphase Nucleus

During mitosis, all the DNA is highly condensed to allow separation of the sister chromatids. This is the only time in the cell cycle when the chromosome structure is visible. Chromosome abnormalities may be assessed on mitotic chromosomes by karyotype analysis (metaphase chromosomes) and by banding techniques (prophase or prometaphase), which identify aneuploidy, translocations, deletions, inversions, and duplications.

Chapter Summary

- Nucleic acids:
    - RNA and DNA
    - Nucleotides (nucleoside monophosphates) linked by phosphodiester bonds
    - Have polarity (3′ end versus 5′ end)
    - Sequence always specified 5′-to-3′ (left to right on page)
- Double-stranded nucleic acids:
    - Two strands associate by hydrogen bonding
    - Sequences are complementary and antiparallel
- Eukaryotic DNA in the nucleus:
    - Packaged with histones (H2a, H2b, H3, H4)$_2$ to form nucleosomes (10-nm fiber)
    - 10-nm fiber associates with H1 (30-nm fiber).
    - 10-nm fiber and 30-nm fiber comprise euchromatin (active gene expression).
    - Higher-order packaging forms heterochromatin (no gene expression).
    - Mitotic DNA most condensed (no gene expression)

Section I • Biochemistry

Review Questions

Select the ONE best answer.

1. A double-stranded RNA genome isolated from a virus in the stool of a child with gastroenteritis was found to contain 15% uracil. What is the percentage of guanine in this genome?

   A. 15
   B. 25
   C. 35
   D. 75
   E. 85

2. What is the structure indicated below?

   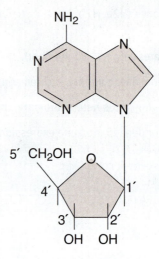

   A. Purine nucleotide
   B. Purine
   C. Pyrimidine nucleoside
   D. Purine nucleoside
   E. Deoxyadenosine

3. Endonuclease activation and chromatin fragmentation are characteristic features of eukaryotic cell death by apoptosis. Which of the following chromosome structures would most likely be degraded first in an apoptotic cell?

   A. Barr body
   B. 10-nm fiber
   C. 30-nm fiber
   D. Centromere
   E. Heterochromatin

4. A medical student working in a molecular biology laboratory is asked by her mentor to determine the base composition of an unlabeled nucleic acid sample left behind by a former research technologist. The results of her analysis show 10% adenine, 40% cytosine, 30% thymine and 20% guanine. What is the most likely source of the nucleic acid in this sample?

   A. Bacterial chromosome
   B. Bacterial plasmid
   C. Mitochondrial chromosome
   D. Nuclear chromosome
   E. Viral genome

Answers

1. **Answer: C.**
   U = A = 15%.
   Since A + G = 50%, G = 35%.
   Alternatively, U = A = 15%, then U + A = 30%
   C + G = 70%, and
   G = 35%.

2. **Answer: D.** A nucleoside consists of a base and a sugar. The figure shows the nucleoside adenosine, which is the base adenine attached to ribose.

3. **Answer: B.** The more "opened" the DNA, the more sensitive it is to enzyme attack. The 10-nm fiber, without the H1, is the most open structure listed. The endonuclease would attack the region of unprotected DNA between the nucleosomes.

4. **Answer: E.** A base compositional analysis that deviates from Chargaff's rules (%A = %T, %C = %G) is indicative of single-stranded, not double-stranded, nucleic acid molecule. All options listed except E are examples of circular (**choices A, B and C**) or linear (**choice D**) DNA double helices. Only a few viruses (e.g. parvovirus) have single-stranded DNA.

DNA Replication and Repair 2

Learning Objectives

- Explain information related to comparison of DNA and RNA synthesis
- Answer questions about steps of DNA replication
- Solve problems concerning DNA repair

OVERVIEW OF DNA REPLICATION

Genetic information is transmitted from parent to progeny by replication of parental DNA, a process in which two daughter DNA molecules are produced that are each identical to the parental DNA molecule. During DNA replication, the two complementary strands of parental DNA are pulled apart. Each of these parental strands is then used as a template for the synthesis of a new complementary strand (semiconservative replication). During cell division, each daughter cell receives one of the two identical DNA molecules.

Replication of Prokaryotic and Eukaryotic Chromosomes

The overall process of DNA replication in prokaryotes and eukaryotes is compared in Figure I-2-1.

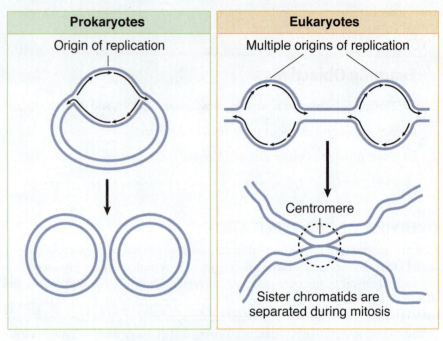

Figure I-2-1. DNA Replication by a Semi-Conservative, Bidirectional Mechanism

The bacterial chromosome is a closed, double-stranded circular DNA molecule having a single origin of replication. Separation of the two parental strands of DNA creates two replication forks that move away from each other in opposite directions around the circle. Replication is, thus, a bidirectional process. The two replication forks eventually meet, resulting in the production of two identical circular molecules of DNA.

Each eukaryotic chromosome contains one linear molecule of dsDNA having multiple origins of replication. Bidirectional replication occurs by means of a pair of replication forks produced at each origin. Completion of the process results in the production of two identical linear molecules of dsDNA (sister chromatids). DNA replication occurs in the nucleus during the S phase of the eukaryotic cell cycle. The two identical sister chromatids are separated from each other when the cell divides during mitosis.

In a Nutshell
Polymerases and Nucleases

- **Polymerases** are enzymes that synthesize nucleic acids by forming phosphodiester (PDE) bonds.
- **Nucleases** are enzymes that hydrolyze PDE bonds.
  - Exonucleases remove nucleotides from either the 5′ or the 3′ end of a nucleic acid.
  - Endonucleases cut within the nucleic acid and release nucleic acid fragments.

The structure of a representative eukaryotic chromosome during the cell cycle is shown in Figure I-2-2 below.

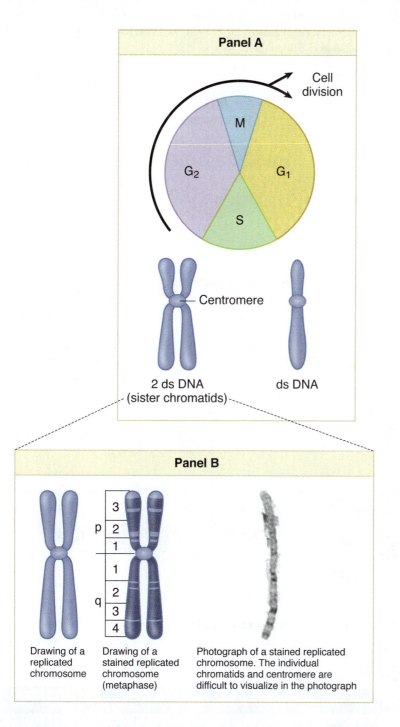

Figure I-2-2. Panel A: Eukaryotic Chromosome Replication During S-Phase
Panel B: Different Representations of a Replicated Eukaryotic Chromosome

Section I • Biochemistry

COMPARISON OF DNA AND RNA SYNTHESIS

The overall process of DNA replication requires the synthesis of both DNA and RNA. These two types of nucleic acids are synthesized by DNA polymerases and RNA polymerases, respectively. DNA synthesis and RNA synthesis are compared in Figure I-2-3 and Table I-2-1.

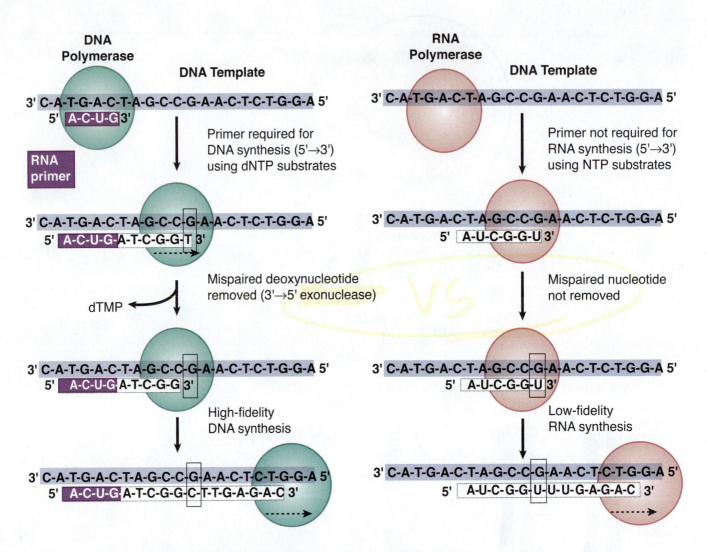

Figure I-2-3. Polymerase Enzymes Synthesize DNA and RNA

Table I-2-1. Comparison of DNA and RNA Polymerases

	DNA Polymerase	RNA Polymerase
Nucleic acid synthesized (5′→3′)	DNA	RNA
Required template (copied 3′→5′)	DNA*	DNA*
Required substrates	dATP, dGTP, dCTP, dTTP	ATP, GTP, CTP, UTP
Required primer	RNA (or DNA)	None
Proofreading activity (3′→5′ exonuclease)	Yes	No

*Certain DNA and RNA polymerases require RNA templates. These enzymes are most commonly associated with viruses.

Similarities include:

- The newly synthesized strand is made in the 5'→3' direction.
- The template strand is scanned in the 3'→5' direction.
- The newly synthesized strand is complementary and antiparallel to the template strand.
- Each new nucleotide is added when the 3' hydroxyl group of the growing strand reacts with a nucleoside triphosphate, which is base-paired with the template strand. Pyrophosphate (PPi, the last two phosphates) is released during this reaction.

Differences include:

- The substrates for DNA synthesis are the dNTPs, whereas the substrates for RNA synthesis are the NTPs.
- DNA contains thymine, whereas RNA contains uracil.
- DNA polymerases require a primer, whereas RNA polymerases do not. That is, DNA polymerases cannot initiate strand synthesis, whereas RNA polymerases can.
- DNA polymerases can correct mistakes ("proofreading"), whereas RNA polymerases cannot. DNA polymerases have 3' → 5' exonuclease activity for proofreading.

STEPS OF DNA REPLICATION

The molecular mechanism of DNA replication is shown in Figure I-2-4. The sequence of events is as follows:

1. The base sequence at the origin of replication is recognized.
2. Helicase breaks the hydrogen bonds holding the base pairs together. This allows the two parental strands of DNA to begin unwinding and forms two replication forks.
3. Single-stranded DNA binding protein (SSB) binds to the single-stranded portion of each DNA strand, preventing them from reassociating and protecting them from degradation by nucleases.
4. Primase synthesizes a short (about 10 nucleotides) RNA primer in the 5'→3' direction, beginning at the origin on each parental strand. The parental strand is used as a template for this process. RNA primers are required because DNA polymerases are unable to initiate synthesis of DNA, and can only extend a strand from the 3' end of a preformed "primer."
5. DNA polymerase III begins synthesizing DNA in the 5'→3' direction, beginning at the 3' end of each RNA primer. The newly synthesized strand is complementary and antiparallel to the parental strand used as a template. This strand can be made continuously in one long piece and is known as the "leading strand."

- The "lagging strand" is synthesized discontinuously as a series of small fragments (about 1,000 nucleotides long) known as Okazaki fragments. Each Okazaki fragment is initiated by the synthesis of an RNA primer by primase, and then completed by the synthesis of DNA using DNA polymerase III. Each fragment is made in the 5'→3' direction.
- There is a leading and a lagging strand for each of the two replication forks on the chromosome.

Section I • Biochemistry

6. RNA primers are removed by RNAase H in eukaryotes and an uncharacterized DNA polymerase fills in the gap with DNA. In prokaryotes DNA polymerase I both removes the primer (5' exonuclease) and synthesizes new DNA, beginning at the 3' end of the neighboring Okazaki fragment.

7. Both eukaryotic and prokaryotic DNA polymerases have the ability to "proofread" their work by means of a 3'→5' exonuclease activity. If DNA polymerase makes a mistake during DNA synthesis, the resulting unpaired base at the 3' end of the growing strand is removed before synthesis continues.

8. DNA ligase seals the "nicks" between Okazaki fragments, converting them to a continuous strand of DNA.

9. DNA gyrase (DNA topoisomerase II) provides a "swivel" in front of each replication fork. As helicase unwinds the DNA at the replication forks, the DNA ahead of it becomes overwound and positive supercoils form. DNA gyrase inserts negative supercoils by nicking both strands of DNA, passing the DNA strands through the nick, and then resealing both strands. Quinolones are a family of drugs that block the action of topoisomerases. Nalidixic acid kills bacteria by inhibiting DNA gyrase. Inhibitors of eukaryotic topoisomerase II (etoposide, teniposide) are becoming useful as anticancer agents.

The mechanism of replication in eukaryotes is believed to be very similar to this. However, the details have not yet been completely worked out. The steps and proteins involved in DNA replication in prokaryotes are compared with those used in eukaryotes in Table I-2-2.

Eukaryotic DNA Polymerases

- DNA α and δ work together to synthesize both the leading and lagging strands.
- DNA polymerase γ replicates mitochondrial DNA.
- DNA polymerases β and ε are thought to participate primarily in DNA repair. DNA polymerase ε may substitute for DNA polymerase δ in certain cases.

Telomerase

Telomeres are repetitive sequences at the ends of linear DNA molecules in eukaryotic chromosomes. With each round of replication in most normal cells, the telomeres are shortened because DNA polymerase cannot complete synthesis of the 5' end of each strand. This contributes to the aging of cells, because eventually the telomeres become so short that the chromosomes cannot function properly and the cells die.

Telomerase is an enzyme in eukaryotes used to maintain the telomeres. It contains a short RNA template complementary to the DNA telomere sequence, as well as telomerase reverse transcriptase activity (hTRT). Telomerase is thus able to replace telomere sequences that would otherwise be lost during replication. Normally telomerase activity is present only in embryonic cells, germ (reproductive) cells, and stem cells, but not in somatic cells.

Cancer cells often have relatively high levels of telomerase, preventing the telomeres from becoming shortened and contributing to the immortality of malignant cells.

Note

Telomerase

- Completes the replication of the telomere sequences at both ends of a eukaryotic chromosome
- Present in embryonic cells, fetal cells, and certain adult stem cells; not present in adult somatic cells
- Inappropriately present in many cancer cells, contributing to their unlimited replication

Table I-2-2. Steps and Proteins Involved in DNA Replication

Step in Replication	Prokaryotic Cells	Eukaryotic Cells (Nuclei)
Origin of replication (ori)	One ori site per chromosome	Multiple ori sites per chromosome
Unwinding of DNA double helix	Helicase	Helicase
Stabilization of unwound template strands	Single-stranded DNA-binding protein (SSB)	Single-stranded DNA-binding protein (SSB)
Synthesis of RNA primers	Primase	Primase

Synthesis of DNA
  Leading strand
  Lagging strand
    (Okazaki fragments)
	DNA polymerase III
	DNA polymerase III
		DNA polymerases $\alpha + \delta$
		DNA polymerases $\alpha + \delta$

Removal of RNA primers	DNA polymerase I ($5'\rightarrow3'$ exonuclease)	RNase H ($5'\rightarrow3'$ exonuclease)
Replacement of RNA with DNA	DNA polymerase I	DNA polymerase δ
Joining of Okazaki fragments	DNA ligase	DNA ligase
Removal of positive supercoils ahead of advancing replication forks	DNA topoisomerase II (DNA gyrase)	DNA topoisomerase II
Synthesis of telomeres	Not required	Telomerase

Reverse Transcriptase

Reverse transcriptase is an RNA-dependent DNA polymerase that requires an RNA template to direct the synthesis of new DNA. Retroviruses, most notably HIV, use this enzyme to replicate their RNA genomes. DNA synthesis by reverse transcriptase in retroviruses can be inhibited by AZT, ddC, and ddI.

Eukaryotic cells also contain reverse transcriptase activity:
- Associated with telomerase (hTRT).
- Encoded by retrotransposons (residual viral genomes permanently maintained in human DNA) that play a role in amplifying certain repetitive sequences in DNA (see Chapter 7).

Bridge to Pharmacology
Quinolones and DNA Gyrase

Quinolones and fluoroquinolones inhibit DNA gyrase (prokaryotic topoisomerase II), preventing DNA replication and transcription. These drugs, which are most active against aerobic gram-negative bacteria, include:

- Levofloxacin
- Ciprofloxacin
- Moxifloxacin

Resistance to the drugs has developed over time; current uses include treatment of gonorrhea and upper and lower urinary tract infections in both sexes.

Bridge to Pharmacology

One chemotherapeutic treatment of HIV is the use of AZT (3'-azido-2',3'-dideoxythymidine) or structurally related compounds. Once AZT enters cells, it can be converted to the triphosphate derivative and used as a substrate for the viral reverse transcriptase in synthesizing DNA from its RNA genome.

The replacement of an azide instead of a normal hydroxyl group at the 3' position of the deoxyribose prevents further replication by effectively causing chain termination. Although it is a DNA polymerase, reverse transcriptase lacks proofreading activity.

Section I • Biochemistry

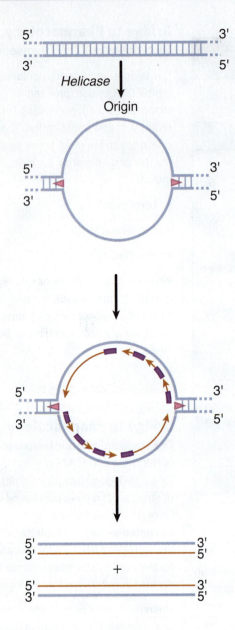

Leading Strand Synthesis (Continuous)

1. *Primase* synthesizes the primer (—) 5' to 3'.
2. *DNA polymerases* α and δ extend the primer, moving **into** the replication fork (Leading strand synthesis).
3. *Helicase* (◄) continues to unwind the DNA.

Lagging Strand Synthesis (Discontinuous)

1. *Primase* synthesizes the primer (—) 5' to 3'.
2. *DNA polymerases* α and δ extend the primer, moving **away from** the replication fork (Lagging strand synthesis)
3. Synthesis stops when *DNA polymerase* encounters the primer of the leading strand on the other side of the diagram (not shown), or the primer of the previous (Okasaki) fragment.
4. As *helicase* opens more of the replication fork, a third Okasaki fragment will be added.

RNase H (5' exoribonuclease activity) digests the RNA primer from fragment 1. In the eukaryotic cell, *DNA polymerase* extends the next fragment (2), to fill in the gap.

In prokaryotic cells *DNA polymerase 1* has both the 5' exonuclease activity to remove primers, and the *DNA polymerase* activity to extend the next fragment (2) to fill in the gap.

In both types of cells *DNA ligase* connects fragments 1 and 2 by making a phosphodiester bond.

This whole process repeats to remove all RNA primers from both the leading and lagging strands.

Figure I-2-4. DNA Replication

DNA REPAIR

The structure of DNA can be damaged in a number of ways through exposure to chemicals or radiation. Incorrect bases can also be incorporated during replication. Multiple repair systems have evolved, allowing cells to maintain the sequence stability of their genomes (Table I-2-3). If cells are allowed to replicate their DNA using a damaged template, there is a high risk of introducing stable mutations into the new DNA. Thus any defect in DNA repair carries an increased risk of cancer. Most DNA repair occurs in the G1 phase of the eukaryotic cell cycle. Mismatch repair occurs in the G2 phase to correct replication errors.

Table I-2-3. DNA Repair

Damage	Cause	Recognition/ Excision Enzyme	Repair Enzymes
Thymine dimers (G_1)	UV radiation	Excision endonuclease (deficient in Xeroderma pigmentosum)	DNA polymerase DNA ligase
Mismatched base (G_2)	DNA replication errors	A mutation on one of two genes, hMSH2 or hMLH1, initiates defective repair of DNA mismatches, resulting in a condition known as hereditary nonpolyposis colorectal cancer—HNPCC.	DNA polymerase DNA ligase
Cytosine deamination G_1	Spontaneous/ heat	Uracil glycosylase AP endonuclease	DNA polymerase DNA ligase

Repair of Thymine Dimers

Ultraviolet light induces the formation of dimers between adjacent thymines in DNA (also occasionally between other adjacent pyrimidines). The formation of thymine dimers interferes with DNA replication and normal gene expression. Thymine dimers are eliminated from DNA by a nucleotide excision-repair mechanism (Figure I-2-5).

Bridge to Pathology
Tumor Suppressor Genes and DNA Repair

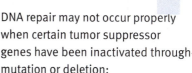

DNA repair may not occur properly when certain tumor suppressor genes have been inactivated through mutation or deletion:

- The *p53* gene encodes a protein that prevents a cell with damaged DNA from entering the S phase. Inactivation or deletion associated with Li Fraumeni syndrome and many solid tumors.

- *ATM* gene encodes a kinase essential for p53 activity. *ATM* is inactivated in ataxia telangiectasia, characterized by hypersensitivity to x-rays and predisposition to lymphomas.

- *BRCA-1* (breast, prostate, and ovarian cancer) and *BRCA-2* (breast cancer).

- *Rb* The retinoblastoma gene was the first tumor suppressor gene cloned, and is a negative regulator of the cell cycle through its ability to bind the transcription factor E2F and repress transcription of genes required for S phase.

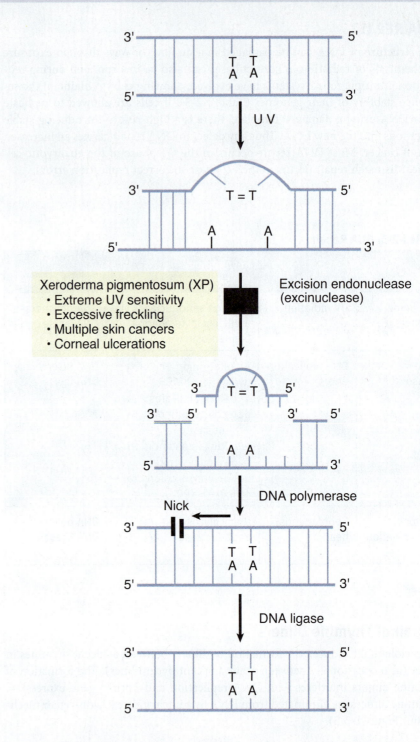

Figure I-2-5. Thymine Dimer Formation and Excision Repair

Steps in nucleotide excision repair:

- An excision endonuclease (excinuclease) makes nicks in the phosphodiester backbone of the damaged strand on both sides of the thymine dimer and removes the defective oligonucleotide.
- DNA polymerase fills in the gap by synthesizing DNA in the 5'→3' direction, using the undamaged strand as a template.
- DNA ligase seals the nick in the repaired strand.

Base excision repair: cytosine deamination

Cytosine deamination (loss of an amino group from cytosine) converts cytosine to uracil. The uracil is recognized and removed (base excision) by a uracil glycosylase enzyme.

- Subsequently this area is recognized by an AP endonuclease that removes the damaged sequence from the DNA.
- DNA polymerase fills in the gap
- DNA ligase seals the nick in the repaired strand

A summary of important genes involved in maintaining DNA fidelity and where they function in the cell cycle is shown in Figure I-2-6.

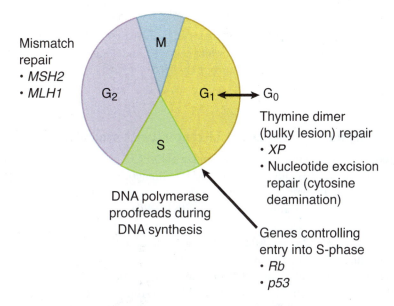

Figure I-2-6. Important Genes Associated with Maintaining Fidelity of Replicating DNA

Diseases Associated with DNA Repair

Inherited mutations that result in defective DNA repair mechanisms are associated with a predisposition to the development of cancer.

Xeroderma pigmentosum is an autosomal recessive disorder, characterized by extreme sensitivity to sunlight, skin freckling and ulcerations, and skin cancer. The most common deficiency occurs in the excinuclease enzyme.

Hereditary nonpolyposis colorectal cancer results from a deficiency in the ability to repair mismatched base pairs in DNA that are accidentally introduced during replication.

Section I • Biochemistry

> #### *Xeroderma pigmentosum*
>
> Xeroderma pigmentosum is an autosomal recessive disorder (incidence 1/250,000) characterized by extreme sensitivity to sunlight, skin freckling, ulcerations, and skin cancer. Carcinomas and melanomas appear early in life, and most patients die of cancer. The most common deficiency occurs in the excision endonuclease.
>
> A 6-year-old child was brought to the clinic because his parents were concerned with excessive lesions and blistering in the facial and neck area. The parents noted that the lesions did not go away with typical ointments and creams and often became worse when the child was exposed to sunlight. The physician noted excessive freckling throughout the child's body, as well as slight stature and poor muscle tone.
>
> Xeroderma pigmentosum can be diagnosed by measurement of the relevant enzyme excision endonuclease in white cells of blood. Patients with the disease should avoid exposure to any source of UV light.

Hereditary nonpolyposis colorectal cancer (Lynch syndrome)

Hereditary nonpolyposis colorectal cancer (HNPCC) results from a mutation in one of the genes (usually *hMLH1* or *hMSH2*) encoding enzymes that carry out DNA mismatch repair. These enzymes detect and remove errors introduced into the DNA during replication. In families with HNPCC, individuals may inherit one nonfunctional, deleted copy of the *hMLH1* gene or one nonfunctional, deleted copy of the *hMSH2* gene. After birth, a somatic mutation in the other copy may occur, causing loss of the mismatch repair function. This causes chromosomes to retain errors (mutations) in many other loci, some of which may contribute to cancer progression. This is manifested in intestinal cells because they are constantly undergoing cell division.

One prominent type of error that accompanies DNA replication is **microsatellite instability**. In a patient with HNPCC, cells from the resected tumor show microsatellite instability, whereas normal cells from the individual (which still retain mismatch repair) do not show microsatellite instability. Along with information from a family pedigree and histologic analysis, microsatellite instability may be used as a diagnostic tool.

Note

Microsatellite Instability

Microsatellites (also known as short tandem repeats) are di-, tri-, and tetranucleotide repeats dispersed throughout the DNA, usually (but not exclusively) in noncoding regions.

For example, TGTGTGTG may occur at a particular locus. If cells lack mismatch repair, the replicated DNA will vary in the number of repeats at that locus, e.g., TGTGTGTGTGTG or TGTGTG. This variation is microsatellite instability.

Chapter Summary

DNA Synthesis

	Prokaryotic	Eukaryotic
Timing	Prior to cell division	S phase
Enzymes	DNA A protein	
	Helicase	Helicase
	ssDNA-binding protein	ssDNA-binding protein
	Primase (an RNA polymerase)	Primase (an RNA polymerase)
	DNA pol III	DNA pol δ
		DNA pol α
	DNA pol I	RNAase H
	DNA ligase	DNA ligase
	DNA gyrase (Topo II)	DNA topoisomerase II
		Telomerase

DNA Repair

- G1 phase of eukaryotic cell cycle:
    - UV radiation: thymine (pyrimidine) dimers; excinuclease
    - Deaminations (C becomes U); uracil glycosylase
    - Loss of purine or pyrimidine; AP endonuclease
- G2 phase of eukaryotic cell cycle:
    - Mismatch repair: *hMSH2, hMLH1* (HNPCC)

Review Questions

Select the ONE best answer.

1. It is now believed that a substantial proportion of the single nucleotide substitutions causing human genetic disease are due to misincorporation of bases during DNA replication. Which proofreading activity is critical in determining the accuracy of nuclear DNA replication and thus the base substitution mutation rate in human chromosomes?

    A. 3′ to 5′ polymerase activity of DNA polymerase δ
    B. 3′ to 5′ exonuclease activity of DNA polymerase γ
    C. Primase activity of DNA polymerase α
    D. 5′ to 3′ polymerase activity of DNA polymerase III
    E. 3′ to 5′ exonuclease activity of DNA polymerase δ

Section I • Biochemistry

2. The proliferation of cytotoxic T-cells is markedly impaired upon infection with a newly discovered human immunodeficiency virus, designated HIV-V. The defect has been traced to the expression of a viral-encoded enzyme that inactivates a host-cell nuclear protein required for DNA replication. Which protein is a potential substrate for the viral enzyme?

   A. TATA-box binding protein (TBP)
   B. Cap binding protein (CBP)
   C. Catabolite activator protein (CAP)
   D. Acyl-carrier protein (ACP)
   E. Single-strand binding protein (SBP)

3. The deficiency of an excision endonuclease may produce an exquisite sensitivity to ultraviolet radiation in xeroderma pigmentosum. Which of the following functions would be absent in a patient deficient in this endonuclease?

   A. Removal of introns
   B. Removal of pyrimidine dimers
   C. Protection against DNA viruses
   D. Repair of mismatched bases during DNA replication
   E. Repair of mismatched bases during transcription

4. The anti-*Pseudomonas* action of norfloxacin is related to its ability to inhibit chromosome duplication in rapidly dividing cells. Which of the following enzymes participates in bacterial DNA replication and is directly inhibited by this antibiotic?

   A. DNA polymerase I
   B. DNA polymerase II
   C. Topoisomerase I
   D. Topoisomerase II
   E. DNA ligase

5. Cytosine arabinoside (araC) is used as an effective chemotherapeutic agent for cancer, although resistance to this drug may eventually develop. In certain cases, resistance is related to an increase in the enzyme cytidine deaminase in the tumor cells. This enzyme would inactivate araC to form

   A. cytosine
   B. cytidylic acid
   C. thymidine arabinoside
   D. uracil arabinoside
   E. cytidine

6. Dyskeratosis congenital (DKC) is a genetically inherited disease in which the proliferative capacity of stem cells is markedly impaired. The defect has been traced to inadequate production of an enzyme needed for chromosome duplication in the nuclei of rapidly dividing cells. Structural analysis has shown that the active site of this protein contains a single-stranded RNA that is required for normal catalytic function. Which step in DNA replication is most likely deficient in DKC patients?

    A. Synthesis of centromeres
    B. Synthesis of Okazaki fragments
    C. Synthesis of RNA primers
    D. Synthesis of telomeres
    E. Removal of RNA primers

7. Single-strand breaks in DNA comprise the single most frequent type of DNA damage. These breaks are frequently due to reactive oxygen species damaging the deoxyribose residues of the sugar phosphate backbone. This type of break is repaired by a series of enzymes that reconstruct the sugar and ultimately reform the phosphodiester bonds between nucleotides. Which class of enzyme catalyses the formation of the phosphodiester bond in DNA repair?

    A. DNA glycosylases
    B. DNA helicases
    C. DNA ligases
    D. DNA phosphodiesterases
    E. DNA polymerases

Answers

1. **Answer: E.** The 3′ to 5′ exonuclease activity of DNA pol δ represents the proofreading activity of an enzyme required for the replication of human chromosomal DNA. DNA pol γ (mitochondrial) and DNA pol III (prokaryotic) do not participate in this process, short RNA primers are replaced with DNA during replication, and new DNA strands are always synthesized in the 5′ to 3′ direction.

2. **Answer: E.** TBP and CBP participate in eukaryotic gene transcription and mRNA translation, respectively. CAP regulates the expression of prokaryotic lactose operons. ACP is involved in fatty acid synthesis.

3. **Answer: B.** Nucleotide excision repair of thymine (pyrimidine) dimers is deficient in XP patients.

4. **Answer: D.** Norfloxacin inhibits DNA gyrase (topoisomerase II).

5. **Answer: D.** Deamination of cytosine would produce uracil.

Section I • Biochemistry

6. **Answer: D.** The enzyme is described as an RNA dependent DNA polymerase required for chromosome duplication in the nuclei of rapidly dividing cells. This enzyme is telomerase, a reverse transcriptase, that replicates the ends (telomeres) of linear chromosomes.

   None of the other options have reverse transcriptase activity.

7. **Answer: C.** All DNA repair systems use a ligase to seal breaks in the sugar phosphate backbone of DNA. Although polymerase enzymes make phosphodiester bonds during DNA synthesis, these enzymes do not ligate strands of DNA.

Transcription and RNA Processing 3

Learning Objectives

- Use knowledge of types of RNA
- Interpret scenarios about production of other classes of RNA
- Answer questions about RNA polymerases
- Demonstrate understanding of transcription terminology
- Answer questions about production of prokaryotic messenger RNA
- Interpret scenarios about production of eukaryotic messenger RNA
- Demonstrate understanding of alternative splicing of eukaryotic primary pre-mRNA transcripts
- Demonstrate understanding of how ribosomal RNA (rRNA) is used to construct ribosomes
- Explain information related to how transfer RNA (tRNA) carries activated amino acids for translation

OVERVIEW OF TRANSCRIPTION

The first stage in the expression of genetic information is transcription of the information in the base sequence of a double-stranded DNA molecule to form the base sequence of a single-stranded molecule of RNA. For any particular gene, only one strand of the DNA molecule, called the template strand, is copied by RNA polymerase as it synthesizes RNA in the 5′ to 3′ direction. Because RNA polymerase moves in the 3′ to 5′ direction along the template strand of DNA, the RNA product is antiparallel and complementary to the template. RNA polymerase recognizes start signals (promoters) and stop signals (terminators) for each of the thousands of transcription units in the genome of an organism. Figure I-3-1 illustrates the arrangement and direction of transcription for several genes on a DNA molecule.

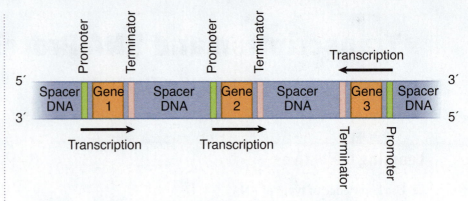

Figure I-3-1. Transcription of Several Genes on a Chromosome

TYPES OF RNA

RNA molecules play a variety of roles in the cell. The major types of RNA are:

- Ribosomal RNA (rRNA), which is the most abundant type of RNA in the cell. It is used as a structural component of the ribosome. Ribosomal RNA associates with ribosomal proteins to form the complete, functional ribosome.

- Transfer RNA (tRNA), which is the second most abundant type of RNA. Its function is to carry amino acids to the ribosome, where they will be linked together during protein synthesis.

- Messenger RNA (mRNA), which carries the information specifying the amino acid sequence of a protein to the ribosome. Messenger RNA is the only type of RNA that is translated. The mRNA population in a cell is very heterogeneous in size and base sequence, as the cell has essentially a different mRNA molecule for each of the thousands of different proteins made by that cell.

- Heterogeneous nuclear RNA (hnRNA or pre-mRNA), which is found only in the nucleus of eukaryotic cells. It represents precursors of mRNA, formed during its posttranscriptional processing.

- Small nuclear RNA (snRNA), which is also only found in the nucleus of eukaryotes. One of its major functions is to participate in splicing (removal of introns) mRNA.

- Ribozymes, which are RNA molecules with enzymatic activity. They are found in both prokaryotes and eukaryotes.

PRODUCTION OF OTHER CLASSES OF RNA

Genes encoding other classes of RNA are also expressed. The RNA products are not translated to produce proteins, but rather serve different roles in the process of translation.

RNA POLYMERASES

There is a single prokaryotic RNA polymerase that synthesizes all types of RNA in the cell. The core polymerase responsible for making the RNA molecule has the subunit structure $\alpha_2\beta\beta'$. A protein factor called sigma (σ) is required for the initiation of transcription at a promoter. Sigma factor is released immediately after initiation of transcription. Termination of transcription sometimes requires a protein called rho (ρ) factor. The prokaryotic RNA polymerase is inhibited by rifampin. Actinomycin D binds to the DNA, preventing transcription.

There are three eukaryotic RNA polymerases, distinguished by the particular types of RNA they produce.

- RNA polymerase I is located in the nucleolus and synthesizes 28S, 18S, and 5.8S rRNAs.
- RNA polymerase II is located in the nucleoplasm and synthesizes hnRNA/mRNA and some snRNA.
- RNA polymerase III is located in the nucleoplasm and synthesizes tRNA, some snRNA, and 5S rRNA.

Transcription factors (such as TFIID for RNA polymerase II) help to initiate transcription. The requirements for termination of transcription in eukaryotes are not well understood. All transcription can be inhibited by actinomycin D. In addition, RNA polymerase II is inhibited by α-amanitin (a toxin from certain mushrooms).

Table I-3-1. Comparison of RNA Polymerases

Prokaryotic	Eukaryotic
Single RNA polymerase ($\alpha_2 \beta\beta'$)	RNAP 1: rRNA (nucleolus) Except 5S rRNA RNAP 2: hnRNA/mRNA and some snRNA RNAP 3: tRNA, 5S rRNA
Requires sigma (σ) to initiate at a promoter	No sigma, but transcription factors (TFIID) bind before RNA polymerase
Sometimes requires rho (ρ) to terminate	No rho required
Inhibited by rifampin Actinomycin D	RNAP 2 inhibited by α-amanitin (mushrooms) Actinomycin D

TRANSCRIPTION: IMPORTANT CONCEPTS AND TERMINOLOGY

RNA is synthesized by a DNA-dependent RNA polymerase (uses DNA as a template for the synthesis of RNA). Important terminology used when discussing transcription is illustrated in Figure I-3-2.

- RNA polymerase locates genes in DNA by searching for promoter regions. The promoter is the binding site for RNA polymerase. Binding establishes where transcription begins, which strand of DNA is used as the template, and in which direction transcription proceeds. No primer is required.

- RNA polymerase moves along the template strand in the 3′ to 5′ direction as it synthesizes the RNA product in the 5′ to 3′ direction using NTPs (ATP, GTP, CTP, UTP) as substrates. RNA polymerase does not proofread its work. The RNA product is complementary and antiparallel to the template strand.

- The coding (antitemplate) strand is not used during transcription. It is identical in sequence to the RNA molecule, except that RNA contains uracil instead of the thymine found in DNA.
- By convention, the base sequence of a gene is given from the coding strand (5′→3′).
- In the vicinity of a gene, a numbering system is used to identify the location of important bases. The first base transcribed as RNA is defined as the +1 base of that gene region.
  - To the left (5′, or upstream) of this starting point for transcription, bases are −1, −2, −3, etc.
  - To the right (3′, or downstream) of this point, bases are +2, +3, etc.
- Transcription ends when RNA polymerase reaches a termination signal.

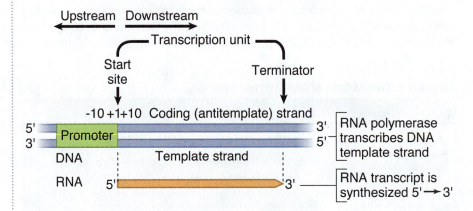

Figure I-3-2. Transcription of DNA

Flow of Genetic Information from DNA to Protein

For the case of a gene coding for a protein, the relationship among the sequences found in double-stranded DNA, single-stranded mRNA, and protein is illustrated in Figure I-3-3. Messenger RNA is synthesized in the 5′ to 3′ direction. It is complementary and antiparallel to the template strand of DNA. The ribosome translates the mRNA in the 5′ to 3′ direction, as it synthesizes the protein from the amino to the carboxyl terminus.

Chapter 3 • Transcription and RNA Processing

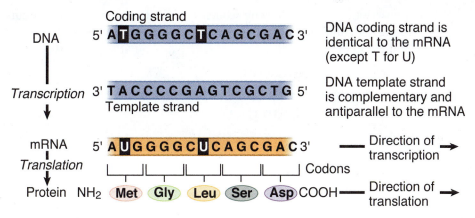

Figure I-3-3. Flow of Genetic Information from DNA to Protein

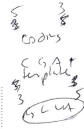

Sample Questions

1. During RNA synthesis, the DNA template sequence TAGC would be transcribed to produce which of the following sequences?

   A. ATCG
   B. GCTA
   C. CGTA
   D. AUCG
   E. GCUA

The answer is E. RNA is antiparallel and complementary to the template strand. Also remember that, by convention, all base sequences are written in the 5′ to 3′ direction regardless of the direction in which the sequence may actually be used in the cell.

Approach:

- Cross out any option with a T (RNA has U).
- Look at the 5′ end of DNA (T in this case).
- What is the complement of this base? (A)

Examine the options given. A correct option will have the complement (A in this example) at the 3′ end. Repeat the procedure for the 3′ end of the DNA. This will usually leave only one or two options.

2. Transcription of the following sequence of the tryptophan operon occurs in the direction indicated by the arrow. What would be the base sequence of the mRNA produced?

   3' CGTCAGC 5'
   Transcription →   Which product?
   5'...GCAGTCG...3'

   A. 5'...GCAGUCG...3'
   B. 5'...CGUGAGC...3'
   C. 5'...GCUGACG...3'
   D. 5'...CGUCAGC...3'
   E. 5'...CGUGAGC...3'

The answer is A. Because all nucleic acids are synthesized in the 5' to 3' direction, mRNA and the coding strand of DNA must each be oriented 5' to 3', i.e., in the direction of transcription. This means that the bottom strand in this example is the coding strand. The top strand is the template strand.

Approach:

- Cross out any option with a T.
- Identify the coding strand of DNA from the direction of transcription.
- Find the option with a sequence identical to the coding strand (remember to substitute U for T, if necessary).
- Alternatively, if you prefer to find the complement of the template strand, you will get the same answer.

PRODUCTION OF PROKARYOTIC MESSENGER RNA

The structure and expression of a typical prokaryotic gene coding for a protein are illustrated in Figure I-3-4. The following events occur during the expression of this gene:

1. With the help of sigma factor, RNA polymerase recognizes and binds to the promoter region. The bacterial promoter contains two "consensus" sequences, called the Pribnow box (or TATA box) and the –35 sequence. The promoter identifies the start site for transcription and orients the enzyme on the template strand. The RNA polymerase separates the two strands of DNA as it reads the base sequence of the template strand.

2. Transcription begins at the +1 base pair. Sigma factor is released as soon as transcription is initiated.

3. The core polymerase continues moving along the template strand in the 3' to 5' direction, synthesizing the mRNA in the 5' to 3' direction.

4. RNA polymerase eventually reaches a transcription termination signal, at which point it will stop transcription and release the completed mRNA molecule. There are two kinds of transcription terminators commonly found in prokaryotic genes:

   - Rho-independent termination occurs when the newly formed RNA folds back on itself to form a GC-rich hairpin loop closely followed by 6–8 U residues. These two structural features of the newly synthesized RNA promote dissociation of the RNA from the DNA template. This is the type of terminator shown in Figure I-3-4.

- Rho-dependent termination requires participation of rho factor. This protein binds to the newly formed RNA and moves toward the RNA polymerase that has paused at a termination site. Rho then displaces RNA polymerase from the 3′ end of the RNA.

5. Transcription and translation can occur simultaneously in bacteria. Because there is no processing of prokaryotic mRNA (no introns), ribosomes can begin translating the message even before transcription is complete. Ribosomes bind to a sequence called the Shine-Dalgarno sequence in the 5′ untranslated region (UTR) of the message. Protein synthesis begins at an AUG codon at the beginning of the coding region and continues until the ribosome reaches a stop codon at the end of the coding region.

6. The ribosome translates the message in the 5′ to 3′ direction, synthesizing the protein from amino terminus to carboxyl terminus.

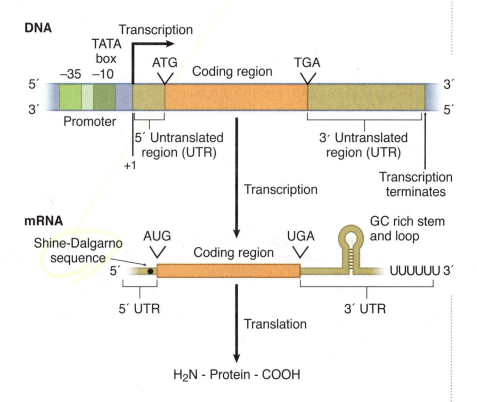

Figure I-3-4. Expression of a Prokaryotic Protein Coding Gene

The mRNA produced by the gene shown in Figure I-3-4 is a monocistronic message. That is, it is transcribed from a single gene and codes for only a single protein. The word cistron is another name for a gene. Some bacterial operons (for example, the lactose operon) produce polycistronic messages. In these cases, related genes grouped together in the DNA are transcribed as one unit. The mRNA in this case contains information from several genes and codes for several different proteins (Figure I-3-5).

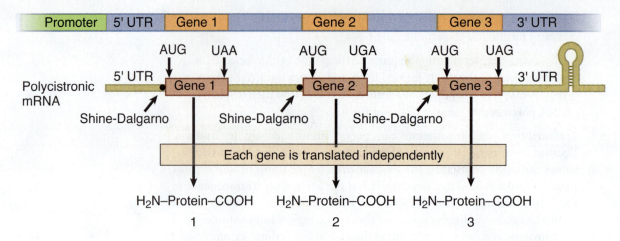

Figure I-3-5. Polycistronic Gene Region Codes for Several Different Proteins

PRODUCTION OF EUKARYOTIC MESSENGER RNA

In eukaryotes, most genes are composed of coding segments (exons) interrupted by noncoding segments (introns). Both exons and introns are transcribed in the nucleus. Introns are removed during processing of the RNA molecule in the nucleus. In eukaryotes, all mRNA is monocistronic. The mature mRNA is translated in the cytoplasm. The structure and transcription of a typical eukaryotic gene coding for a protein is illustrated in Figure I-3-6. Transcription of this gene occurs as follows:

1. With the help of proteins called transcription factors, RNA polymerase II recognizes and binds to the promoter region. The basal promoter region of eukaryotic genes usually has two consensus sequences called the TATA box (also called Hogness box) and the CAAT box.

2. RNA polymerase II separates the strands of the DNA over a short region to initiate transcription and read the DNA sequence. The template strand is read in the 3′ to 5′ direction as the RNA product (the primary transcript) is synthesized in the 5′ to 3′ direction. Both exons and introns are transcribed.

3. RNA polymerase II ends transcription when it reaches a termination signal. These signals are not well understood in eukaryotes.

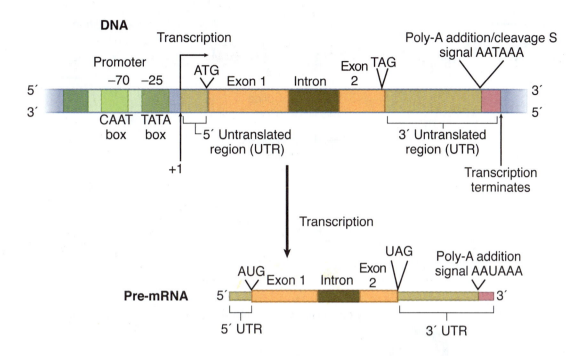

Figure I-3-6. A Eukaryotic Transcription Unit

Processing of Eukaryotic Pre-Messenger RNA

The primary transcript must undergo extensive posttranscriptional processing inside the nucleus to form the mature mRNA molecule (Figure I-3-7). These processing steps include the following:

1. A 7-methylguanosine cap is added to the 5′ end while the RNA molecule is still being synthesized. The cap structure serves as a ribosome-binding site and also helps to protect the mRNA chain from degradation.

2. A poly-A tail is attached to the 3′ end. In this process, an endonuclease cuts the molecule on the 3′ side of the sequence AAUAAA (poly-A addition signal), then poly-A polymerase adds the poly-A tail (about 200 As) to the new 3′ end. The poly-A tail protects the message against rapid degradation and aids in its transport to the cytoplasm. A few mRNAs (for example, histone mRNAs) have no poly-A tails.

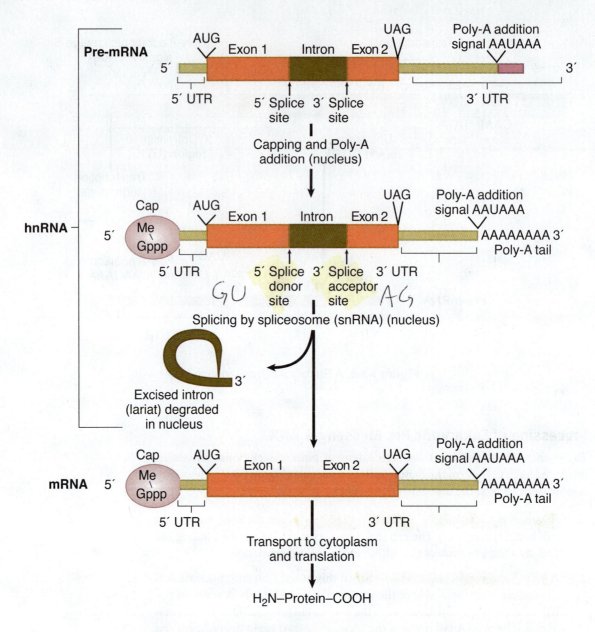

Figure I-3-7. Processing Eukaryotic Pre-mRNA

Note

Mutations in splice sites can lead to abnormal proteins. For example, mutations that interfere with proper splicing of β-globin mRNA are responsible for some cases of β-thalassemia.

3. Introns are removed from hnRNA by splicing, accomplished by spliceosomes (also known as an snRNP, or snurp), which are complexes of snRNA and protein. The hnRNA molecule is cut at splice sites at the 5′ (donor) and 3′ (acceptor) ends of the intron. The intron is excised in the form of a lariat structure and degraded. Neighboring exons are joined together to assemble the coding region of the mature mRNA.

4. All of the intermediates in this processing pathway are collectively known as hnRNA.

5. The mature mRNA molecule is transported to the cytoplasm, where it is translated to form a protein.

ALTERNATIVE SPLICING OF EUKARYOTIC PRIMARY PRE-mRNA TRANSCRIPTS

For some genes, the primary transcript is spliced differently to produce two or more variants of a protein from the same gene. This process is known as alternative splicing and is illustrated in Figure I-3-8. Variants of the muscle proteins tropomyosin and troponin T are produced in this way. The synthesis of membrane-bound immunoglobulins by unstimulated B lymphocytes, as opposed to secreted immunoglobulins by antigen-stimulated B lymphocytes, also involves alternative splicing.

The primary transcripts from a large percentage of genes undergo alternative splicing. This may occur within the same cell, or the primary transcript of a gene may be alternatively spliced in different tissues, giving rise to tissue-specific protein products. By alternative splicing, an organism can make many more different proteins than it has genes to encode. A current estimate of the number of human proteins is at least 100,000, whereas the current estimate of human genes is about only 20,000 to 25,000. These figures should not be memorized because they may change upon more research. Alternative splicing can be detected by Northern blot, a technique discussed in Chapter 7.

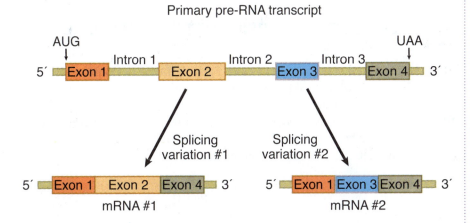

Figure I-3-8. Alternative Splicing of Eukaryotic hnRNA (Pre-mRNA) to Produce Different Proteins

RIBOSOMAL RNA (rRNA) IS USED TO CONSTRUCT RIBOSOMES

Figure I-3-9 shows the components of prokaryotic and eukaryotic ribosomes.

Eukaryotic ribosomal RNA is transcribed in the nucleolus by RNA polymerase I as a single piece of 45S RNA, which is subsequently cleaved to yield 28S rRNA, 18S rRNA, and 5.8S rRNA. RNA polymerase III transcribes the 5S rRNA unit from a separate gene. The ribosomal subunits assemble in the nucleolus as the rRNA pieces combine with ribosomal proteins. Eukaryotic ribosomal subunits are 60S and 40S. They join during protein synthesis to form the whole 80S ribosome.

Bridge to Microbiology

Shiga toxin (*Shigella dysenteriae*) and Verotoxin, a shiga-like toxin (enterohemorrhagic *E. coli*), inactivate the 28S rRNA in the 60S subunit of the eukaryotic ribosome. The A subunits of these toxins are RNA glycosylases that remove a single adenine residue from the 28S rRNA. This prevents aminoacyl-tRNA binding to the ribosome, halting protein synthesis.

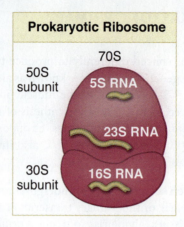
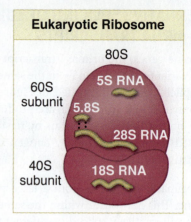

Figure I-3-9. The Composition of Prokaryotic and Eukaryotic Ribosomes

The large and small prokaryotic ribosomal subunits are 50S and 30S, respectively. The complete prokaryotic ribosome is a 70S particle. (Note: The S values are determined by behavior of the particles in an ultracentrifuge. They are a function of both size and shape, and therefore the numbers are not additive.)

TRANSFER RNA (TRNA) CARRIES ACTIVATED AMINO ACIDS FOR TRANSLATION

There are many different specific tRNAs. Each tRNA carries only one type of activated amino acid for making proteins during translation. The genes encoding these tRNAs in eukaryotic cells are transcribed by RNA polymerase III. The tRNAs enter the cytoplasm where they combine with their appropriate amino acids. Although all tRNAs have the same general shape shown in Figure I-3-10, small structural features distinguish among them.

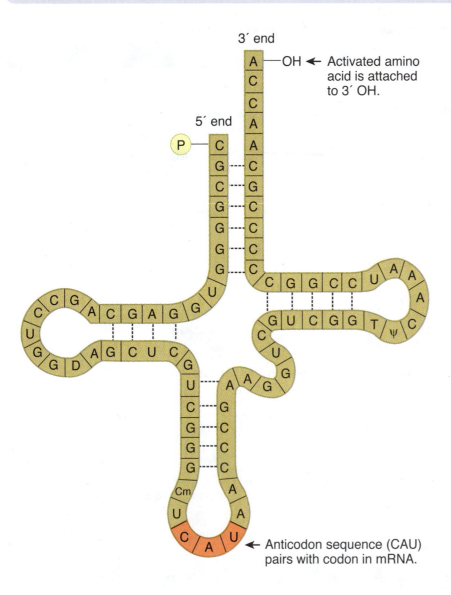

Figure I-3-10. Transfer RNA (tRNA)

RNA Editing

RNA editing is a process by which some cells make discrete changes to specific nucleotide sequences within a RNA molecule after its gene has been transcribed by RNA polymerase. Posttranscription editing events may include insertion, deletion, and base alterations of nucleotides (such as adenine deamination) within the edited RNA molecule. RNA editing has been observed in some mRNA, rRNA, mRNA, or tRNA molecules in humans. An important example is cytosine-to-uracil deamination in the apoprotein B gene. Apoprotein B100 is expressed in the liver, and apoprotein B48 is expressed in the intestines. In the intestines, the mRNA is edited from a CAA sequence to be UAA, a stop codon, thus producing the shorter apoprotein B48 form.

Section I • Biochemistry

Table I-3-2. Summary of Important Points About Transcription and RNA Processing

	Prokaryotic	Eukaryotic
Gene regions	May be polycistronic Genes are continuous coding regions Very little spacer (noncoding) DNA between genes	Always monocistronic Genes have exons and introns Large spacer (noncoding) DNA between genes
RNA polymerase	Core enzyme: $\alpha_2\beta\beta'$	RNA polymerase I: rRNA RNA polymerase II: mRNA; snRNA RNA polymerase III: tRNA, 5S RNA
Initiation of transcription	Promoter (−10) TATAAT and (−35) sequence Sigma initiation subunit required to recognize promoter	Promoter (−25) TATA and (−70) CAAT Transcription factors (TFIID) bind promoter
mRNA synthesis	Template read 3′ to 5′; mRNA synthesized 5′ to 3′; gene sequence specified from coding strand 5′ to 3′; transcription begins at +1 base	
Termination of transcription	Stem and loop + UUUUU Stem and loop + rho factor	Not well characterized
Relationship of RNA transcript to DNA	RNA is antiparallel and complementary to DNA template strand; RNA is identical (except U substitutes for T) to DNA coding strand	
Posttranscriptional processing of hnRNA (pre-mRNA)	None	In nucleus: 5′ cap (7-MeG) 3′ tail (poly-A sequence) Removal of introns from pre-RNA • Alternative splicing yields variants of protein product
Ribosomes	70S (30S and 50S) rRNA and protein	80S (40S and 60S) rRNA and protein
tRNA	Cloverleaf secondary structure • Acceptor arm (CCA) carries amino acid • Anticodon arm; anticodon complementary and antiparallel to codon in mRNA	

Chapter 3 • Transcription and RNA Processing

Review Questions

Select the ONE best answer.

1. The base sequence of codons 57-58 in the cytochrome β5 reductase gene is CAGCGC. The mRNA produced upon transcription of this gene will contain the sequence:

    A. GCGCTG
    B. CUGCGC
    C. GCGCUG
    D. CAGCGC
    E. GUCGCG

2. A gene encodes a protein with 150 amino acids. There is one intron of 1,000 bps, a 5′-untranslated region of 100 bp, and a 3′-untranslated region of 200 bp. In the final processed mRNA, how many bases lie between the start AUG codon and the final termination codon?

    A. 1,750
    B. 750
    C. 650
    D. 450
    E. 150

Items 3–5: Identify the nuclear location.

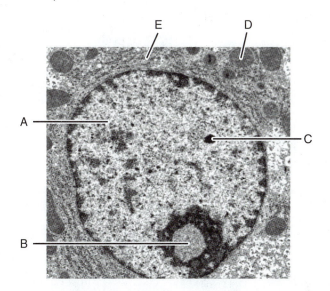

3. Transcription of genes by RNA polymerase 1
4. Euchromatin
5. Polyadenylation of pre-mRNA by poly-A polymerase

Section I • Biochemistry

Answers

1. **Answer: D.** Since the sequence in the stem represents the coding strand, the mRNA sequence must be identical (except U for T). No T in the DNA means no U in the mRNA.

2. **Answer: D.** Only the coding region remains to be calculated 3 × 150 = 450.

3. **Answer: B.** rRNA genes are transcribed by this enzyme in the nucleolus.

4. **Answer: A.** Less condensed chromatin, lighter areas in the nucleus. Darker areas are heterochromatin.

5. **Answer: A.** Polyadenylation of pre-mRNA occurs in the nucleoplasm. Generally associated with active gene expression in euchromatin.

The Genetic Code, Mutations, and Translation 4

Learning Objectives

❏ Demonstrate understanding of the Genetic Code
❏ Solve problems concerning mutations
❏ Interpret scenarios about amino acid activation and codon translation by tRNAs
❏ Demonstrate understanding of translation (protein synthesis)
❏ Interpret scenarios about polysomes
❏ Explain information related to inhibitors of protein synthesis
❏ Interpret scenarios about protein folding and subunit assembly
❏ Answer questions about how translation occurs on free ribosomes and on the rough endoplasmic reticulum
❏ Demonstrate understanding of co- and posttranslational covalent modifications
❏ Solve problems concerning posttranslational modifications of collagen

OVERVIEW OF TRANSLATION

The second stage in gene expression is translating the nucleotide sequence of a messenger RNA molecule into the amino acid sequence of a protein. The genetic code is defined as the relationship between the sequence of nucleotides in DNA (or its RNA transcripts) and the sequence of amino acids in a protein. Each amino acid is specified by one or more nucleotide triplets (codons) in the DNA.

During translation, mRNA acts as a working copy of the gene in which the codons for each amino acid in the protein have been transcribed from DNA to mRNA. tRNAs serve as adapter molecules that couple the codons in mRNA with the amino acids they each specify, thus aligning them in the appropriate sequence before peptide bond formation. Translation takes place on ribosomes, complexes of protein and rRNA that serve as the molecular machines coordinating the interactions between mRNA, tRNA, the enzymes, and the protein factors required for protein synthesis. Many proteins undergo posttranslational modifications as they prepare to assume their ultimate roles in the cell.

Section I • Biochemistry

THE GENETIC CODE

Most genetic code tables designate the codons for amino acids as mRNA sequences (Figure I-4-1). Important features of the genetic code include:

- Each codon consists of three bases (triplet). There are 64 codons. They are all written in the 5′ to 3′ direction.

- 61 codons code for amino acids. The other three (UAA, UGA, UAG) are stop codons (or nonsense codons) that terminate translation.

- There is one start codon (initiation codon), AUG, coding for methionine. Protein synthesis begins with methionine (Met) in eukaryotes, and formylmethionine (fmet) in prokaryotes.

- The code is unambiguous. Each codon specifies no more than one amino acid.

- The code is degenerate. More than one codon can specify a single amino acid. All amino acids, except Met and tryptophan (Trp), have more than one codon.

- For those amino acids having more than one codon, the first two bases in the codon are usually the same. The base in the third position often varies.

- The code is universal (the same in all organisms). Some minor exceptions to this occur in mitochondria.

- The code is commaless (contiguous). There are no spacers or "commas" between codons on an mRNA.

- Neighboring codons on a message are nonoverlapping.

First Position (5' End)	Second Position U	C	A	G	Third Position (3' End)
U	UUU UUC } Phe UUA UUG } Leu	UCU UCC UCA UCG } Ser	UAU UAC } Tyr UAA UAG } Stop	UGU UGC } Cys UGA Stop UGG Trp	U C A G
C	CUU CUC CUA CUG } Leu	CCU CCC CCA CCG } Pro	CAU CAC } His CAA CAG } Gln	CGU CGC CGA CGG } Arg	U C A G
A	AUU AUC } Ile AUA AUG Met	ACU ACC ACA ACG } Thr	AAU AAC } Asn AAA AAG } Lys	AGU AGC } Ser AGA AGG } Arg	U C A G
G	GUU GUC GUA GUG } Val	GCU GCC GCA GCG } Ala	GAU GAC } Asp GAA GAG } Glu	GGU GGC GGA GGG } Gly	U C A G

Figure I-4-1. The Genetic Code

MUTATIONS

A mutation is any permanent, heritable change in the DNA base sequence of an organism. This altered DNA sequence can be reflected by changes in the base sequence of mRNA, and, sometimes, by changes in the amino acid sequence of a protein. Mutations can cause genetic diseases. They can also cause changes in enzyme activity, nutritional requirements, antibiotic susceptibility, morphology, antigenicity, and many other properties of cells.

A very common type of mutation is a single base alteration or point mutation.

- A transition is a point mutation that replaces a purine-pyrimidine base pair with a different purine-pyrimidine base pair. For example, an A-T base pair becomes a G-C base pair.

- A transversion is a point mutation that replaces a purine-pyrimidine base pair with a pyrimidine-purine base pair. For example, an A-T base pair becomes a T-A or a C-G base pair.

Mutations are often classified according to the effect they have on the structure of the gene's protein product. This change in protein structure can be predicted using the genetic code table in conjunction with the base sequence of DNA or mRNA. A variety of such mutations is listed in Table I-4-1. Point mutations and frameshifts are illustrated in more detail in Figure I-4-2.

Table I-4-1. Effects of Some Common Types of Mutations on Protein Structure

Type of Mutation	Effect on Protein
Silent: new codon specifies same amino acid	None
Missense: new codon specifies different amino acid	Possible decrease in function; variable effects
Nonsense: new codon is stop codon	Shorter than normal; usually nonfunctional
Frameshift/in-frame: addition or deletion of base(s)	Usually nonfunctional; often shorter than normal
Large segment deletion (unequal crossover in meiosis)	Loss of function; shorter than normal or entirely missing
5′ splice site (donor) or 3′ splice site (acceptor)	Variable effects ranging from addition or deletion of a few amino acids to deletion of an entire exon
Trinucleotide repeat expansion	Expansions in coding regions cause protein product to be longer than normal and unstable. Disease often shows anticipation in pedigree.

Section I • Biochemistry

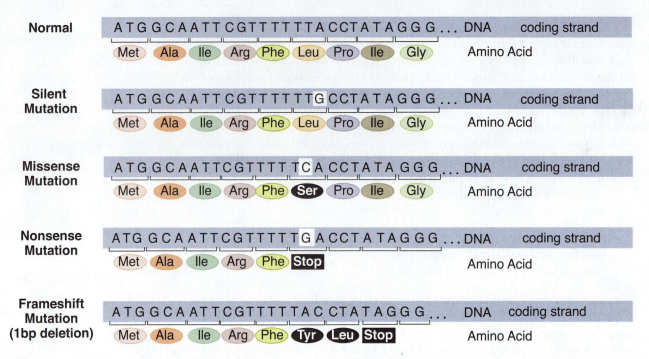

Figure I-4-2. Some Common Types of Mutations in DNA

Large Segment Deletions

Large segments of DNA can be deleted from a chromosome during an unequal crossover in meiosis. Crossover or recombination between homologous chromosomes is a normal part of meiosis I that generates genetic diversity in reproductive cells (egg and sperm), a largely beneficial result. In a normal crossover event, the homologous maternal and paternal chromosomes exchange equivalent segments, and although the resultant chromosomes are mosaics of maternal and paternal alleles, no genetic information has been lost from either one. On rare occasions, a crossover can be unequal and one of the two homologs loses some of its genetic information.

α-thalassemia is a well-known example of a genetic disease in which unequal crossover has deleted one or more α-globin genes from chromosome 16. Cri-du-chat (mental retardation, microcephaly, wide-set eyes, and a characteristic kittenlike cry) results from a terminal deletion of the short arm of chromosome 5.

Mutations in Splice Sites

Mutations in splice sites affect the accuracy of intron removal from hnRNA during posttranscriptional processing. If a splice site is lost through mutation, spliceosomes may:

- Delete nucleotides from the adjacent exon.
- Leave nucleotides of the intron in the processed mRNA.
- Use the next normal upstream or downstream splice site, deleting an exon from the processed mRNA.

Mutations in splice sites have now been documented in many different diseases, including β-thalassemia, Gaucher disease, and Tay-Sachs.

β-Thalassemia

There are two genes for the beta chain of hemoglobin. In β-thalassemia, there is a deficiency of β-globin protein compared with α-globin. A large number of β-globin mutations have been described, including gene deletions, mutations that slow the transcriptional process, and translational defects involving nonsense and frameshift mutations. Other mutations involve β-globin mRNA processing (more than 70% of the β-globin gene is not encoding information and eventually must be spliced out), such as splice site mutations at the consensus sequences. Also, mutations within intron 1 create a new splice site, resulting in an abnormally long mRNA.

A 9-month-old infant of Greek descent was brought to the hospital by his parents because he became pale, listless, and frequently irritable. The attending physician noted that the spleen was enlarged and that the infant was severely anemic. His face had "rat-like" features due to deformities in the skull.

β-thalassemias are found primarily in Mediterranean areas. It is believed that, similar to sickle cell anemia and glucose-6-phosphate dehydrogenase deficiency, the abnormality of red blood cells in β-thalassemia may protect against malaria. Splenomegaly is due to the role of the spleen in clearing damaged red cells from the bloodstream. The excessive activity of the bone marrow produces bone deformities of the face and other areas. The long bones of the arms and legs are abnormally weak and fracture easily. The most common treatment is blood transfusions every 2–3 weeks, but iron overload is a serious consequence.

Trinucleotide Repeat Expansion

The mutant alleles in certain diseases, such as Huntington disease, fragile X syndrome, and myotonic dystrophy, differ from their normal counterparts only in the number of tandem copies of a trinucleotide. In these diseases, the number of repeats often increases with successive generations and correlates with increasing severity and decreasing age of onset, a phenomenon called anticipation. For example, in the normal Huntington allele, there are five tandem repeats of CAG in the coding region. Affected family members may have 30 to 60 of these CAG repeats. The normal protein contains five adjacent glutamine residues, whereas the proteins encoded by the disease-associated alleles have 30 or more adjacent glutamines. The long glutamine tract makes the abnormal proteins extremely unstable. A major clinical manifestation of the trinucleotide repeat expansion disorders is neurodegeneration of specific neurons.

The expansion of the trinucleotide repeat in the mutant allele can be in a coding region or in an untranslated region of the gene. A summary of the important trinucleotide repeat expansion diseases is shown in Table I-4-2:

Table I-4-2. Two Classes of Trinucleotide Repeat Expansion Diseases

Translation repeat disorders (polyglutamine disorders)	Untranslated repeat disorders
Huntington disease: (CAG)n	Fragile X syndrome: (CGG)n
Spinobulbar muscular atrophy: (CAG)n	Myotonic dystrophy: (CTG)n
	Friedreich's ataxia: (GAA)n

Clinical Correlate

Huntington disease, an autosomal dominant disorder, has a mean age-of-onset of 43–48 years. Symptoms appear gradually and worsen over a period of about 15 years until death occurs. Mood disturbance, impaired memory, and hyperreflexia are often the first signs, followed by abnormal gait, chorea (loss of motor control), dystonia, dementia, and dysphagia.

Cases of juvenile onset (<10 years old) are more severe and most frequently occur when the defective allele is inherited paternally. About 25% of cases have late onset, slower progression, and milder symptoms.

AMINO ACID ACTIVATION AND CODON TRANSLATION BY TRNAs

Inasmuch as amino acids have no direct affinity for mRNA, an adapter molecule, which recognizes an amino acid on one end and its corresponding codon on the other, is required for translation. This adapter molecule is tRNA.

Amino Acid Activation

As tRNAs enter the cytoplasm, each combines with its cognate amino acid in a process called amino acid activation (Figure I-4-3).

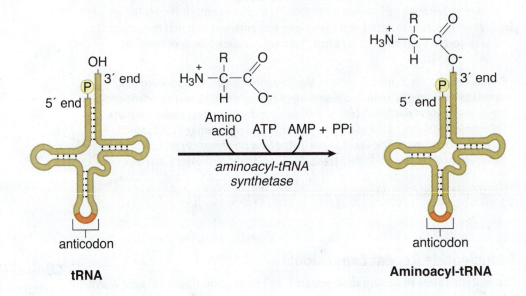

Figure I-4-3. Activation of Amino Acid for Protein Synthesis

- Each type of amino acid is activated by a different aminoacyl tRNA synthetase.
- Two high-energy bonds from an ATP are required.
- The aminoacyl tRNA synthetase transfers the activated amino acid to the 3′ end of the correct tRNA.
- The amino acid is linked to its cognate tRNA with an energy-rich bond.
- This bond will later supply energy to make a peptide bond linking the amino acid into a protein.

Aminoacyl tRNA synthetases have self-checking functions to prevent incorrectly paired aminoacyl tRNAs from forming. If, however, an aminoacyl tRNA synthetase does release an incorrectly paired product (ala-tRNA^{ser}), there is no mechanism during translation to detect the error and an incorrect amino acid will be introduced into some protein.

Each tRNA has an anticodon sequence that allows it to pair with the codon for its cognate amino acid in the mRNA. Because base pairing is involved, the orientation of this interaction will be complementary and antiparallel. For example, the amino acyl tRNA arg-tRNA^{arg} has an anticodon sequence, UCG, allowing it to pair with the arginine codon CGA.

Chapter 4 • The Genetic Code, Mutations, and Translation

TRANSLATION (PROTEIN SYNTHESIS)

Protein synthesis occurs by peptide bond formation between successive amino acids whose order is specified by a gene and thus by an mRNA. The formation of a peptide bond between the carboxyl group on one amino acid and the amino group of another is illustrated in Figure I-4-4.

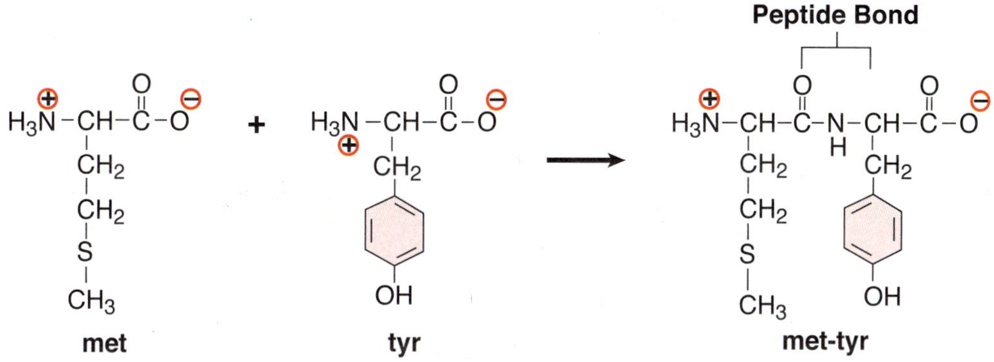

Figure I-4-4. Peptide Bond Formation

During translation, the amino acids are attached to the 3′ ends of their respective tRNAs. The aminoacyl–tRNAs are situated in the P and A sites of the ribosome as shown in Figure I-4-5. Notice that the peptide bond forms between the carboxyl group of the amino acid (or growing peptide) in the P site and the amino group of the next amino acid in the A site. Proteins are synthesized from the amino to the carboxyl terminus.

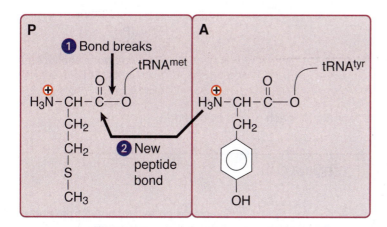

Figure I-4-5. Formation of a Peptide Bond by a Ribosome During Translation

Steps of Translation

Translation occurs in the cytoplasm of both prokaryotic (Pr) and eukaryotic (Eu) cells. In prokaryotes, ribosomes can begin translating the mRNA even before RNA polymerase completes its transcription. In eukaryotes, translation

Section I • Biochemistry

and transcription are completely separated in time and space with transcription in the nucleus and translation in the cytoplasm. The process of protein synthesis occurs in 3 stages: initiation, elongation, and termination (Figure I-4-6). Special protein factors for initiation (IF), elongation (EF), and termination (release factors), as well as GTP, are required for each of these stages.

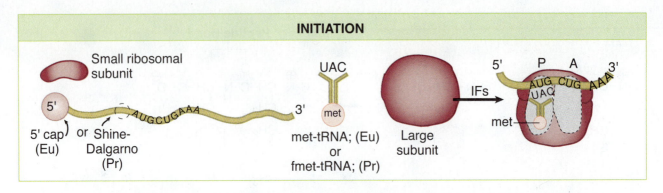

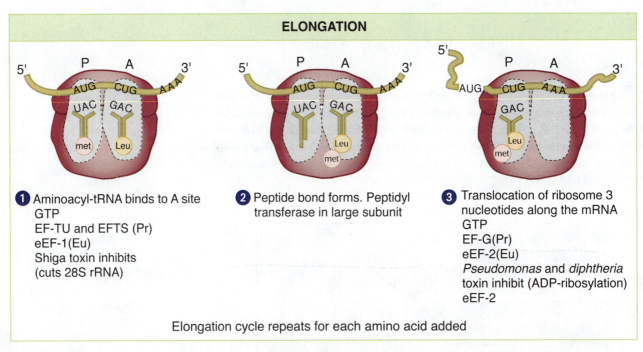

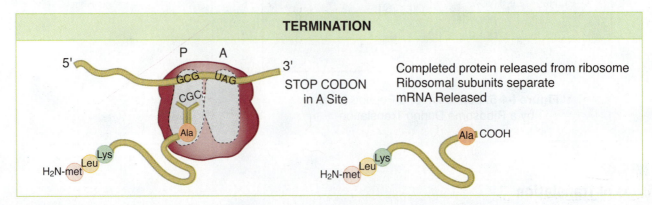

Figure I-4-6. Steps in Translation

Initiation

The small ribosomal subunit binds to the mRNA. In prokaryotes, the 16S rRNA of the small subunit binds to the Shine-Dalgarno sequence in the 5′ untranslated region of the mRNA. In eukaryotes, the small subunit binds to the 5′ cap structure and slides down the message to the first AUG.

The charged initiator tRNA becomes bound to the AUG start codon on the message through base pairing with its anticodon. The initiator tRNA in prokaryotes carries fmet, whereas the initiator tRNA in eukaryotes carries Met.

The large subunit binds to the small subunit, forming the completed initiation complex.

There are 2 important binding sites on the ribosome called the P site and the A site.

- The peptidyl site (P site) is the site on the ribosome where (f)met–tRNA$_i$ initially binds. After formation of the first peptide bond, the P site is a binding site for the growing peptide chain.
- The aminoacyl site (A site) binds each new incoming tRNA molecule carrying an activated amino acid.

Elongation

Elongation is a 3-step cycle that is repeated for each amino acid added to the protein after the initiator methionine. Each cycle uses 4 high-energy bonds (2 from the ATP used in amino acid activation to charge the tRNA, and 2 from GTP). During elongation, the ribosome moves in the 5′ to 3′ direction along the mRNA, synthesizing the protein from amino to carboxyl terminus. The 3 steps are:

- A charged tRNA binds in the A site. The particular aminoacyl–tRNA is determined by the mRNA codon aligned with the A site.
- Peptidyl transferase, an enzyme that is part of the large subunit, forms the peptide bond between the new amino acid and the carboxyl end of the growing polypeptide chain. The bond linking the growing peptide to the tRNA in the P site is broken, and the growing peptide attaches to the tRNA located in the A site.
- In the translocation step, the ribosome moves exactly three nucleotides (one codon) along the message. This moves the growing peptidyl–tRNA into the P site and aligns the next codon to be translated with the empty A site.

In eukaryotic cells, elongation factor-2 (eEF-2) used in translocation is inactivated through ADP-ribosylation by *Pseudomonas* and *Diphtheria* toxins.

Shiga and Shiga-like toxins clip an adenine residue from the 28S rRNA in the 60S subunit stopping protein synthesis in eukaryotic cells.

Termination

When any of the 3 stop (termination or nonsense) codons moves into the A site, peptidyl transferase (with the help of release factor) hydrolyzes the completed protein from the final tRNA in the P site. The mRNA, ribosome, tRNA, and factors can all be reused for additional protein synthesis.

POLYSOMES

Messenger RNA molecules are very long compared with the size of a ribosome, allowing room for several ribosomes to translate a message at the same time. Because ribosomes translate mRNA in the 5′ to 3′ direction, the ribosome closest to the 3′ end has the longest nascent peptide. Polysomes are found free in the cytoplasm or attached to the rough endoplasmic reticulum (RER), depending on the protein being translated.

INHIBITORS OF PROTEIN SYNTHESIS

Some well-known inhibitors of prokaryotic translation include streptomycin, erythromycin, tetracycline, and chloramphenicol. Inhibitors of eukaryotic translation include cycloheximide and *Diphtheria* and *Pseudomonas* toxins.

Certain antibiotics (for example, chloramphenicol) inhibit mitochondrial protein synthesis, but not cytoplasmic protein synthesis, because mitochondrial ribosomes are similar to prokaryotic ribosomes.

PROTEIN FOLDING AND SUBUNIT ASSEMBLY

As proteins emerge from ribosomes, they fold into three-dimensional conformations that are essential for their subsequent biologic activity. Generally, four levels of protein shape are distinguished:

Primary—sequence of amino acids specified in the gene.

Secondary—folding of the amino acid chain into an energetically stable structure. Two common examples are the α-helix and the β-pleated sheet. These shapes are reinforced by hydrogen bonds. An individual protein may contain both types of secondary structures. Some proteins, like collagen, contain neither but have their own more characteristic secondary structures.

Tertiary—positioning of the secondary structures in relation to each other to generate higher-order three-dimensional shapes (the domains of the IgG molecule are examples). Tertiary structure also includes the shape of the protein as a whole (globular, fibrous). Tertiary structures are stabilized by weak bonds (hydrogen, hydrophobic, ionic) and, in some proteins, strong, covalent disulfide bonds. Agents such as heat or urea disrupt tertiary structure to denature proteins, causing loss of function.

Quaternary—in proteins such as hemoglobin that have multiple subunits, quaternary structure describes the interactions among subunits.

TRANSLATION OCCURS ON FREE RIBOSOMES AND ON THE ROUGH ENDOPLASMIC RETICULUM

Although all translation of eukaryotic nuclear genes begins on ribosomes free in the cytoplasm, the proteins being translated may belong in other locations. For example, certain proteins are translated on ribosomes associated with the rough endoplasmic reticulum (RER), including:

Clinical Correlate
Gray Baby Syndrome

Gray syndrome is a dangerous condition that occurs in newborns (especially premature babies) who are given the drug chloramphenicol. Chloramphenicol is a drug used to fight bacterial infections, including meningitis. If given to a newborn, however, this drug can trigger a potentially deadly reaction. Babies do not have sufficient UDP-glucuronyl transferase activity needed to allow excretion of this drug. The drug builds up in the baby's bloodstream and can lead to:

- Blue lips, nail beds, and skin (cyanosis)
- Death
- Low blood pressure

- Secreted proteins
- Proteins inserted into the cell membrane
- Lysosomal enzymes

Proteins translated on free cytoplasmic ribosomes include:
- Cytoplasmic proteins
- Mitochondrial proteins (encoded by nuclear genes)

Molecular Chaperones and Proteasomes

Protein folding is an essential step in the final synthesis of any protein. There is a class of specialized proteins, **chaperones**, whose function is to assist in this process. Molecular chaperones function in many cell compartments, including the endoplasmic reticulum, where extensive protein synthesis occurs. Failure to fold correctly usually results in eventual destruction of the protein.

Proteasomes and Ubiquitin

Whenever protein synthesis occurs in a cell, a few copies of a particular protein may not fold correctly. These defective copies are covalently marked for destruction by the addition of multiple copies of ubiquitin. Polyubiquinated proteins are directed to proteasomes for destruction. Proteasomes are large, cytoplasmic complexes that have multiple protease activities capable of digesting damaged proteins to peptides, as shown in Figure I-4-7. Proteasomes also play a role in producing antigenic peptides for presentation by class I MHC molecules.

Clinical Correlate
Cystic Fibrosis

The majority of cases of cystic fibrosis result from the deletion of phenylalanine at position 508 (ΔF508), which interferes with proper protein folding and the posttranslational processing of oligosaccharide side chains. The abnormal chloride channel protein (CFTR) is degraded by the cytosolic proteasome complex rather than being translocated to the cell membrane. Other functional defects in CFTR protein reaching the cell membrane may also contribute to the pathogenesis of cystic fibrosis.

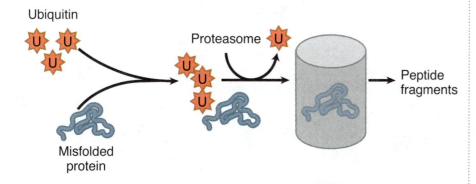

Figure I-4-7. Degradation of Misfolded Proteins by Proteasomes

Many proteins require signals to ensure delivery to the appropriate organelles. Especially important among these signals are:
- The *N*-terminal hydrophobic signal sequence used to ensure translation on the RER
- Phosphorylation of mannose residues important for directing an enzyme to a lysosome

The targeting process for these proteins is illustrated in Figure I-4-8.

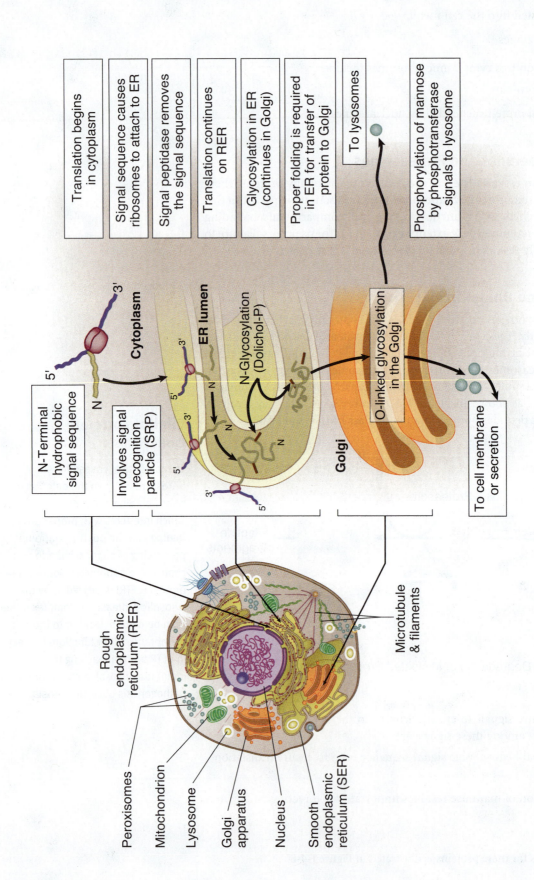

Figure 1-4-8. Synthesis of Secretory, Membrane, and Lysosomal Proteins

N-Terminal Hydrophobic Signal Sequence

This sequence is found on proteins destined to be secreted (insulin), placed in the cell membrane (Na^+-K^+ ATPase), or ultimately directed to the lysosome (sphingomyelinase). These proteins all require N-terminal hydrophobic signal sequences as part of their primary structure. Translation begins on free cytoplasmic ribosomes, but after translation of the signal sequence, the ribosome is positioned on the ER (now RER) with the help of a signal recognition particle. During translation, the nascent protein is fed through the membrane of the RER and captured in the lumen. The signal sequence is cleaved off in the ER, and then the protein passes into the Golgi for further modification and sorting.

In transit through the ER and Golgi, most proteins acquire oligosaccharide side chains, becoming glycoproteins. N-glycosylation refers to the addition of sugar chains to the nitrogen of asparagine residues (N-linked). The attachment of sugars in N-glycosylation begins in the ER (cotranslational modification) and requires the participation of a special lipid called dolichol phosphate. The N-linked sugar chain can further be modified upon entry in the Golgi (posttranslational modification). O-glycosylation refers to the addition of sugar chains to the hydroxyl group of either serine or threonine residues of the protein, and it occurs exclusively in the Golgi (posttranslational modification). Depending of the particular glycoprotein, some proteins are solely N-glycosylated (for example, transferrin); some are solely O-glycosylated (for example, heparin); and some are both N- and O-glycosylated (for example, LDL receptor). Significantly, the structure and sequence of the oligosaccharide chains on proteins and lipids (glycolipids) are the basis of the A, B, O blood groups.

Accumulation or ineffective targeting of misfolded proteins

Proteins synthesized in the endoplasmic reticulum must fold correctly for transport to the Golgi and then to their final destinations. In certain genetic diseases, the mutation may cause all copies of the protein to fold incorrectly. The result is loss of protein function and, in some cases, accumulation of the misfolded protein in the endoplasmic reticulum.

α_1-Antitrypsin Deficiency

A 70-year-old woman with elevated liver function tests was being evaluated for cirrhosis. Her serum α_1-antitrypsin level was 25 mg/dL (normal: 90–225 mg/dL). A liver biopsy showed micronodular cirrhosis and prominent fibrosis. Immunohistochemical studies showed intense staining with α_1-antitrypsin antibody. The patient was tested for likely mutations in the α_1-antitrypsin gene and found to be homozygous for the Z mutation (ZZ). This mutation causes the α_1-antitrypsin protein to misfold and aggregate in the endoplastic reticulum, where it damages cells, eventually leading to cirrhosis. She had no evidence of pulmonary disease.

α_1-antitrypsin is a protein synthesized primarily by the liver and secreted in the bloodstream. Its function is to protect cells by serving as an inhibitor of proteases released during a normal inflammatory response. Among the more than 90 allelic variants of the α_1-antitrypsin gene, the Z and S variants are most often encountered with α_1-antitrypsin deficiency. Both are the result of point mutations, which can be detected with the polymerase chain reaction (PCR) technique.

Section I • Biochemistry

Bridge to Anatomy
Lysosomes

- Organelles whose major function is to digest materials that the cell has ingested by endocytosis.
- Contain multiple enzymes that, collectively, digest carbohydrates (glycosylases), lipids (lipases), and proteins (proteases).
- Especially prominent in cells such as neutrophils and macrophages, though they serve this essential role in almost all cells.

When a lysosomal enzyme is missing (for instance in a genetic disease such as Tay-Sachs), the undigested substrate accumulates in the cell, often leading to serious consequences.

Lysosomal Enzymes and Phosphorylation of Mannose

Lysosomal enzymes are glycosylated and modified in a characteristic way. Most importantly, when they arrive in the Golgi apparatus, specific mannose residues located in their N-linked oligosaccharide chains are phosphorylated by N-acetyl-glucosamine-1 phosphotransferase, forming a critical mannose-6-phosphate in the oligosaccharide chain. This phosphorylation is the critical event that removes them from the secretion pathway and directs them to lysosomes. Genetic defects affecting this phosphorylation produce I-cell disease in which lysosomal enzymes are released into the extracellular space, and inclusion bodies accumulate in the cell, compromising its function.

Major Symptoms of I-Cell Disease

A child aged 5 months was referred to a specialist. The child had been born with dislocated hips and a coarse featured face. He had been suffering repeated upper respiratory tract infections and did not seem to be developing his motor abilities, Clinical examination revealed hyperplasia of the gums, restriction of joint mobility and hepatosplenomegaly. On listening to the heart a mitral valve murmur could be detected. Further investigation involved cell culture of the child's fibroblasts obtained from a skin biopsy. Examination of the fibroblasts under the microscope revealed the presence of numerous intracellular inclusions, which on electron microscopy were revealed to be large lysosomes. Biochemical analysis showed decreased levels of the lysosomal hydrolase ß-glucuronidase within the fibroblasts, but elevated levels of this enzyme within the culture medium. A diagnosis of I-cell disease was made.

- Coarse facial features, gingival hyperplasia, macroglossia
- Craniofacial abnormalities, joint immobility, clubfoot, claw-hand, scoliosis
- Psychomotor retardation, growth retardation
- Cardiorespiratory failure, death in first decade
- Bone fracture and deformities
- Mitral valve defect
- Secretion of active lysosomal enzymes into blood and extracellular fluid

CO- AND POSTTRANSLATIONAL COVALENT MODIFICATIONS

In addition to disulfide bond formation while proteins are folding, other covalent modifications include:

- Glycosylation: addition of oligosaccharide as proteins pass through the ER and Golgi apparatus
- Proteolysis: cleavage of peptide bonds to remodel proteins and activate them (proinsulin, trypsinogen, prothrombin)
- Phosphorylation: addition of phosphate by protein kinases

- γ-Carboxylation: produces Ca^{2+} binding sites
- Prenylation: addition of farnesyl or geranylgeranyl lipid groups to certain membrane-associated proteins

POSTTRANSLATIONAL MODIFICATIONS OF COLLAGEN

Collagen is an example of a protein that undergoes several important co- and posttranslational modifications. It has a somewhat unique primary structure in that much of its length is composed of a repeating tripeptide Gly-X-Y-Gly-X-Y-etc. Hydroxyproline is an amino acid unique to collagen. The hydroxyproline is produced by hydroxylation of prolyl residues at the Y positions in procollagen chains as they pass through the RER. Important points about collagen synthesis are summarized below and in Figure I-4-9.

1. Prepro-α chains containing a hydrophobic signal sequence are synthesized by ribosomes attached to the RER.
2. The hydrophobic signal sequence is removed by signal peptidase in the RER to form pro-α chains.
3. Selected prolines and lysines are hydroxylated by prolyl and lysyl hydroxylases. These enzymes, located in the RER, require ascorbate (vitamin C), deficiency of which produces scurvy.
4. Selected hydroxylysines are glycosylated.
5. Three pro-α chains assemble to form a triple helical structure (procollagen), which can now be transferred to the Golgi. Modification of oligosaccharide continues in the Golgi.
6. Procollagen is secreted from the cell.
7. The propeptides are cleaved from the ends of procollagen by proteases to form collagen molecules (also called tropocollagen).
8. Collagen molecules assemble into fibrils. Cross-linking involves lysyl oxidase, an enzyme that requires O_2 and copper.
9. Fibrils aggregate and cross-link to form collagen fibers.

Table I-4-3. Collagen

Collagen Type	Characteristics	Tissue Distribution	Associated Diseases
I	Bundles of fibers High tensile strength	Bone, skin, tendons	Osteogenesis imperfecta Ehlers-Danlos (various)
II	Thin fibrils Structural	Cartilage Vitreous humor	----------
III	Thin fibrils Pliable	Blood vessels Granulation tissue	Ehlers-Danlos Type IV Keloid formation
IV	Amorphous	Basement membranes	Goodpasture syndrome Alport disease Epidermolysis bullosa

Section I • Biochemistry

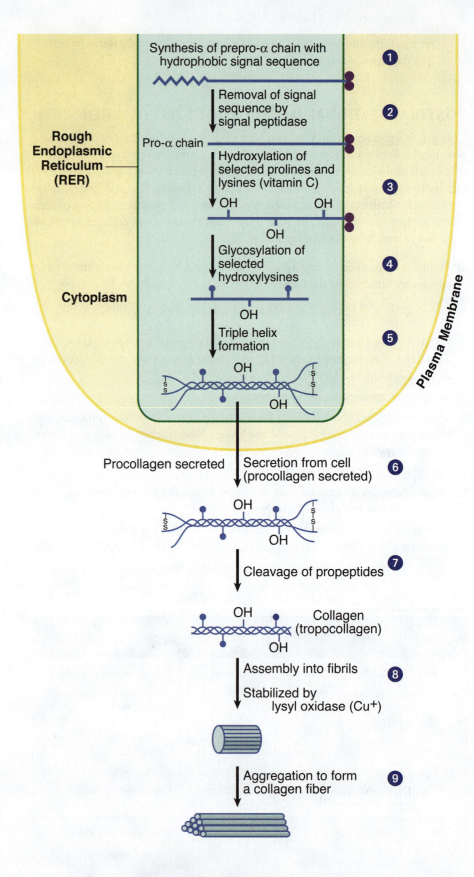

Figure I-4-9. Synthesis of Collagen

Several important diseases associated with defective collagen production are shown in Table I-4-4.

Table I-4-4. Disorders of Collagen Biosynthesis

Disease	Defect	Major Symptoms
Scurvy	Deficient hydroxylation secondary to ascorbate deficiency	Petechiae, ecchymoses Loose teeth, bleeding gums Poor wound healing Poor bone development
Osteogenesis imperfecta	Mutations in collagen genes	Skeletal deformities Fractures, blue sclera
Ehlers-Danlos syndromes	Mutations in collagen genes and proline and lysyl hydroxylases	Hyperextensible, fragile skin Hypermobile joints, dislocations, varicose veins, ecchymoses, arterial, intestinal ruptures
Menkes disease	Deficient cross-linking secondary to functional copper deficiency	Depigmented (steely) hair Arterial tortuosity, rupture Cerebral degeneration Osteoporosis, anemia

Clinical Correlate

Ehlers-Danlos (ED) Syndromes represent a collection of defects in the normal synthesis and processing of collagen. Like osteogenesis imperfecta, these syndromes are a result of locus heterogeneity in which defects in several different genes (loci) can result in similar symptoms.

ED Type IV, the vascular type, is an autosomal dominant disease caused by mutations in the gene for type-3 procollagen. Characteristic features include thin, translucent skin; arterial, intestinal, or uterine rupture; and easy bruising.

Also see Section II, Chapter 1; Locus Heterogeneity.

Menkes Disease

A 4-month-old infant who failed to grow and appeared to be mentally retarded was brought to the clinic for testing. The physician noted that the infant had abnormally kinky and hypopigmented hair. An arteriogram showed elongation and tortuosity of the major arteries. Additional tests revealed bladder diverticula and subdural hematomas. A blood test showed that the infant had low serum ceruloplasmin and only 10% of normal serum copper levels.

This infant has Menkes disease, which is also known as Ehlers-Danlos syndrome type IX (kinky hair syndrome). It is an X-linked recessive disease that has an incidence of 1/100,000 newborns. Common with Ehlers-Danlos diseases, Menkes disease has a symptomology due, in part, to weak collagen.

The disease is caused by mutations in the gene ATP7A, which encodes an ATP-dependent copper efflux protein in the intestine. Copper can be absorbed into the mucosal cell, but it cannot be transported into the bloodstream. Consequently, an affected individual will have severe copper deficiency and all copper-requiring enzymes will be adversely affected. Lysyl oxidase requires copper and plays a direct role in collagen formation by catalyzing the cross-linking of collagen fibrils. A deficiency in the activity of this enzyme and other copper-dependent enzymes would be directly responsible for the described symptoms in this infant.

Table I-4-5. Important Points About the Genetic Code, Mutations, and Translation

	Prokaryotic	Eukaryotic
Genetic code	Start: AUG (also codes for Met) Stop: UAG, UGA, UAA Unambiguous (1 codon = 1 amino acid) Redundant (1 amino acid >1 codon); often differ at base 3	
Mutations	Point mutations: silent, missense, nonsense Frameshift (delete 1 or 2 nucleotides; not multiple of 3) Large segment deletion	
		Mutation in splice site Trinucleotide repeat expansion
Amino acid activation	Aminoacyl-tRNA synthetase: two high-energy bonds (ATP) to link amino acid to tRNA	
Translation: Initiation	30S subunit binds to Shine-Dalgarno sequence on mRNA fMet–tRNA$_i$ binds to P site GTP required	40S subunit associates with 5′ cap on mRNA Met–tRNA$_i$ binds to P site GTP required
Translation: Elongation	Charged aminoacyl–tRNA binds to A site (GTP) Peptide bond forms (two high-energy bonds from amino acid activation) Peptidyl synthase (50S subunit) Translocation: GTP required	Charged aminoacyl–tRNA binds to A site (GTP) 28S rRNA is cut by Shiga and Shiga-like toxins removing an adenine residue. Prevents protein synthesis. Peptide bond forms (two high-energy bonds from amino acid activation) Peptidyl synthase (60S subunit) Translocation: GTP required eEF-2 inhibited by *Diphtheria* and *Pseudomonas* toxins
Termination	Release of protein; protein synthesized N to C	
Protein targeting		Secreted or membrane proteins: N-terminal hydrophobic signal sequence Lysosomal enzymes: phosphorylation of mannose by phosphotransferase in Golgi I-cell disease
Other important disease associations		Scurvy (prolyl hydroxylase, Vit C) Menke Disease (Cu deficiency, lysyl oxidase)

Review Questions

Select the ONE best answer.

1. In the genetic code of human nuclear DNA, one of the codons specifying the amino acid tyrosine is UAC. Another codon specifying this same amino acid is

    A. AAC
    B. UAG
    C. UCC
    D. AUG
    E. UAU

Items 2 and 3

   A. ATGCAA...→ ATG**T**AA
   B. ATGAAA...→ **G**TGAAA
   C. TATAAG...→ T**C**TAAG
   D. CTTAAG...→ **G**TTAAG
   E. ATGAAT ...→ ATG**C**AT

The options above represent mutations in the DNA with base changes indicated in boldface type. For each mutation described in the questions below, choose the most closely related sequence change in the options above.

2. Nonsense mutation

3. Mutation decreasing the initiation of transcription

4. Accumulation of heme in reticulocytes can regulate globin synthesis by indirectly inactivating eIF-2. Which of the following steps is most directly affected by this mechanism?

    A. Attachment of spliceosomes to pre-mRNA
    B. Attachment of the ribosome to the endoplasmic reticulum
    C. Met-tRNAmet binding to the P-site
    D. Translocation of mRNA on the ribosome
    E. Attachment of RNA polymerase II to the promoter

Section I • Biochemistry

5. A nasopharyngeal swab obtained from a 4-month-old infant with rhinitis and paroxysmal coughing tested positive upon culture for *Bordetella pertussis*. He was admitted to the hospital for therapy with an antibiotic that inhibits the translocation of the 70S ribosomes on the mRNA. This patient was most likely treated with

    A. erythromycin
    B. tetracycline
    C. chloramphenicol
    D. rifamycin
    E. levofloxacin

6. A 25-month-old Caucasian girl has coarse facial features and gingival hyperplasia and, at 2 months of age, began developing multiple, progressive symptoms of mental retardation, joint contractures, hepatomegaly, and cardiomegaly. Levels of lysosomal enzymes are elevated in her serum, and fibroblasts show phase-dense inclusions in the cytoplasm. Which of the following enzyme deficiencies is most consistent with these observations?

    A. Golgi-associated phosphotransferase
    B. Lysosomal α-1,4-glucosidase
    C. Endoplasmic reticulum–associated signal peptidase
    D. Cytoplasmic α-1,4-phosphorylase
    E. Lysosomal hexosaminidase A

7. Parahemophilia is an autosomal recessive bleeding disorder characterized by a reduced plasma concentration of the Factor V blood coagulation protein. Deficiency arises from a 12 base-pair deletion in the Factor V gene that impairs the secretion of Factor V by hepatocytes and results in an abnormal accumulation of immunoreactive Factor V antigen in the cytoplasm. In which region of the Factor V gene would this mutation most likely be located?

    A. 5′ Untranslated region
    B. First exon
    C. Middle intron
    D. Last exon
    E. 3′ Untranslated region

8. Collagen, the most abundant protein in the human body, is present in varying amounts in many tissues. If one wished to compare the collagen content of several tissues, one could measure their content of

   A. glycine
   B. proline
   C. hydroxyproline
   D. cysteine
   E. lysine

9. A 6-month-old infant is seen in the emergency room with a fractured rib and subdural hematoma. The child's hair is thin, colorless, and tangled. His serum copper level is 5.5 nM (normal for age, 11–12 nM). Developmental delay is prominent. A deficiency of which enzyme activity most closely relates to these symptoms?

   A. Lysyl oxidase
   B. Prolyl hydroxylase
   C. γ-Glutamyl carboxylase
   D. Phosphotransferase in Golgi
   E. α-1,4-glucosidase

10. Respiratory tract infections caused by *Pseudomonas aeruginosa* are associated with the secretion of exotoxin A by this organism. What effect will this toxin most likely have on eukaryotic cells?

    A. Stimulation of nitric oxide (NO) synthesis
    B. ADP-ribosylation of a Gs protein
    C. ADP-ribosylation of eEF-2
    D. ADP-ribosylation of a Gi protein
    E. Stimulation of histamine release

11. A 4-year-old toddler with cystic fibrosis (CF) is seen by his physician for an upper respiratory infection with *Pseudomonas aeruginosa*. He is started on oral ciprofloxacin and is referred to a CF center as a potential candidate for gene therapy. Prior genetic testing of the patient identified the mutation causing cystic fibrosis as a 3-base-pair deletion in exon 10 of the CF gene. The nucleotide sequences of codons 506–511 in this region of the normal and mutant alleles are compared below.

Codon Number	506	507	508	509	510	511
Normal Gene	ATC	ATC	TTT	GGT	GTT	TCC
Mutant Gene	ATC	AT•	••T	GGT	GTT	TCC

3-base deletion (between codons 507 and 508)

What effect will this patient's mutation have on the amino acid sequence of the protein encoded by the CF gene?

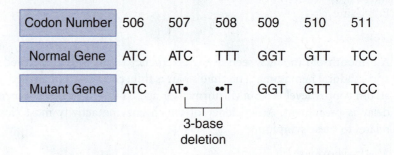

A. Deletion of a phenylalanine residue with no change in C-terminal sequence

B. Deletion of a leucine residue causing a change in the C-terminal sequence

C. Deletion of a phenylalanine residue causing a change in the C-terminal sequence

D. Deletion of a leucine residue with no change in C-terminal sequence

12. A 10-year-old boy with severe progressive skin ulceration, decreased resistance to infection, and impaired cognitive ability has been diagnosed with a genetic deficiency of the enzyme prolidase. Mutation analysis has identified a single base substitution at the 3' end of intron 6 of the mutant allele as well as deletion of a 45-base exon (exon 7) in the prolidase cDNA. Which type of gene mutation was most likely inherited by this boy?

    A. Frameshift mutation
    B. In-frame mutation
    C. Missense mutation
    D. Nonsense mutation
    E. Splice site mutation

Answers

1. **Answer: E.** Because of wobble codons for the same amino acid often differ in the third base. Option B would be acceptable, except that it is a stop codon.

2. **Answer: A.** The sequence now contains TAA which will be transcribed to UAA in the mRNA.

3. **Answer: C.** The transcription promoter TATA has been changed to TCTA. Don't choose the distractor B. The question is not about translation.

4. **Answer: C.** eIF-2 designates a protein factor of the initiation phase in eukaryotic translation. The only event listed that would occur during this phase is placement of initiator tRNA in the P-site.

5. **Answer: A.** Erythromycin is the antibiotic of choice for pertussis. It inhibits translocation.

6. **Answer: A.** Characteristic symptoms of I-cell disease. Note release of lysosomal enzymes into serum, which would not be seen in the other deficiencies.

7. **Answer: B.** Decreased factor V secretion and a corresponding accumulation of cytoplasmic antigen suggest a defect in the translocation of the nascent protein to the endoplasmic reticulum. This implies a mutation in the N-terminal amino acid signal sequence required for targeting to the ER and encoded by the first exon of the gene.

8. **Answer: C.** Hydroxyproline is found uniquely in collagen. Although collagen is also rich in glycine, many other proteins contain significant amounts of glycine.

9. **Answer: A.** The child has Menkes disease, in which cellular copper transport is abnormal and produces a functional copper deficiency. Lysyl oxidase in collagen metabolism requires copper. His fragile bones and blood vessels result from weak, poorly crosslinked connective tissue.

Section I • Biochemistry

10. **Answer: C.** *Pseudomonas* and diphtheria toxins inhibit eEF-2, the translocation factor in eukaryotic translation.

11. **Answer: A.** Deletion of CTT results only in the loss of phe 508; ile 507 and the C-terminal sequence are unaltered because ATC and ATT both code for ile (the coding sequence is unchanged).

12. **Answer: E.** A base *substitution* at an intron-exon junction, which leads to the deletion of an entire exon is indicative of a splice site mutation.

Regulation of Eukaryotic Gene Expression   5

Learning Objectives

❑ Demonstrate understanding of regulation of eukaryotic gene expression

OVERVIEW OF GENETIC REGULATION

Regulation of gene expression is an essential feature in maintaining the functional integrity of a cell. Increasing or decreasing the expression of a gene can occur through a variety of mechanisms, but many of the important ones involve regulating the rate of transcription. In addition to the basic transcription proteins, RNA polymerase and TFIID in eukaryotes activator and repressor proteins help control the rate of the process. These regulatory proteins bind to specific DNA sequences (enhancer or silencer elements) associated with eukaryotic gene regions.

Other mechanisms are important, and gene expression is controlled at multiple levels.

REGULATION OF EUKARYOTIC GENE EXPRESSION

In eukaryotic cells, DNA is packaged in chromatin structures, and gene expression typically requires chromatin remodeling (Figure I-5-1) in order to make the desired gene region accessible to RNA polymerase and other proteins (transcription factors) required for gene expression. Important aspects of chromatin remodeling include:

- Transcription factors that bind to the DNA and recruit other coactivators such as histone acetylases

- Histone acetylases (favor gene expression) and deacetylases (favor inactive chromatin)

- Certain lysyl residues in the histones are acetylated decreasing the positive charge and weakening the interaction with DNA.

- A chromatin remodeling engine that binds to acetylated lysyl residues and reconfigures the DNA to expose the promoter region.

- Additional transcription factors bind in the promoter region and recruit RNA polymerase.

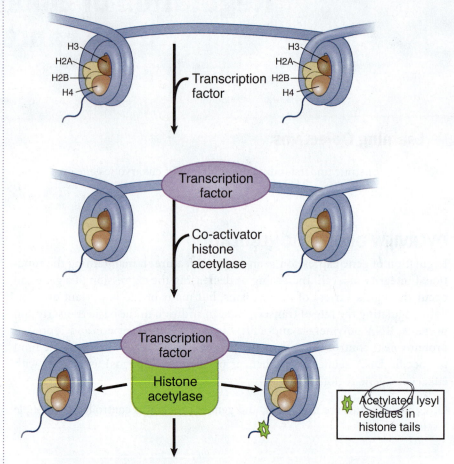

Figure I-5-1.

Once the transcription complex is formed, basal (low level) transcription occurs, maintaining moderate, but adequete, levels of the protein encoded by this gene in the cell. The transcription factors assembled in this complex are referred to as general transcription factors.

There are times when the expression of the gene should be increased in response to specific signals such as hormones, growth factors, intracellular conditions. In this case there are DNA sequences referred to as response elements that bind specific transcription factors. Several of these response elements may be grouped together to form an enhancer that allows control of gene expression by multiple signals (Figure I-5-2).

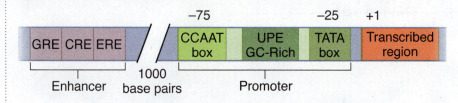

Figure I-5-2. Enhancers and Upstream Promoter Elements

Upstream Promoter Elements

Only the proximity of the upstream promoter element to the −25 sequence distinguishes it from an enhancer. Upstream promoter elements include:

- A CCAAT box (around −75) that binds a transcription factor NF-1
- A GC-rich sequence that binds a general transcription factor SP-1

Enhancers

Enhancers in the DNA are binding sites for activator proteins. Enhancers have the following characteristics:

- They may be up to 1,000 base pairs away from the gene.
- They may be located upstream, downstream, or within an intron of the gene they control.
- The orientation of the enhancer sequence with respect to the gene is not important.
- Enhancers can appear to act in a tissue-specific manner if the DNA-binding proteins that interact with them are present only in certain tissues.
- Enhancers may be brought close to the basal promoter region in space by bending of the DNA molecule (Figure I-5-3).

Similar sequences that bind repressor proteins in eukaryotes are called silencers. There are fewer examples of these sequences known.

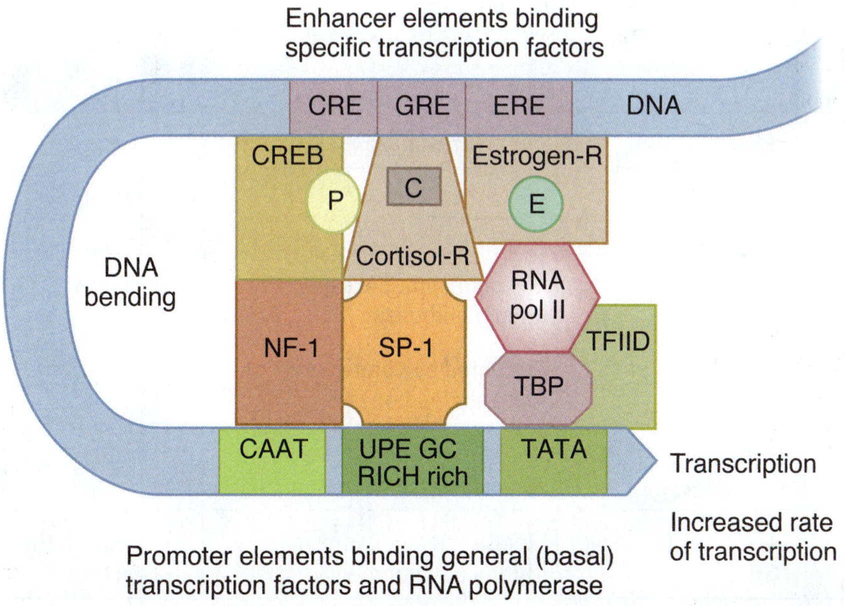

Note

The Ig heavy chain locus has an enhancer in the large intron separating the coding regions for the variable domain from the coding regions for the constant domains.

Note

Cis and Trans Regulatory Elements

The DNA regulatory base sequences (e.g., promoters, enhancers, response elements, and UPEs) in the vicinity of genes that serve as binding sites for proteins are often called "*cis*" regulators.

Transcription factors (and the genes that code for them) are called "*trans*" regulators. *Trans* regulatory proteins can diffuse through the cell to their point of action.

Figure I-5-3. Stimulation of Transcription by an Enhancer and Its Associated Transcription Factors

Section I • Biochemistry

Transcription Factors

The activator proteins that bind response elements are often referred to as transcription factors. Typically, transcription factors contain at least 2 recognizable domains, a DNA-binding domain and an activation domain.

1. The DNA-binding domain binds to a specific nucleotide sequence in the promoter or response element. Several types of DNA-binding domain motifs have been characterized and have been used to define certain families of transcription factors. Some common DNA-binding domains include:

   - Zinc fingers (steroid hormone receptors)
   - Leucine zippers (cAMP-dependent transcription factor)
   - Helix-loop-helix
   - Helix-turn-helix (homeodomain proteins encoded by homeotic/homeobox genes)

2. The activation domain allows the transcription factor to:

   - Bind to other transcription factors and coregulators
   - Interact with RNA polymerase II to stabilize the formation of the initiation complex
   - Recruit chromatin-modifying proteins such as histone acetylases or deacetylases

Two types can be distinguished: general transcription factors and specific transcription factors. Examples are listed in Table I-5-1.

Table I-5-1. Properties of Important Specific Transcription Factors

Transcription Factor (DNA-Binding Protein)	Response Element (Binding Site)	Function	Protein Class
Steroid receptors	HRE	Steroid response	Zinc finger
cAMP response element binding (CREB) protein	CRE	Response to cAMP	Leucine zipper
Peroxisome proliferator-activated receptors (PPARs)	PPREs	Regulate multiple aspects of lipid metabolism Activated by fibrates and thiazolidinediones	Zinc finger
NFkB (nuclear factor kappa-B)	kB elements	Regulates expression of many genes in immune system	Rel domains
Homeodomain proteins	—	Regulate gene expression during development	Helix-turn-helix

General Transcription Factors

In eukaryotes, general transcription factors must bind to the promoter to allow RNA polymerase II to bind and form the initiation complex at the start site for transcription. General transcription factors are common to most genes. The general transcription factor TFIID with its TATA box-binding protein subunit (TBP) must bind to the TATA box before RNA polymerase II can bind. Other examples include SP-1 and NF-1 that modulate basal transcription of many genes.

Specific Transcription Factors

Specific transcription factors bind to enhancer regions or, in a few cases, to silencers and modulate the formation of the initiation complex, thus regulating the rate of initiation of transcription. Each gene contains a variety of enhancer or silencer sequences in its regulatory region. The exact combination of specific transcription factors available (and active) in a particular cell at a particular time determines which genes will be transcribed at what rates. Because specific transcription factors are proteins, their expression can be cell-type specific. Additionally, hormones may regulate the activity of some specific transcription factors. Examples include steroid receptors and the CREB protein.

Peroxisome proliferator-activated receptors (PPARs) are transcription factors that bind to DNA response elements (PPREs) and control multiple aspects of lipid metabolism. Individual members of this family of zinc-finger proteins are activated by a variety of natural and xenobiotic ligands, including:

- Fatty acids
- Prostaglandin derivatives
- Fibrates
- Thiazolidinediones

The improvement in insulin resistance seen with thiazolidinediones is thought to be mediated through their interaction with PPARγ. Clofibrate binds PPARα, affecting different aspects of lipid metabolism than the thiazolidinediones.

Bridge to Pathology
Zellweger Syndrome

Zellweger syndrome is a genetic disease caused by a mutation in any one of several genes (locus heterogeneity) involved in peroxisome biogenesis. The disease is characterized by a deficiency of peroxisomes that causes an accumulation of very long chain fatty acids and several unusual fatty acids, such as hydroxylated and branched fatty acids.

Mechanism: a defect in fatty acid efflux from peroxisomes. The most common features are enlarged liver, high blood levels of Cu and Fe, and vision problems. In affected infants, there is failure to grow, mental retardation, abnormal muscle tone, and multiple developmental abnormalities. Infants usually die within their first year.

Peroxisomes: Hypertriglyceridemia and Fibrates

A 50-year-old man sees his physician for increasingly frequent episodes of acute pain in his upper abdomen and back after meals. The physician orders fasting blood tests and the results are notable for mild hypocalcemia (8.4 mg/dL; normal: 8.9–10.3 mg/dL) and hypertriglyceridemia (500 mg/dL; normal: <200 mg/mL) with increased VLDL. Total cholesterol (170 mg/dL; normal: <200 mg/dL), LDL cholesterol (100 mg/dL; normal: <130 mg/dL), and HDL (34 mg/dL; normal: 34–86 mg/dL) are within normal ranges. The patient is put on a low-fat diet and given a prescription for gemfibrozil.

Peroxisomes are single-membrane organelles that accomplish β-oxidation of long and very long chain fatty acids similar to the mitochondrial β-oxidation pathway. One notable difference of the peroxisome pathway is that peroxisomes generate hydrogen peroxide from fatty acid oxidation. They also conduct oxidation of branched fatty acids and ω-oxidation of ordinary fatty acids. Gemfibrozil is a hypolipidemic drug that is prescribed to treat certain types of hyperlipoproteinemia, notably patients with elevated blood triglyercides but normal cholesterol and LDL levels. This drug acts by stimulating proliferation of peroxisomes and increasing gene expression of lipoprotein lipase, resulting in the induction of the fatty acid oxidation pathway in these organelles.

Section I • Biochemistry

Control of Gluconeogenesis by Response Elements

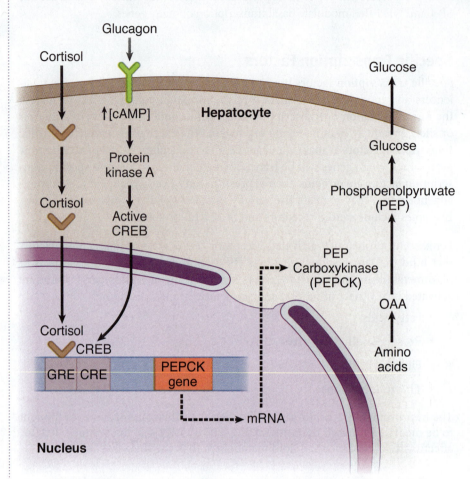

Figure I-5-4. Cortisol and Glucagon Stimulate Gluconeogenesis Through Enhancer Mechanisms

An example of how response elements affect metabolism can be seen in the pathway of gluconeogenesis (Figure I-5-4). Gluconeogenesis is a hepatic pathway whose major function is to maintain adequate glucose in the blood for tissues such as the nerves (brain) and red blood cells during fasting. It also provides glucose during periods of stress. Hormones that activate the pathway include:

- Glucagon secreted in response to hypoglycemia and functioning via a membrane-associated receptor that increases cAMP concentration

- Cortisol secreted in response to stress is permissive for glucagon in hypoglycemia and acts through an intracellular receptor, which, like other steroid receptors, is a zinc-finger DNA binding protein.

Phosphoenolpyruvate carboxykinase (PEPCK) catalyzes a critical reaction in gluconeogenesis, which under many conditions is the rate-limiting step in the pathway. A cAMP response element (CRE) and a glucocorticoid response element (GRE) are each located upstream from the transcription start site.

Cortisol induces PEPCK gene expression by the following sequence:

- Cortisol diffuses into the hepatocyte, where it
- Binds to its receptor.
- The complex enters the nucleus, and
- Binds (through the zinc fingers) to the glucocorticoid response element (GRE) associated with the PEPCK gene, which
- Increases gene expression.
- PEPCK concentration increases in the cell.
- The rate of gluconeogenesis increases.

Glucagon induces PEPCK gene expression by the following sequence:

- Glucagon binds to a receptor in the cell membrane (Chapter 9).
- cAMP concentration increases.
- Protein kinase A becomes active, and then
- Phosphorylates and activates CREB.
- Activated CREB enters the nucleus and binds to the CRE associated with the PEPCK gene, which
- Increases gene expression.
- PEPCK concentration increases in the cell.
- The rate of gluconeogenesis increases.

These effects of CREB and the cortisol-receptor complex are not entirely independent of each other. Each contributes, along with several other transcription factors, to assembling a complex of activator proteins that ultimately determine the level of PEPCK gene expression.

Control of Cell Differentiation by Homeodomain Proteins During Development *In Utero*

Sequential and coordinated gene expression is necessary for proper tissue and cell differentiation during embryonic life. Groups of regulatory proteins called homeodomain proteins are major factors in controlling this embryonic gene expression. Each regulatory protein is responsible for activating a different set of genes at the proper time in development.

The regulatory proteins themselves are encoded by genes called homeobox (HOX) or homeotic genes. Another closely related set of genes is the PAX (paired-box) genes. Mutations in HOX or PAX genes might be expected to produce developmental errors. Klein-Waardenburg syndrome (WS-III) is one such developmental disorder resulting from a mutation in a PAX gene.

Clinical Correlate
Klein-Waardenburg Syndrome

All of the tissues affected in Klein-Waardenburg syndrome are derived from embryonic tissue in which PAX-3 is expressed. Symptoms include:

- Dystopia canthorum (lateral displacement of the inner corner of the eye)
- Pigmentary abnormalities (frontal white blaze of hair, patchy hypopigmentation of the skin, heterochromia irides)
- Congenital deafness
- Limb abnormalities

Section I • Biochemistry

Clinical Correlate
Mutations in Sonic Hedgehog (SHH) Gene

Holoprosencephaly (HPE) is a common developmental anomaly of the human forebrain and midface where the cerebral hemispheres fail to separate into distinct left and right halves. Haploinsufficiency for Sonic Hedgehog (*SHH*) is a cause of HPE.

Bridge to Medical Genetics
Genetic Imprinting in Prader-Willi Syndrome

Genetic imprinting of a few gene regions results in monoallelic expression. In some cases, this imprinting is according to the parent of origin. The gene involved in Prader-Willi syndrome is on chromosome 15 and is imprinted so that it is normally expressed only from the paternal, not the maternal, chromosome.

In such a case, if one inherits a paternal chromosome in which this region has been deleted, Prader-Willi syndrome results. It can also result from uniparental (maternal) disomy of chromosome 15. Symptoms of Prader-Willi include:

- Childhood obesity and hyperphagia
- Hypogonadotrophic hypogonadism
- Small hands and feet
- Mental retardation
- Hypotonia

Co-Expression of Genes

Most eukaryotic cells are diploid, each chromosome being present in two homologous copies. The alleles of a gene on the two homologous chromosomes are usually co-expressed. In a person heterozygous for the alleles of a particular gene, for example a carrier of sickle cell trait, two different versions of the protein will be present in cells that express the gene. In the person heterozygous for the normal and sickle alleles, about 50% of the β-globin chains will contain glutamate and 50% valine at the variable position (specified by codon 6).

Major exceptions to this rule of codominant expression include genes:

- On the Barr body (inactivated X chromosome) in women
- In the immunoglobulin heavy and light chain loci (ensuring that one B cell makes only one specificity of antibody)
- In the T-cell receptor loci

Other Mechanisms for Controlling Gene Expression in Eukaryotes

Table I-5-2 summarizes some of the mechanisms that control gene expression in eukaryotic cells.

Table I-5-2. Control of Eukaryotic Gene Expression and Protein Levels

Control Point	Example
Inactivation of specific chromosomes or chromosomal regions during development	One X chromosome in each cell of a woman is inactivated by condensation to heterochromatin (Barr bodies)
Local chromatin-modifying activities	Acetylation of histones increases gene expression (many genes) Methylation of DNA silences genes in genetic imprinting (Prader-Willi and Angelman syndromes)
Gene amplification	Many oncogenes are present in multiple copies: *erbB* amplified in certain breast cancers Dihydrofolate reductase genes are amplified in some tumors, leading to drug resistance
Specific transcription factors	Steroid hormone receptors, CREB, and homeodomain proteins
Processing mRNA	Alternative splicing of mRNA in the production of membrane-bound vs. secreted antibodies
Rate of translation	Heme increases the initiation of β-globin translation
Protein modification	Proinsulin is cleaved to form active insulin
Protein degradation rate	ALA synthase has a half-life of 1 hour in the hepatocyte

Chapter Summary

Eukaryotic

- Repressers bind silencer elements.
- Activators (transcription factors) bind:
  - Upstream promoter elements (general transcription factors)
  - Enhancer response elements (specific transcription factors)
- Specific transcription factors include:
  - Steroid receptors (zinc finger)
  - cAMP-dependent activator protein, CREB (leucine zipper)
  - PPARs (zinc finger)
  - Homeodomain proteins: pHOX, pPAX (helix-turn-helix)
  - Sonic Hedgehog protein (holoprosencephaly)
  - NFkB (immune responses)

Review Questions

Select the ONE best answer.

1. Klein-Waardenburg syndrome is a single-gene disorder that includes dystopia canthorum (lateral displacement of the inner corner of the eye), impaired hearing, and pigmentary abnormalities. The gene involved is most likely to be a

    A. pseudogene
    B. proto-oncogene
    C. transgene
    D. homeotic gene
    E. tumor suppressor gene

2. Enhancers are transcriptional regulatory sequences that function by enhancing the activity of

    A. general transcriptional factors
    B. RNA polymerase to enable the enzyme to transcribe through the terminating region of a gene
    C. transcription factors that bind to the promoter but not to RNA polymerase
    D. RNA polymerase at a single promoter site
    E. spliceosomes

Section I • Biochemistry

3. A pharmacologist employed by a pharmaceutical company is investigating the mechanism of action of a new drug that significantly inhibits the division of tumor cells obtained from patients with acute myelogenous leukemia. He has determined that the drug serves as a potent inactivator of chromatin-modifying activity that up-regulates the expression of a cluster of oncogenes in these tumor cells. Which type of chromatin-modifying activity is most likely stimulated by the enzyme target of this drug?

   A. Acetylation of core histones
   B. Binding of histone H1 to nucleosomes
   C. Deacetylation of core histone H4
   D. Deamination of cytosine bases in DNA
   E. Methylation of cytosine bases in DNA

Answers

1. **Answer: D.** Multiple developmental abnormalities due to mutation in a single gene.

2. **Answer: D.** Specific transcription factors (e.g., any steroid receptor) bind to specific DNA sequences (enhancers) and to RNA polymerase at a single promoter sequence and enable the RNA polymerase to transcribe the gene more efficiently.

3. **Answer: A.** Acetylation of nucleosome core histones is strongly associated with transcriptionally active chromatin. Other modifications (**choices B, C and E**) are associated with down-regulation of gene expression. Deamination of cytosine in DNA (**choice D**) is not related to chromatin remodeling and increased gene expression.

Genetic Strategies in Therapeutics 6

Learning Objectives

❏ Demonstrate understanding of the Human Genome Project

❏ Solve problems concerning cloning genes as cDNA produced by reverse transcription of cellular mRNA

❏ Answer questions about medical applications of recombinant DNA

OVERVIEW OF RECOMBINANT DNA TECHNOLOGY

Recombinant DNA technology allows a DNA fragment from any source to be joined *in vitro* with a nucleic acid vector that can replicate autonomously in microorganisms. This provides a means of analyzing and altering genes and proteins. It also provides the reagents necessary for genetic testing for carrier detection and prenatal diagnosis of genetic diseases and for gene therapy. Additionally, this technology can provide a source of a specific protein, such as recombinant human insulin, in almost unlimited quantities.

Section I • Biochemistry

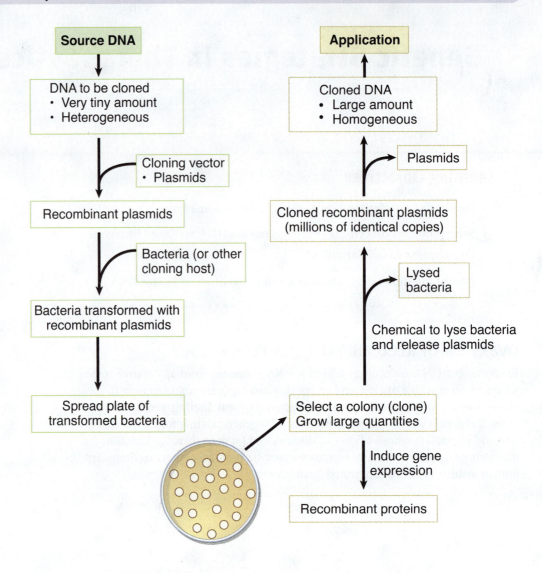

Figure I-6-1. Cloning Recombinant DNA

The DNA to be cloned is usually present in a small quantity and is part of a heterogeneous mixture containing other DNA sequences. The goal is to produce a large quantity of homogeneous DNA for one of the above applications. The general strategy for cloning DNA and isolating the cloned material is shown in Figure I-6-1. The steps include:

- Ligate the DNA into a piece of nucleic acid (the vector) that can be autonomously replicated in a living organism. The vector containing the new DNA is referred to as a recombinant vector.
- Transfer the recombinant vectors into host cells.
- Grow the host cells in isolated colonies so that each colony contains only one recombinant vector.
- Each cultured colony is a clone; all members are genetically identical.
- Select a colony for study.
- Grow a large quantity of that colony.
- Lyse the host cells and re-isolate the replicated recombinant vectors.
- Remove (by restriction enzyme cutting) the cloned DNA from the vector.

CLONING RESTRICTION FRAGMENTS OF DNA: THE HUMAN GENOME PROJECT

The Human Genome Project, initiated in 1991, involved the identification of the entire 3 billion–base-pair human DNA sequence. This project has now been completed. Although humans appear to be quite different from each other, the sequence of our DNA is, in reality, highly conserved. On average, 2 unrelated individuals share over 99.9% of their DNA sequences. For the Human Genome Project, DNA was obtained from a relatively small number of individuals. Although the variety of techniques involved is well beyond this review, the basic effort required cloning DNA restriction fragments, determining their sequences, and identifying overlaps to align the fragments properly. The major points to be understood include:

- Restriction endonucleases cut DNA specifically at palindrome sequences, yielding restriction fragments of chromosomes.
- The restriction fragments are cloned in vectors.
- The cloned fragments are re-isolated from the cloned recombinant vectors.
- The restriction fragments from each clone are sequenced.

Producing Restriction Fragments: Restriction Endonucleases

Chromosomes obtained from the DNA donors were cut with restriction endonucleases to produce restriction fragments, as shown in Figure I-6-2. These enzymes are isolated from bacteria, their natural source. There are many different restriction endonucleases isolated from a variety of bacteria that are now readily available commercially. In bacteria, they act as part of a restriction/modification system that protects the bacteria from infection by DNA viruses.

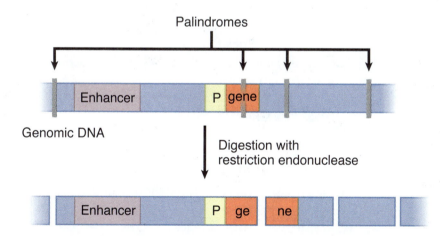

Figure I-6-2. DNA Digestion with a Restriction Endonuclease

Note
Human Genome Project data can be used to identify:

- Protein-coding genes
- Regulatory sequences in noncoding DNA
- Polymorphic genetic markers (restriction endonuclease sites, short tandem repeats, and single nucleotide polymorphisms) dispersed throughout chromosomes in coding and noncoding DNA

Restriction endonucleases recognize double-stranded DNA sequences called palindromes (inverted repeats) usually of four to eight base pairs in length. For example, Figure I-6-3 shows the recognition site for *Eco*RI, a restriction endonuclease isolated from *Escherichia coli*. A palindrome can be identified by examining the sequence of only one strand. Draw a line through the center of the sequence (through the central base for palindromes with an odd number of nucleotides). If the sequence is folded along this line, the bases should pair.

DNA sequence recognized by the restriction endonuclease *Eco*RI

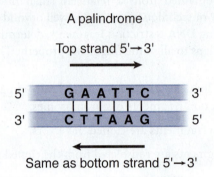

Figure I-6-3. EcoRI Recognition Sequence

DNA from a source to be cloned is mixed with a particular restriction endonuclease, such as *Eco*RI, producing DNA restriction fragments. Some restriction endonucleases, such as *Eco*RI, produce offset cuts within the palindrome, yielding "sticky ends" on the fragments. Sticky ends are advantageous in facilitating the recombination of a restriction fragment with the vector DNA. An example is shown in Figure I-6-4.

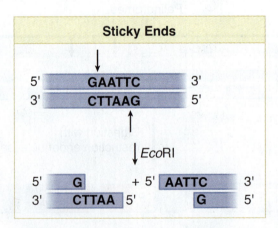

Figure I-6-4. Example of a Restriction Endonuclease

Cloning Restriction Fragments Using Vectors

Each restriction fragment (which may include a gene) must be inserted into a vector to be cloned. A vector is a piece of DNA (plasmid, viral chromosome, yeast chromosome) capable of autonomous replication in a host cell—for instance, the plasmid pBR322 shown in Figure I-6-5. The DNA used as a vector usually has:

- At least one type of palindrome recognized by a restriction endonuclease
- An origin for autonomous replication
- At least one gene for resistance to an antibiotic (allows selection for colonies with recombinant plasmids)

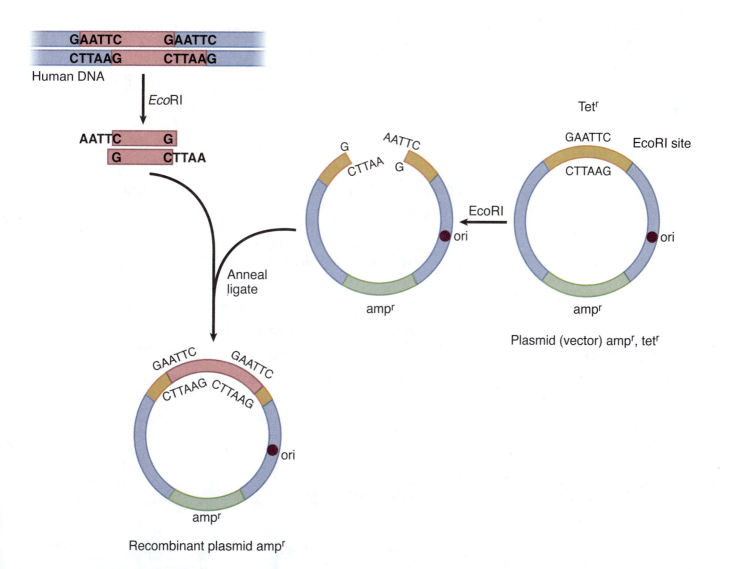

Figure I-6-5. Formation of a Recombinant Plasmid

Section I • Biochemistry

Note

The major goal of the **Human Genome Project**, initiated in 1991, was the identification of the entire 3 billion–base-pair human DNA sequence. This project has now been completed. Because the entire human DNA sequence has been identified, it will be easier to identify each of the estimated 20,000 to 25,000 protein-coding genes located within the sequence. Additionally, important regulatory sequences, which are located outside of coding DNA, will be identified.

Bridge to Medical Genetics
Restriction Maps

- Line drawings of DNA identifying sites cut by restriction endonucleases
- Identify potential RFLP markers for genetic diagnosis

Genomic Libraries

Genomic libraries have been used to sequence DNA as accomplished in the Human Genome Project. These sequences can be used to identify

- Protein-coding genes
- Restriction endonuclease sites (see Margin Note: Restriction Maps)
- Other genetic markers (short tandem repeats, single nucleotide polymorphisms)
- Non-expressed DNA (enhancers, promoters, introns, noncoding DNA between gene regions)

CLONING GENES AS CDNA PRODUCED BY REVERSE TRANSCRIPTION OF CELLULAR mRNA

If the end goal of cloning is to have a cloned gene expressed in a cell, the entire coding sequence must be cloned intact. Furthermore, if a cloned eukaryotic gene is to be expressed in bacteria (to make recombinant proteins), the gene must not contain introns, which could not be processed in a prokaryotic cell. In these cases, it is more convenient to clone cDNA rather than DNA restriction fragments.

Producing cDNA by Reverse Transcription of mRNA

Cytoplasmic mRNA is isolated from a cell known to express the desired gene. Reverse transcriptase, along with other components (Figure I-6-6), is used *in vitro* to produce double-stranded cDNA that is subsequently recombined with a chosen vector to produce the recombinant DNA for cloning. In this approach:

- All genes expressed will be cloned along with the desired gene.
- None of the non-expressed DNA in the cell will be cloned.
- Each cDNA represents the complete coding sequence of a gene.
- The cDNAs have no introns.
- An expression library is produced at the end of the cloning procedure.

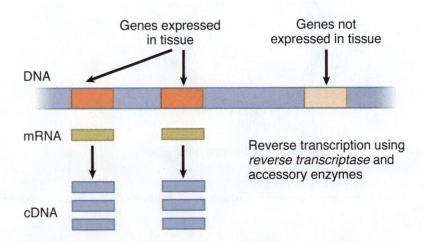

Figure I-6-6. Cloning Expressed Genes by Producing cDNAs

cDNA (Expression) Libraries

Once the recombinant expression vectors containing the cDNA inserts are produced, they are cloned in bacteria (or other host cells) and produce cDNA (expression) libraries. These libraries can be used to:

- Sequence specific genes and identify disease-causing mutations
- Produce recombinant proteins (insulin, factor VIII, HBsAg for vaccination)
- Conduct gene replacement therapy
- Produce transgenic animals

Several of these applications are discussed in more detail in subsequent sections of this chapter.

Table I-6-1. Comparison of Genomic and cDNA (Expression) Libraries

	Genomic Libraries	cDNA (Expression) Library
Source of DNA	Chromosomal DNA	mRNA (cDNA)
Enzymes to make library	Restriction endonuclease DNA ligase	Reverse transcriptase DNA ligase
Contains nonexpressed sequences of chromosomes	Yes	No
Cloned genes are complete sequences	Not necessarily	Yes
Cloned genes contain introns	Yes	No
Promoter and enhancer sequences present	Yes, but not necessarily in same clone	No
Gene can be expressed in cloning host (recombinant proteins)	No	Yes
Can be used for gene therapy or constructing transgenic animals	No	Yes

MEDICAL APPLICATIONS OF RECOMBINANT DNA

Recombinant DNA can be used as follows:

1. To produce recombinant proteins, used variously in:
   a. Replacement therapy (e.g., insulin in diabetes)
   b. Disease prevention (e.g., vaccines)
   c. Diagnostic tests (e.g., monoclonal antibodies)

2. To conduct gene therapy in the treatment of genetic diseases.

Recombinant Proteins

Recombinant proteins can be made by cloning the relevant gene for the protein in a host organism, growing large quantities of the organism, and inducing it to express the gene (as indicated in the lower right of Figure I-6-1). Many therapeutics proteins are now mass-produced as recombinant proteins. Some important examples are shown in Table I-6-2.

Table I-6-2. Examples of Protein Products of Recombinant DNA Technology

Product	Produced in	Use
Insulin	*E. coli*	Diabetes
Growth factor	*E. coli*	Growth defects
Epidermal growth factor	*E. coli*	Burns, ulcers
Hepatitis B vaccine	*Saccharomyces cerevisae*	Prevention of viral hepatitis
Erythropoietin	Mammalian cells	Anemia
Factor VIII	Mammalian cells	Hemophilia

Gene Therapy

Gene therapy now offers potential cures for individuals with inherited diseases. The initial goal is to introduce a normal copy of the gene that is defective into the tissues that give rise to the pathology of the genetic disease. For instance, about 50% of the children with severe combined immunodeficiency have a mutation in the gene encoding the γ chain common to several of the interleukin receptors. Recently, cDNA from a normal γ-chain gene was used to transduce autologous cells from infants with X-linked severe combined immunodeficiency (SCID) with subsequent correction of the defects in their T cells and natural killer cells.

- Gene transfer requires a delivery vector (retrovirus, adenovirus, liposome).
- Only tissues giving rise to the disease pathology are targeted for gene therapy.
- The normal gene is not inherited by offspring.

Gene delivery vectors

For gene replacement therapy to be a realistic possibility, efficient gene delivery vectors must be used to transfer the cloned gene into the target cells' DNA. Because viruses naturally infect cells to insert their own genetic material, most gene delivery vectors now in use are modified viruses. A portion of the viral genome is replaced with the cloned gene (as either DNA or RNA) such that the virus can infect but not complete its replication cycle. Steps in the production of a retrovirus for gene replacement therapy are illustrated in Figure I-6-7.

Retroviruses and adenoviruses were early vectors used in gene delivery. However, newer strategies take advantage of vectors with better properties, such as

Note

Ex Vivo

Cells modified outside the body, then transplanted back in

In Vivo

Gene changed in cells still in body

adeno-associated viruses (AAV). Major advantages of AAV include having no disease association in humans and limited innate immunity. In addition, AAV restricts expression to specific tissues: A tissue-specific promoter in the AAV is genetically engineered to control transcription of the inserted transgene. Viruses used as vectors are compared in Table I-6-3.

Table I-6-3. Vectors Used in Gene Therapy

Viral Vector	Retroviruses	Adenovirus	Adeno-Associated Virus (AAV)
Family	Retroviridae	Adenoviridae	Parvoviridae
Genome	ssRNA	dsDNA	ssDNA
Disease association?	Yes	Yes	No
Inserts into chromosome?	Yes	No	No (episomal)
Innate immunity?	Yes	Yes	Limited

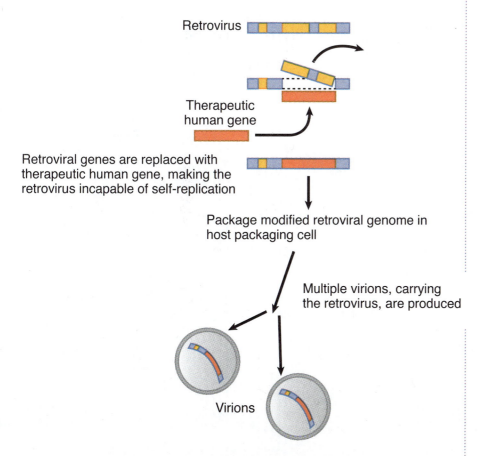

Figure I-6-7. Preparation of a Retrovirus for Gene Replacement Therapy

There are two strategies for delivering a therapeutic gene (transgene) into an individual. *In vivo* gene replacement therapy involves the direct delivery of a therapeutic gene into a patient's body. Upon entry into the target cells, the inserted transgene is expressed into a therapeutic protein. *Ex vivo* gene replacement therapy involves the genetic manipulation of a patient's target cells outside the body. Target cells are infected with a recombinant virus harboring the therapeutic transgene. The genetically modified target cells, harboring and expressing the therapeutic protein, are then reintroduced into the same patient. Both gene replacement strategies are shown in Figure I-6-8.

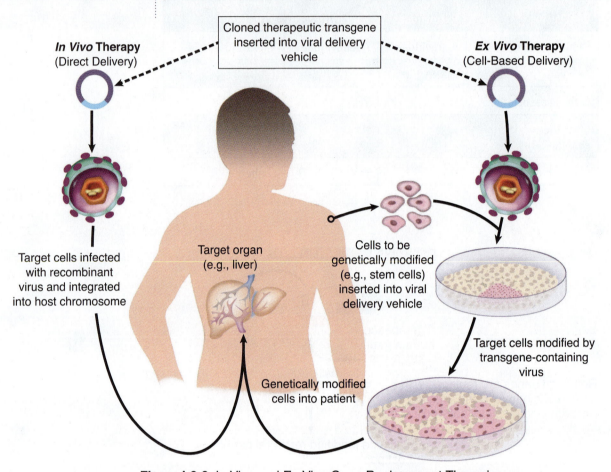

Figure I-6-8. In Vivo and Ex Vivo Gene Replacement Therapies

Gene replacement therapy (*in vivo* therapy) for cystic fibrosis illustrates one important example of direct delivery of a transgene (Figure I-6-9).

Chapter 6 • Genetic Strategies in Therapeutics

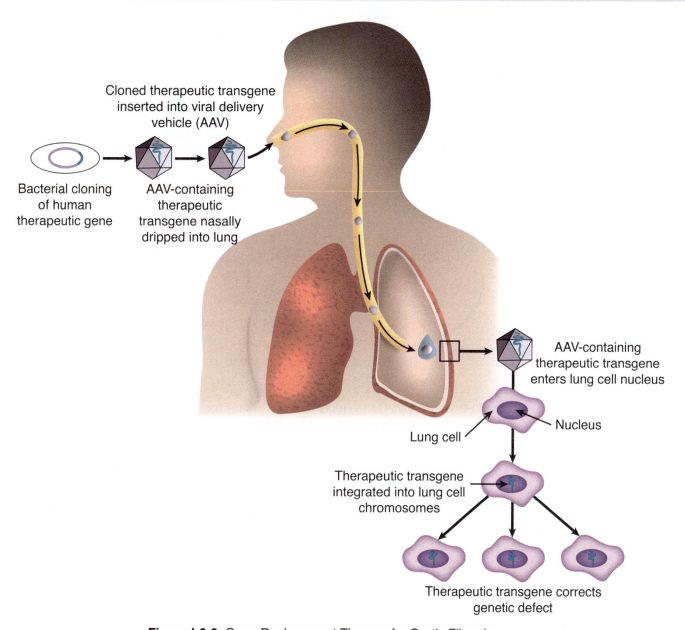

Figure I-6-9. Gene Replacement Therapy for Cystic Fibrosis

An important example of *ex vivo* gene replacement therapy is illustrated in Figure I-6-10.

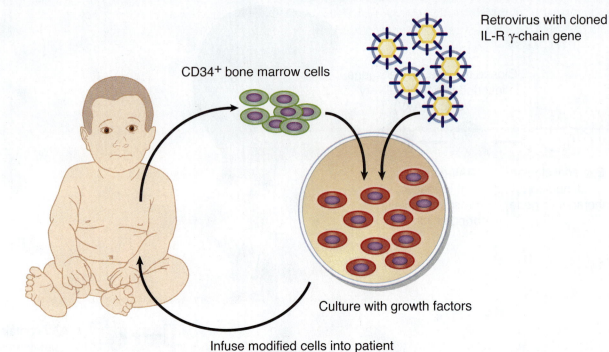

Figure I-6-10. *Ex Vivo* Gene Replacement Therapy for X-Linked Severe Combined Immunodeficiency

Remaining challenges to gene replacement therapy

Although much progress has been made in gene replacement therapy, significant challenges still remain. These challenges include:

- Targeting the therapeutic gene to the appropriate tissues
- Low-level or transient expression of the therapeutic gene
- Problems caused by random insertion of the therapeutic gene into the host DNA.

RNA Interference

RNA interference (RNAi) refers to downregulation of gene expression through the use of small RNA molecules, which mediate gene expression by either inhibiting translation or causing premature degradation of the genes' mRNAs. Two types of small RNA molecules are involved in RNA interference: microRNA (miRNA) and small interfering RNA (siRNA). The RNAi pathway occurs in many eukaryotes, including humans, and plays a central role in defending cells against viruses and transposons (discussed in Microbiology).

The RNAi process begins when an enzyme known as dicer cleaves long double-stranded RNA into small double-stranded RNA fragments (siRNA) approximately 20 nucleotides in length. The double-stranded siRNA then unwinds into two single-stranded RNAs: the passenger strand (sense strand), which subsequently degrades, and the guide strand (antisense strand), which associates into the RNA-induced silencing complex (RISC). Next, the guide strand pairs with a complementary sequence in a messenger RNA molecule and induces cleavage using argonaute, the catalytic component of the RISC complex. Since the mRNA is degraded, its encoded protein is not produced. The result is posttranscriptional gene silencing. This effect is often referred to as "knockdown" because gene expression continues, though in greatly reduced extent. In "knockout," by contrast, gene expression is entirely absent. Figure I-6-11 shows the RNAi pathway.

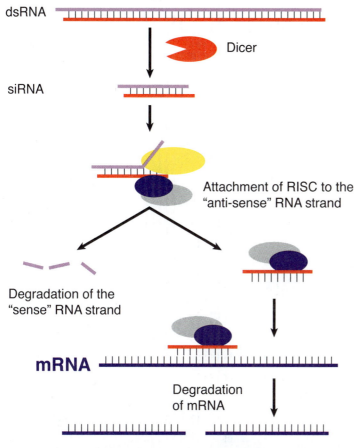

Figure I-6-11. RNAi Pathway

To time-limit the effects of RNAi, siRNAs can be administered as stabilized RNAs conjugated to targeting compounds or enclosed in lipid vesicles. A single RNAi treatment can silence expression of a particular gene for 2 weeks. siRNAs can be stabilized against endogenous RNases in blood or cells by modifying the 2' hydroxyl with a methyl or fluorine group.

RNA interference technology is being explored as a treatment for cancer and many neurodegenerative diseases and for use in antiviral therapies. Clinical trials are also exploring the use of RNAi in other clinical applications, such as therapy for age-related macular degeneration.

Section I • Biochemistry

Table I-6-4. Summary of Important Points About Recombinant DNA

Restriction endonucleases	Recognize palindromes in dsDNA: 5'---GAATTC---3' 3'---CTTAAG---5' Cut leaving sticky ends: 5'---GAATTC---3' 3'---CTTAAG---5' Used to make restriction maps of DNA Produce fragments for genetic analysis Produce fragments for making recombinant DNA and cloning DNA sequences
Vectors for recombinant DNA and cloning	Plasmid: • Restriction site • Replication origin • Resistance to antibiotic(s) Expression vector also requires: • Promoter • Shine-Dalgarno sequence Other vectors: phage, YACs
Approaches to cloning DNA	Genomic DNA • Restriction endonucleases fragment DNA • Total nuclear DNA cloned • Genes contain introns cDNA • Reverse transcription of mRNAs from cell • Genes expressed cloned • Genes have no introns
Uses of cloned genes	Produce recombinant proteins Gene therapy (somatic) Transgenic animals (germline) Produce cDNA probes for blots

Review Questions

1. If a patient with cystic fibrosis were to be treated by gene therapy, which type of cells should be targeted as host cells?

    (A) Germ cells

    (B) Epithelial cells

    (C) T cells

    (D) Hemopoietic stem cells

2. A pharmaceutical firm is interested in the bacterial production of thymidylate synthase in large quantities for drug-targeting studies. An important step in the overall cloning strategy involves the ligation of synthase cDNA into a plasmid vector containing a replication origin, an antibiotic resistance gene, and a promoter sequence. Which additional nucleotide sequence should be included in this vector to ensure optimal production of the thymidylate synthase?

    (A) Operator sequence

    (B) PolyA sequence

    (C) Shine-Dalgarno sequence

    (D) Attenuator sequence

    (E) 3′-splice acceptor sequence

3. Restriction fragment length polymorphisms may be produced by mutations in the sites for restriction endonucleases. For instance, a single base change in the site for the nuclear *Sal*I produces the sequence GTGGAC, which can no longer be recognized by the enzyme. What was the original sequence recognized by *Sal*I?

    (A) GTAGAC

    (B) GCGGAC

    (C) CTGGAC

    (D) GTCGAC

    (E) GTGTAC

Answers

1. **Answer: B.** The pathogenesis of cystic fibrosis is related to defective chloride transport in epithelial cells.

2. **Answer: C.** Incorporation of a Shine-Dalgarno sequence into the expression vector will promote ribosome binding to the translation start site on the mRNA produced by transcription of the cDNA insert.

3. **Answer: D.** All options represent single-base changes in the mutant sequence in the stem, but only choice D reestablishes a palindrome.

Techniques of Genetic Analysis 7

Learning Objectives

❏ Interpret scenarios about blotting technique

❏ Explain information related to polymerase chain reaction

Techniques of genetic analysis are assuming an increasingly larger role in medical diagnosis. These techniques, which once were a specialized part of medical genetics, are now becoming essential tools for every physician to understand. Blotting techniques allow testing for genetic diseases, gene expression profiling, and routine testing for antigens and antibodies. The polymerase chain reaction (PCR) is now an essential tool in many aspects of genetic testing, forensic medicine, and paternity testing. These techniques are discussed in this chapter, but their applications will be further explored in Medical Genetics (Section II of this book).

BLOTTING TECHNIQUES

Blotting techniques have been developed to detect and visualize specific DNA, RNA, and protein among complex mixtures of contaminating molecules. These techniques have allowed the identification and characterization of the genes involved in numerous inherited diseases. The general method for performing a blotting technique is illustrated in Figure I-7-1.

The fragments in the material to be analyzed (DNA, RNA, or protein) are separated by gel electrophoresis. The smaller molecules travel faster and appear nearer the bottom of the gel. The bands of material in the gel are transferred, or blotted, to the surface of a membrane. The membrane is incubated with a (usually radioactive) labeled probe that will specifically bind to the molecules of interest. Visualization of the labeled probe (usually by autoradiography) will reveal which band(s) interacted with the probe. The most common types of blots are compared in Table I-7-1. Most typically, DNA restriction fragments are analyzed on a Southern blot.

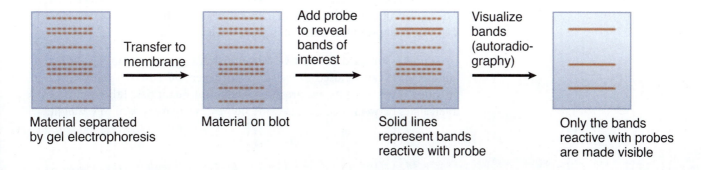

Figure I-7-1. Blotting Technique

Section I • Biochemistry

Table I-7-1. Types of Blots

Blot Type	Material Analyzed	Electro-phoresis Required	Probe Used	Purpose
Southern	DNA	Yes	^{32}P-DNA	To determine which restriction fragments of DNA are associated with a particular gene
Northern	RNA	Yes	^{32}P-DNA	To measure sizes and amounts of specific mRNA molecules to answer questions about gene expression
Western	Protein	Yes	^{125}I- or enzyme-linked antibody	To measure amount of antigen (proteins) or antibody
Dot (slot) (Figure II-6-1)	RNA, DNA, or protein	No	Same as for blots above	To detect specific DNA, RNA, protein, or antibody

Probes

DNA probes are radioactively labeled single-stranded DNA molecules that are able to specifically hybridize (anneal) to particular denatured DNA sequences. Examples include:

- Probes that bind to part of a specific gene region. These are often produced by cloning cDNA transcribed from the gene and labeling it with ^{32}P, a radioactive isotope of phosphorus.

- Probes that bind to markers known to be in close proximity (closely linked) to a gene

- Probes that bind specifically to a single allele of a gene—allele-specific oligonucleotide (ASO) probes (Figure II-6-2, Section II)

When protein is separated and analyzed on a Western blot, ^{125}I-labeled antibody specific for the protein of interest is used as a probe.

The probe is an important part of analyzing any blot because the only bands that will appear on the final autoradiogram are those to which the probe has hybridized. An example of this concept is given in Figure I-7-2.

DNA probes are used to selectively detect DNA fragments. Staining with ethidium bromide can be used to visualize and detect *all* DNA fragments in a gel, provided the fragments are present in sufficient quantities. Ethidium bromide intercalates between stacked bases and fluoresces when exposed to UV light.

Southern Blots and Restriction Fragment Length Polymorphisms (RFLPs)

Although unrelated individuals share over 99.9% of their DNA sequences, the fact that the human genome contains over 3 billion base pairs means that two unrelated individuals' DNA will differ at over a million base pairs (0.1% of a billion equals a million). These differences include mutations in restriction endonuclease sites that can be analyzed as RFLPs on Southern blots. An example is shown in Figure I-7-2.

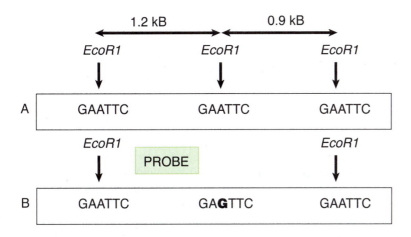

QUESTION: Only one blot below correctly corresponds to the genotypes displayed. Which blot is correct?

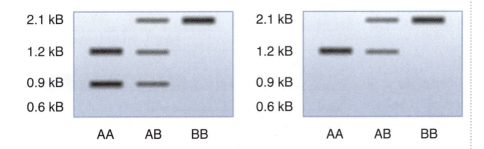

Figure I-7-2. Restriction Fragment Length Polymorphism Analysis on a Southern Blot

A pair of homologous chromosomes is shown in Figure I-7-2. They are designated chromosomes A and B. The figure shows the same region on both chromosomes and identifies sites (GAATTC) cut by the restriction endonuclease EcoR1. The probe used on the Southern blot binds to the area of the chromosomes indicated in the diagram. DNA samples from three individuals are tested: AA (homozygous for A at this region), AB (heterozygous at this region), and BB (homozygous for B at this region). At the bottom, the figure also presents two blots, only one of which correctly represents the results seen on the autoradiogram. Which blot is correct?

(Answer: The blot on the right is correct.)

Repetitive sequences known as VNTRs (variable number of tandem repeats) make some contribution to RFLPs, predominantly in the centromeric and telomeric regions of chromosomes (see margin note: VNTR Sequences and RFLP).

RFLPs and genetic testing

RFLPs may be used in genetic testing to infer the presence of a disease-causing allele of a gene in a family with a genetic disease. For instance, if chromosome A in a family also carried a disease-producing allele of a gene in this region and chromosome B carried a normal allele, finding a 1.2 kilobase (kb) band would indicate that the disease-producing allele was also present (both characteristics of chromosome A). Conversely, finding a 2.1-kb fragment would indicate that the normal allele of the gene was present (both characteristics of chromosome B). This type of genetic analysis is more fully discussed in Medical Genetics, Chapter 6. A simple example is illustrated by the following case.

A phenotypically normal man and woman have an 8-year-old son with sickle cell anemia. They also have a 5-year-old daughter who does not have sickle cell anemia but has not been tested for carrier status. The mother is in her 16th week of pregnancy and wishes to know whether the fetus that she is carrying will develop sickle cell disease. The mutation causing sickle cell anemia (G6V) also destroys a restriction site for the restriction endonuclease MstII. DNA from each of the family members is cut with MstII, Southern blotted, and probed with a ^{32}P-labeled cDNA probe for the 5′UTR of the β-globin gene. The results are shown below in Figure I-7-3, along with the family pedigree. What is the best conclusion about the fetus?

> **Note**
> **VNTR Sequences and RFLP**
>
> Variable number of tandem repeat (VNTR) sequences contribute to some restriction fragment length polymorphisms (RFLPs). A VNTR sequence designates a unit of nucleotides usually between 15 and 60 bp that is repeated in tandem multiple times at a particular location in the DNA. Although the repeated sequence is shared by all individuals, the number of repeated units is variable from person to person.
>
> These VNTR sequences (boxes) can be flanked by restriction endonuclease sites (arrows). The probe used to detect the RFLP would bind to the repeated unit.
>
>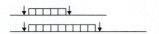

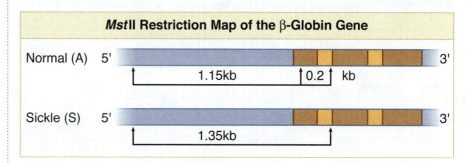

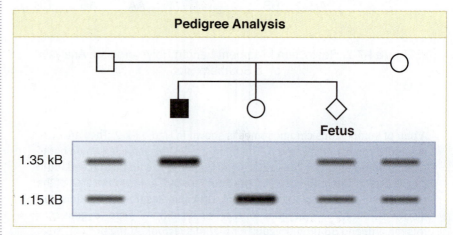

Figure I-7-3. RFLP Diagnosis of Sickle Cell Disease

(Answer: Fetus is heterozygous, or a carrier, for the mutation.)

In the case presented in Figure I-7-3, both the mother and the father have the same size restriction fragments marking the chromosome with the sickle allele. Because they are genetically unrelated, coming from different families this is not always the case. (See question 5 at the end of this chapter). Additional examples will be discussed in Medical Genetics.

Northern Blots

Northern blots analyze RNA extracted from a tissue and are typically used to determine which genes are being expressed. One example is shown in Figure I-7-4. The goal is to determine which tissues express the *FMR1* gene involved in fragile X syndrome. RNA samples from multiple tissues have been separated by electrophoresis, blotted, and probed with a ^{32}P-cDNA probe from the *FMR1* gene. The results are consistent with high-level expression (a 4.4-kb transcript) of this gene in brain and testis and lower-level expression in the lung. In the heart, the gene is also expressed, but the transcripts are only 1.4 kb long. Variability in the lengths of the mRNAs transcribed from a single gene may be the result of alternative splicing as discussed in Chapter 3, Transcription and RNA Processing.

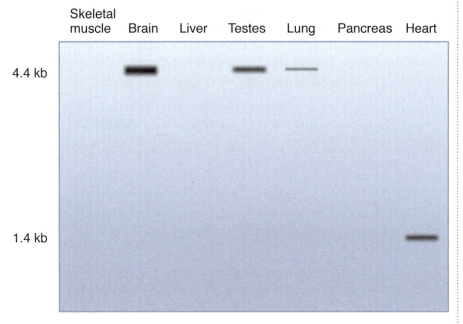

Figure I-7-4. Northern Blot to Determine Pattern of *FMR1* Expression

Clinical Correlate
Fragile X Syndrome

Fragile X syndrome is the leading known cause of inherited mental retardation. Other symptoms include large ears, elongated face, hypermobile joints, and macroorchidism in postpubertal males. The gene involved, *FMR1*, maps to the long arm of the X chromosome. See Section II, Chapter 1, for a further discussion of this single-gene disorder.

Gene expression profiling (microarrays)

It is now possible to embed probes for many different mRNA in a multi-well gel or even on a chip to simultaneously determine whether hundreds of genes are expressed in a particular tissue. This is referred to as gene expression profiling or microarray analysis. For example, previous research has suggested that cells from a breast cancer express a variety of genes that are either not expressed or expressed only at a low level in normal cells. Probes for the corresponding mRNAs can be embedded on a solid support and total mRNA from a particular woman's breast tumor tested with each probe. The pattern of gene expression (gene expression profiling) may give information about the prognosis for that particular woman, aiding in making choices about the appropriate treatment protocol.

Section I • Biochemistry

Western Blots

Western blots separate proteins by gel electrophoresis and use ^{125}I-labeled probe antibodies to detect the proteins (antigens). For this reason, Western blots are also referred to as immunoblots. One important application of Western blotting is to detect the presence of antibodies to the HIV virus in HIV testing. This application is discussed in Immunology. Western blots may also be used to identify whether a particular protein is in a cell and therefore represent a way to test for gene expression at the level of translation.

POLYMERASE CHAIN REACTION (PCR)

The polymerase chain reaction (PCR) is a technique in which a selected region of a chromosome can be amplified more than a million-fold within a few hours. The technique allows extremely small samples of DNA to be used for further testing. The PCR has many different applications.

The region of a chromosome to be amplified by a PCR is referred to as the target sequence and may be an area containing a suspected mutation, a short tandem repeat (STR, or microsatellite sequence), or really any area of interest. The major constraint in performing a PCR is that one must know the nucleotide sequence bordering (flanking) the target region at each of its 3′ ends. This is no longer an obstacle because of the sequence data from the Human Genome Project. The steps of the PCR are illustrated in Figure I-7-5 and include the following:

- Add the sample containing DNA to be amplified.
- Add excess amounts of primers complementary to both 3′ flanks of the target sequence. This selects the region to be amplified.
- Add a heat-stable DNA polymerase (*Taq* DNA polymerase) and deoxyribonucleotides (dNTPs) for DNA synthesis.
- Heat the sample to melt the DNA (convert dsDNA to ssDNA).
- Cool the sample to re-anneal the DNA. Because the ratio of primers to complementary strands is extremely high, primers bind at the 3′ flanking regions.
- Heat the sample to increase the activity of the *Taq* DNA polymerase. Primer elongation occurs, and new complementary strands are synthesized.

This process is repeated for approximately 20 cycles, producing over a million double-stranded copies of the target sequence.

Note
Uses of the PCR

The PCR can be used for:
- Comparing DNA samples in forensic cases
- Paternity testing
- Direct mutation testing
- Diagnosing bacterial and viral infections
- HIV testing in situations where antibody tests are uninformative (importantly, infants whose mothers are HIV positive)

Note
Short Tandem Repeats (STRs, or Microsatellites)

STRs are repeats of a di- to tetranucleotide sequence. These repeats occur both in the spacer regions between genes and within gene regions and are often useful in genetic testing. STRs in noncoding regions show some variability in length as mutations have expanded or contracted the number of repeats throughout evolution. The positions of these STRs are known and documented in chromosome maps, where they are often used in genetic testing.

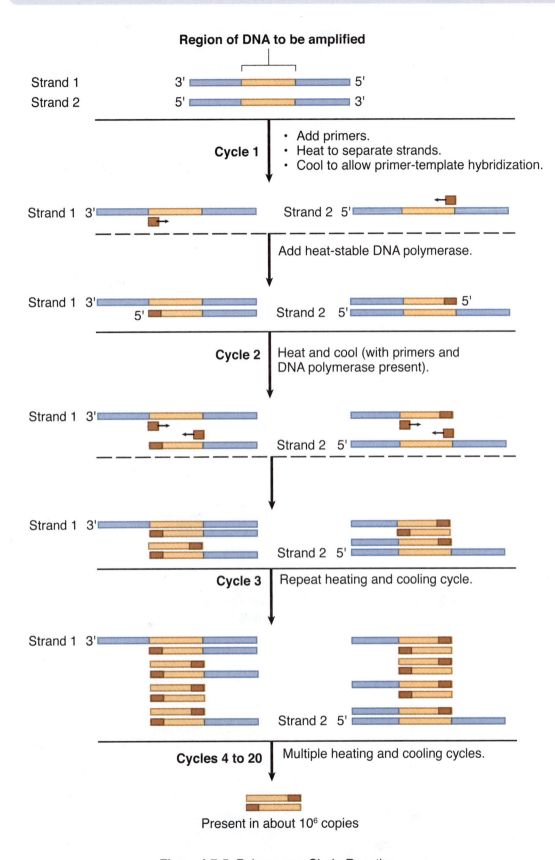

Figure I-7-5. Polymerase Chain Reaction

Section I • Biochemistry

Agarose gel electrophoresis of PCR products

If the known mutation changes the length of the gene (e.g., microsatellite repeats), this difference can be detected in the PCR-amplified DNA by electrophoresis on agarose gel.

A 59-year-old man with increasing clumsiness, loss of balance, and irregular tremor and jerkiness in both arms seeks medical attention. The physician also notes impaired visual tracking. The patient has one sister, who is 53 years old. His father and mother died in an automobile accident at ages 45 and 43, respectively. There is no known history of neurologic dysfunction in his family. He takes a multiple vitamin tablet daily but no prescription drugs or supplements. An MRI reveals visible atrophy of the caudate and total basal ganglia, and a tentative diagnosis of Huntington disease is made. To confirm the diagnosis, a sample of blood is sent for molecular genetic testing. PCR amplification is carried out on a region on 4p16.3 suspected to contain a mutation. The results are shown below in Figure I-7-6 along with results from a normal, healthy, age-matched control. Is this result consistent with the diagnosis?

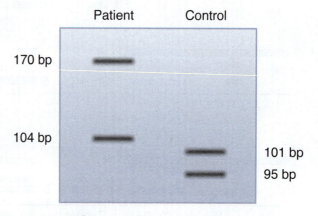

Figure I-7-6. Direct Genetic Diagnosis of Neurodegenerative Disease Using PCR

(Ans: Yes, the results are consistent with Huntington disease. In comparison with the normal control PCR products, one of the patient's PCR products (170 bp) is well out of the normal range. This is consistent with a triplet repeat expansion in that allele of the huntingtin gene. The two bands from the Control are 95 base pairs and 101 base pairs, a difference of two triplet repeats. The Patient sample shows a 104 base pair band, a difference of one triplet repeat from the larger Control band. Significantly, there is a difference of 69 base pairs between the Patient's two bands: 104 base pairs versus 170 base pairs. This is equivalent to 23 triplet repeats.)

Genetic Fingerprinting Using PCR Amplification of Microsatellite Sequences

Most repetitive sequences are not in coding regions. Because expansion of these sequences in spacer DNA rarely affects any function, they become highly polymorphic in the population and can be used to develop a genetic fingerprint. Such fingerprints are important in paternity testing and forensic medicine. Very small samples containing dried tissue can be analyzed by this technique. PCR amplification of repetitive sequences such as VNTR and STR sequences can be used for genetic fingerprinting.

Paternity testing using PCR amplification of microsatellite sequences

Although microsatellite sequences are distributed throughout the DNA, a single region may be selectively amplified by using primers that overlap the 3′-flanking regions adjacent to the repeat analyzed. Such primers amplify "single-locus" sequences, which are highly polymorphic within the population. Because humans have pairs of chromosomes, each individual will have a maximum of two bands, one from the father and one from the mother. An example is shown in Figure I-7-6.

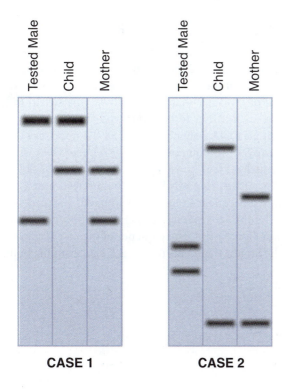

Figure I-7-7. Paternity Testing

Are the tested males (Figure I-7-7) in case 1 and case 2 the fathers of the children? Approach:

- Identify the child's band in common with the mother. The other band must be from the father.
- Does the tested male have a band matching the band from the child? Draw a conclusion.

Case 1: The tested male in case 1 may be the father, as he shares a band with the child. We cannot be certain, however, because many other men in the population could have this same band. Matches are required at several different loci to indicate with high probability that a tested male is the father.

Case 2: The tested male in case 2 cannot be the father, as neither of his bands is shared with the child.

In practice, 9 to 10 different polymorphisms are necessary to indicate a match.

PCR in Direct Mutation Testing

If the mutation(s) causing a specific disease is known, the loci involved can be amplified with a PCR and further analyzed to determine whether the mutation(s) is present. Mutations causing a length difference can be detected by gel electrophoresis as a length difference in the PCR product. Mutations causing a sequence difference can be detected by testing the PCR products with ASOs.

This topic is explored further in Medical Genetics, Chapter 6, Genetic Diagnosis.

Sequencing DNA for direct mutation testing

If a mutation has been mapped to a particular region of a chromosome, one can use the PCR to amplify the region and sequence one of the two strands to determine whether it harbors a mutation. Double-stranded DNA is used along with many copies of a primer that binds only to one strand (often the coding strand). A sample of the DNA to be sequenced is put in each of four reaction mixtures containing a DNA polymerase and all the necessary deoxyribonucleotide triphosphates(dNTPs) required to synthesize new DNA. In each test tube a different dideoxynucleotide triphosphate (ddNTP) which lack both the 3' and 2' hydroxyl groups is added. The ddNTPs can be inserted into a growing chain of DNA, but then any subsequent elongation is stopped. The pieces of newly synthesized DNA in each tube are separated by gel electrophoresis in a different lane of the gel as shown in Figure I-7-8. The sequence of the new strand can be read from the smallest to the largest fragments on the gel, e.g., from the bottom to the top.

Note

Comparison of dATP and ddATP

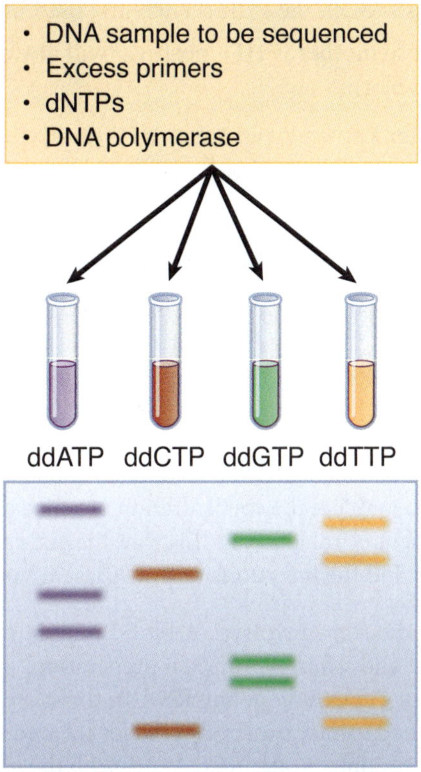

Figure I-7-8. DNA Sequencing

The sequence of the newly synthesized DNA strand in this example is:
5'CTTGGAACTGTA 3'

If one wants the sequence of the original strand, serving as the template in the sequencing procedure, it would be complementary and anti-parallel to the sequence read from the gel. In this example the original strand sequence would be:
5'TACAGTTCCAAG 3'

PCR in HIV Testing

The enzyme-linked immunosorbent assay (ELISA) is currently used to screen individuals for antibodies to the HIV virus. The test has high sensitivity but somewhat lower specificity. A positive result in an ELISA must be confirmed by a Western blot for antibodies that are reactive with specific HIV protein antigens. These tests are described in Immunology.

In certain instances, ELISA/Western blot is not useful and a PCR is the test of choice to detect HIV infection. The PCR is designed to test for the integrated proviral genome, not for antibodies to HIV protein antigens. Primers that are specific for the HIV provirus are used for the PCR. If the person is infected, the proviral genome will be amplified and detected. If the person is not infected, there will be no PCR product detected. A PCR for the HIV provirus has two important advantages over the ELISA/Western blot. The PCR

- Is positive much earlier after infection
- Does not rely on an antibody response by the individual

Important situations in which the PCR is currently used include HIV testing in

- A newborn whose mother is HIV positive (will always be positive in ELISA/Western blot)
- Early testing after known exposure to HIV-positive blood (for example, needlesticks) or other fluids/tissue

Reverse Transcriptase PCR (RT-PCR)

An RT-PCR detects and can quantify a specific RNA rather than DNA in a sample. This test is useful in detecting RNA viruses such as HIV and, in situations similar to the Northern blot, determining whether a gene is transcribed.

Measuring viral load in AIDS patients

The RT-PCR is used to measure the concentration of active circulating virus in the blood of an AIDS patient (viral load). In this way, the test can be used to monitor the status of infection and the infection's response to antiviral drugs.

Figure I-7-9A shows the steps involved. A blood sample from an HIV-infected individual is obtained and, after appropriate preparation, is treated with reverse transcriptase to produce cDNA from any RNA in the sample. The cDNA is subsequently PCR-amplified using primers specific for the end sequences of the HIV cDNA. The amplified product is quantitated and, with the use of a standard curve (Figure I-7-9B), can be related to the original amount of HIV RNA present.

Clinical Correlate

In chronic myelogenous leukemia (CML), the presence of the Philadelphia chromosome translocation (t[9;22]) produces a BCR-ABL, an abnormal fusion protein with tyrosine kinase activity. It has been shown that monitoring the level of BCR-ABL mRNA with an RT-PCR in CML patients during therapy with Imatinib (a tyrosine kinase inhibitor) is helpful for both prognosis and management of therapy.

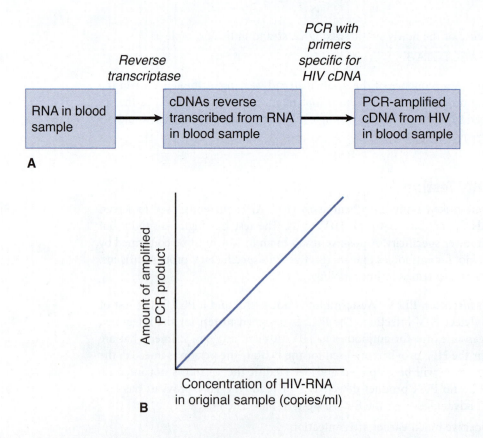

Figure I-7-9. Quantifying Viral Load in HIV Infection Using a Reverse Transcriptase PCR (RT-PCR). (A) RT-PCR technique. (B) Standard curve for quantifying HIV-RNA in blood sample.

Review Questions

1. Two sets of parents were friends in a small town and had babies on the same day. The wristbands of the two similar-looking infants (A and B) were inadvertently mixed at the pediatric care unit. In order to accurately identify the parents of the respective infants, PCR analysis was performed on samples of blood taken from the two infants and both sets of parents (Father 1 and Mother 1 versus Father 2 and Mother 2). Shown below is the analysis of the PCR products by gel electrophoresis.

   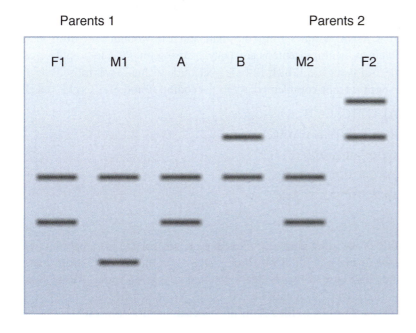

   What is the best conclusion from the analysis?

   (A) A is the child of Parents 1.
   (B) A is the child of Parents 2.
   (C) B is the child of Parents 1.
   (D) Father 1 (F1) could be the father of both infants.
   (E) Father 2 (F2) could be the father of both infants.

2. Paternal relationship between a man and infant can be best determined by the technique commonly referred to as DNA fingerprinting. Which of the following sequences is most conveniently analyzed in a DNA fingerprint?

   (A) Histocompatibility loci
   (B) Centromeres
   (C) Microsatellite tandem repeats (STRs)
   (D) Restriction enzyme sites
   (E) Single-copy sequences

Section I • Biochemistry

3. Sickle cell anemia is caused by a missense mutation in codon 6 of the β-globin gene.

   Codon number

	5	6	7	8
Normal allele	CCT	GAG	GAG	AAG
Mutant allele	CCT	GTG	GAG	AAG

   A man with sickle cell disease and his phenotypically normal wife request genetic testing because they are concerned about the risk for their unborn child. DNA samples from the man and the woman and from fetal cells obtained by amniocentesis are analyzed using the PCR to amplify exon 1 of the β-globin gene. Which 12-base nucleotide sequence was most likely used as a specific probe complementary to the coding strand of the sickle cell allele?

   (A) CCTCACCTCAGG
   (B) CCTGTGGAGAAG
   (C) GGACACCTCTTC
   (D) CTTCTCCACAGG
   (E) CTTCTCCTCAGG

4. mRNA encoding glucose 6-phosphatase was isolated from baboon liver and used to make a ^{32}P-cDNA probe. DNA was then isolated from marmoset and from human tissue, digested with a restriction endonuclease, Southern blotted, and probed with the ^{32}P-cDNA. Which of the following conclusions can be drawn from the results of this analysis shown below?

   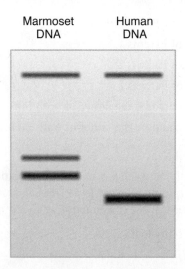

   (A) The glucose 6-phosphatase gene is present in baboon, marmoset and human liver.
   (B) Both marmoset and human liver express the glucose 6-phosphatase gene.
   (C) There are two glucose 6-phosphatase genes in the human liver.
   (D) The glucose 6-phosphatase gene is on different chromosomes in the marmoset and in the human.
   (E) The human and marmoset tissue used in this experiment is from liver.

5. A couple seeks genetic counseling because both the man and the woman (unrelated to each other) are carriers of a mutation causing β-thalassemia, an autosomal recessive condition. The couple has one son who is phenotypically normal and has been shown by DNA analysis to be homozygous for the normal allele. They wish to know whether the fetus in the current pregnancy will have β-thalassemia. Using a probe for the β-globin gene that detects a *Bam*HI RFLP, the following results are obtained. What is the best conclusion about the fetus?

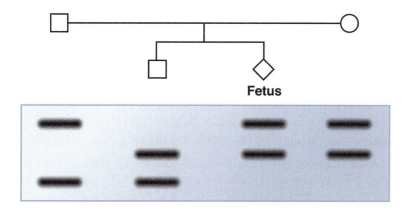

(A) The fetus has inherited the mutation from both parents.
(B) The fetus has inherited the mutation from the mother but not from the father.
(C) The fetus has inherited the mutation from the father but not from the mother.
(D) The fetus has not inherited the mutation from either parent.
(E) The results are inconclusive.

Answers

1. **Answer: A.** Among the conclusions offered, only A is consistent with the results on the blot. Infant A's pattern shows a PCR product (lower on the blot) matching F1 and another PCR product (higher on the blot) matching M1. Neither of infant A's PCR products match F2 (**choices B and E**). The upper PCR product in infant B's pattern does not match with either F1 or M1 (**choices C and D**). Although unlikely given the situation, another possibility is consistent with the blot. Infant A could be the child of M2 and F1, although this is not offered as an option.

2. **Answer: C.** STR sequences are amplified using a PCR and analyzed by gel electrophoresis. Although RFLP analysis could potentially be used for this purpose, it is not the method of choice.

3. **Answer: D.** The complementary probe will be antiparallel to the coding strand of the mutant allele, with all sequences written 5′ → 3′.

4. **Answer: A.** All three tissues contain the gene (the probe was produced from baboon mRNA, implying the gene is also there).

5. **Answer: C.** Knowing the son is homozygous for the normal allele, one can conclude that the two restriction fragments shown in his pattern derived from chromosomes without the mutation. It is also clear that the upper (larger) fragment came from his mother's chromosome and the lower (smaller) fragment came from his father's chromosome. The fetus has the fragment from his mother's normal chromosome. The other fragment (top one on the blot) must have come from the father's chromosome with the mutation. The fetus therefore is heterozygous for the mutation and the normal allele of the β-globin gene.

Amino Acids, Proteins, and Enzymes 8

Learning Objectives

❏ Explain information related to amino acids

❏ Answer questions about protein turnover and amino acid nutrition

❏ Answer questions about biochemical reactions

AMINO ACIDS

General Structure

All amino acids have a central carbon atom attached to a carboxyl group, an amino group, and a hydrogen atom, as shown in Figure I-8-1. The amino acids differ from one another only in the chemical nature of the side chain (R). There are hundreds of amino acids in nature, but only 20 are used as building blocks of proteins in humans.

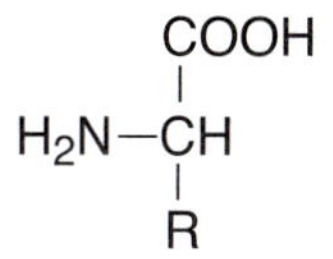

Figure I-8-1. Generalized Structure of Amino Acids

Classification

The amino acids can be classified as either hydrophobic or hydrophilic, depending on the ease with which their side chains interact with water. In general, proteins fold so that amino acids with hydrophobic side chains are in the interior of the molecule where they are protected from water and those with hydrophilic side chains are on the surface.

Hydrophobic amino acids are shown in Figure I-8-2. Additional points about some of these amino acids include:

- Phenylalanine and tyrosine are precursors for catecholamines.
- Tryptophan can form serotonin and niacin.
- Valine, leucine, and isoleucine are branched-chain amino acids whose metabolism is abnormal in maple syrup urine disease (discussed in Chapter 17).
- Proline is a secondary amine whose presence in a protein disrupts normal secondary structure.

Hydrophilic amino acids have side chains that contain O or N atoms. Some of the hydrophilic side chains are charged at physiologic pH. The acidic amino acids (aspartic and glutamic acids) have carboxyl groups that are negatively charged, whereas the basic amino acids (lysine, arginine, and histidine) have nitrogen atoms that are positively charged. The structures of the hydrophilic amino acids are shown in Figure I-8-3. Additional points about some of these amino acids include:

Section I • Biochemistry

- Serine and threonine are sites for O-linked glycosylation of proteins, a posttranslational modification that should be associated with the Golgi apparatus.

- Asparagine is a site for N-linked glycosylation of proteins, a cotranslational modification that should be associated with the endoplasmic reticulum.

- Cysteine contains sulfur and can form disulfide bonds to stabilize the shape (tertiary structure) of proteins. Destroying disulfide bonds denatures proteins.

- Methionine, another sulfur-containing amino acid, is part of S-adenosylmethionine (SAM), a methyl donor in biochemical pathways.

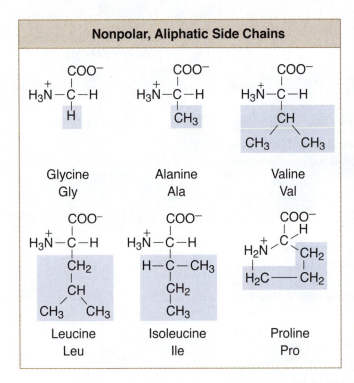
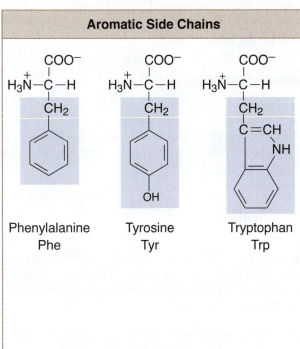

Figure I-8-2. The Hydrophobic Amino Acids

Note: Tyrosine can be considered either nonpolar or polar because of the ability of the -OH group to form a hydrogen bond.

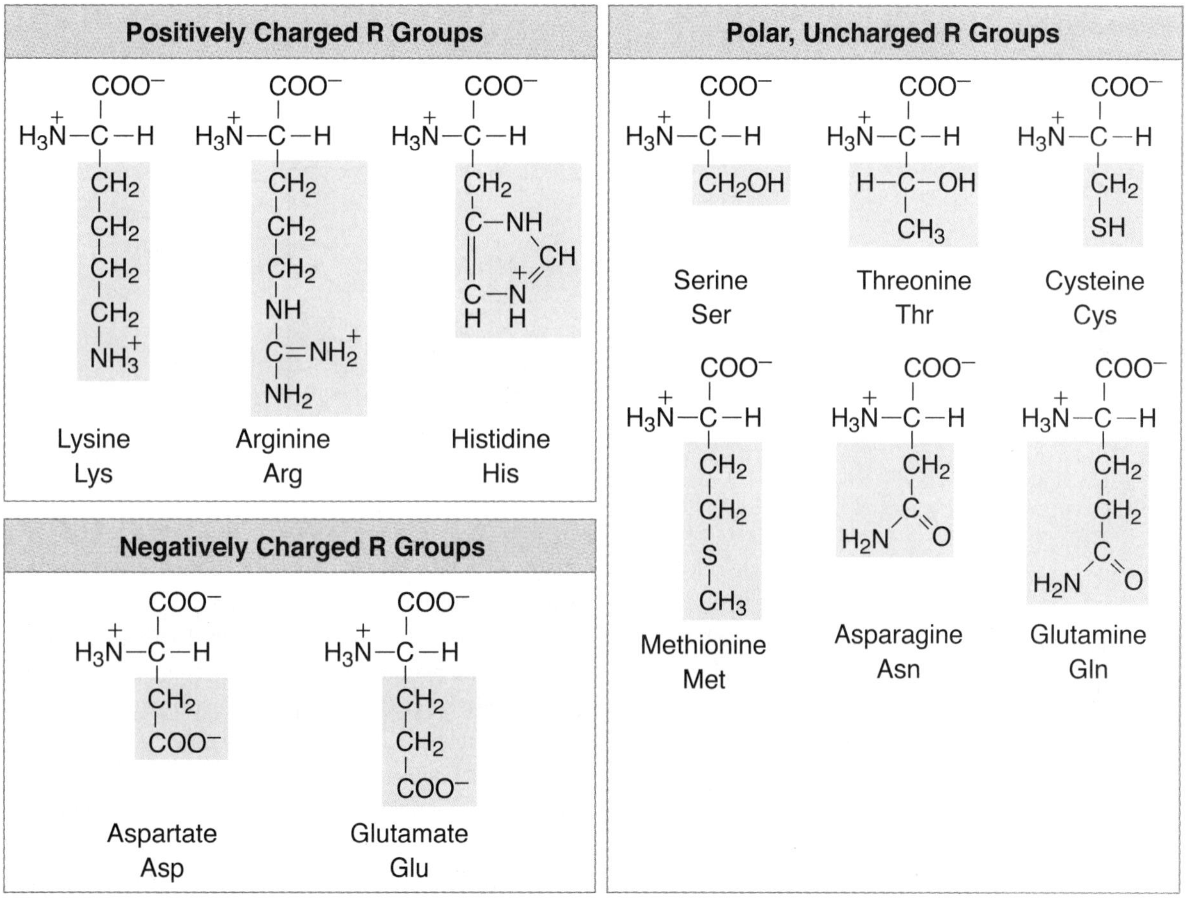

Chapter 8 • Amino Acids, Proteins, and Enzymes

Figure I-8-3. The Hydrophilic Amino Acids

Note: Methionine can be considered nonpolar or polar because it contains a sulfur.

Hemoglobinopathy

An 8-year-old African American boy was experiencing pain in the chest and back. He was taken to the hospital, where he was found to have mild anemia, splenomegaly, and rod-shaped crystals in the erythrocytes. A preliminary diagnosis of sickle cell anemia was made. To validate the diagnosis, a small aliquot of his blood was subjected to electrophoresis to determine the identity of the hemoglobin in his erythrocytes. After reviewing the data, the physician concluded that he did not have sickle cell anemia, but rather a sickle cell anemia–like hemoglobinopathy with the relatively common mutation of HbC.

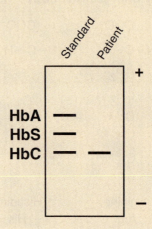

Sickle cell anemia is characterized by severe pain in the bones, abdomen, and chest, along with periods of hemolytic problems. Episodes of vaso-occlusive pain lasting approximately 1 week are a frequent problem. These crises are often precipitated by dehydration or infection. A widely used method to analyze hemoglobins found in various hemoglobinopathies is electrophoresis at pH 8.4, where single amino acid substitutions can be easily detected. In sickle cell anemia, there is a substitution of valine for glutamate at position 6 in Hb, meaning that the HbS will have one less negative charge overall compared with HbA. In HbC, there is a substitution of lysine for glutamate at position 6, meaning that HbC will have two additional positive charges compared with HbA. These three hemoglobins can be resolved by electrophoresis, as shown in the figure.

PROTEIN TURNOVER AND AMINO ACID NUTRITION

When older proteins are broken down in the body, they must be replaced. This concept is called protein turnover, and different types of proteins have very different turnover rates. Protein synthesis occurs during the process of translation on ribosomes. Protein breakdown occurs generally in two cellular locations:

- Lysosomal proteases digest endocytosed proteins.
- Large cytoplasmic complexes, called proteasomes, digest older or abnormal proteins that have been covalently tagged with a protein (called ubiquitin) for destruction.

Essential Amino Acids

All 20 types of amino acids are required for protein synthesis. These amino acids can be derived from digesting dietary protein and absorbing their constituent amino acids or, alternatively, by synthesizing them *de novo*.

The 10 amino acids listed in Table I-8-1 cannot be synthesized in humans and therefore must be provided from dietary sources. These are called the essential amino acids. Arginine is required only during periods of growth, or positive nitrogen balance.

Table I-8-1. Essential Amino Acids

Arginine*	Methionine
Histidine	Phenylalanine
Isoleucine	Threonine
Leucine	Tryptophan
Lysine	Valine

*Essential only during periods of positive nitrogen balance.

Nitrogen Balance

Nitrogen balance is the (normal) condition in which the amount of nitrogen incorporated into the body each day exactly equals the amount excreted.

Negative nitrogen balance occurs when nitrogen loss exceeds incorporation and is associated with:

- Protein malnutrition (kwashiorkor)
- A dietary deficiency of even one essential amino acid
- Starvation
- Uncontrolled diabetes
- Infection

Positive nitrogen balance occurs when the amount of nitrogen incorporated exceeds the amount excreted and is associated with:

- Growth
- Pregnancy
- Convalescence (recovery phase of injury or surgery)
- Recovery from condition associated with negative nitrogen balance

Note
Do not confuse kwashiorkor with marasmus, which is a chronic deficiency of calories. Patients with marasmus do not present with edema as patients do with kwashiorkor.

BIOCHEMICAL REACTIONS

Chemical reactions have two independent properties, their energy and their rate. Table I-8-2 compares these two properties. ΔG represents the amount of energy released or required per mole of reactant. The amount or sign of ΔG indicates nothing about the rate of the reaction.

Section I • Biochemistry

Note

Hydrolysis of high-energy bonds in ATP or GTP provide energy to drive reactions in which $\Delta G > 0$.

Table I-8-2. Comparison of Energy and Rate

Energy (ΔG)	Rate (v)
Not affected by enzymes	Increased by enzymes
$\Delta G < 0$, thermodynamically spontaneous (energy released, often irreversible)	Decrease energy of activation, $\Delta G^\ddagger$
$\Delta G > 0$, thermodynamically nonspontaneous (energy required)	
$\Delta G = 0$, reaction at equilibrium (freely reversible)	
ΔG^0 = energy involved under standardized conditions	

The rate of the reaction is determined by the energy of activation ($\Delta G^\ddagger$), which is the energy required to initiate the reaction. ΔG and $\Delta G^\ddagger$ are represented in Figure I-8-4. Enzymes lower the energy of activation for a reaction; they do not affect the value of ΔG or the equilibrium constant for the reaction, K_{eq}.

— Enzyme catalyzed
— Uncatalyzed

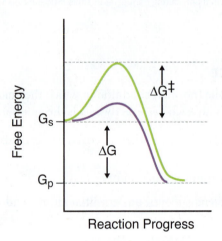

Figure I-8-4. Energy Profile for a Catalyzed and Uncatalyzed Reaction

Michaelis-Menten Equation

The Michaelis-Menten equation describes how the rate of the reaction, V, depends on the concentration of both the enzyme [E] and the substrate [S], which forms product [P].

$$E + S \rightleftharpoons E\text{-}S \rightarrow E + P$$

$$V = \frac{k_2[E][S]}{K_m + [S]} \quad \text{or, with [E] held constant,} \quad V = \frac{V_{max}[S]}{K_m + [S]}$$

Note: $V_{max} = k_2[E]$

V_{max} is the maximum rate possible to achieve with a given amount of enzyme. The only way to increase V_{max} is by increasing the [E]. In the cell, this can be accomplished by inducing the expression of the gene encoding the enzyme.

The other constant in the equation, K_m is often used to compare enzymes. K_m is the substrate concentration required to produce half the maximum velocity. Under certain conditions, K_m is a measure of the affinity of the enzyme for its substrate. When comparing two enzymes, the one with the higher K_m has a lower affinity for its substrate. The K_m value is an intrinsic property of the enzyme-substrate system and cannot be altered by changing [S] or [E].

When the relationship between [S] and V is determined in the presence of constant enzyme, many enzymes yield the graph shown in Figure I-8-5, a hyperbola.

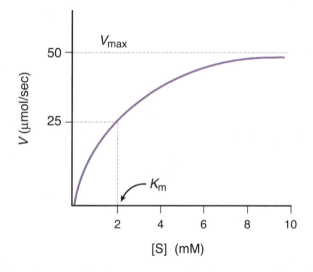

Figure I-8-5. Michaelis-Menten Plot

Bridge to Medical Genetics
A missense mutation in the coding region of a gene may yield an enzyme with a different K_m.

Lineweaver-Burk Equation

The Lineweaver-Burk equation is a reciprocal form of the Michaelis-Menten equation. The same data graphed in this way yield a straight line as shown in Figure I-8-6. The actual data are represented by the portion of the graph to the right of the y-axis, but the line is extrapolated into the left quadrant to determine its intercept with the x-axis. The intercept of the line with the x-axis gives the value of $-1/K_m$. The intercept of the line with the y-axis gives the value of $1/V_{max}$.

$$\frac{1}{V} = \frac{K_m}{V_{max}} \frac{1}{[S]} + \frac{1}{V_{max}}$$

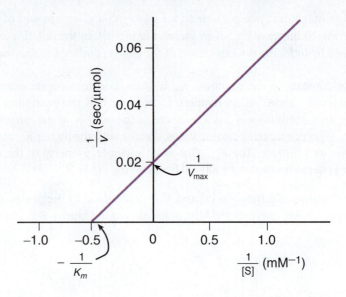

Figure I-8-6. Lineweaver-Burk Plot

Inhibitors and Activators

Two important classes of inhibitors are shown in Table I-8-3. Competitive inhibitors resemble the substrate and compete for binding to the active site of the enzyme. Noncompetitive inhibitors do not bind at the active site. They bind to regulatory sites on the enzyme.

Table I-8-3. Important Classes of Enzyme Inhibitors

Class of Inhibitor	K_m	V_{max}
Competitive	Increase	No effect
Noncompetitive	No effect	Decrease

The effects of these classes of inhibitors on Lineweaver-Burk kinetics are shown in Figures I-8-7 and I-8-8. Notice that on a Lineweaver-Burk graph, inhibitors always lie above the control on the right side of the y-axis.

Note

Drugs That Competitively Inhibit Enzymes

Many drugs are competitive inhibitors of key enzymes in pathways. The statin drugs (lovastatin, simvastatin), used to control blood cholesterol levels, competitively inhibit 3-hydroxy-3-methylglutaryl coenzyme A (HMG CoA) reductase in cholesterol biosynthesis.

Methotrexate, an antineoplastic drug, competitively inhibits dihydrofolate reductase, depriving the cell of active folate needed for purine and deoxythymidine synthesis, thus interfering with DNA replication during S phase.

Drugs That Noncompetitively Inhibit Enzymes

An example of a noncompetitive inhibitor is allopurinol, which noncompetitively inhibits xanthine oxidase.

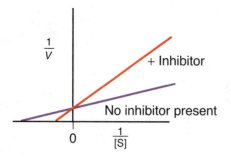

Figure I-8-7. Lineweaver-Burk Plot of Competitive Inhibition

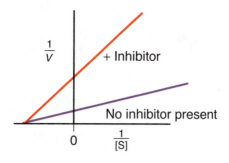

Figure I-8-8. Lineweaver-Burk Plot of Noncompetitive Inhibition

Figure I-8-9 shows the effect on a Lineweaver-Burk plot of adding more enzyme. It might also represent adding an activator to the existing enzyme or a covalent modification of the enzyme. An enzyme activator is a molecule that binds to an enzyme and increases its activity. In these latter two cases the K_m might decrease and/or the V_{max} might increase but the curve would always be below the control curve in the right-hand quadrant of the graph.

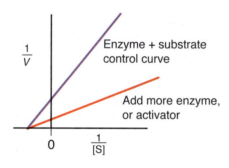

Figure I-8-9. Lineweaver-Burk Plot Showing the Addition of More Enzyme or the Addition of an Activator

Cooperative Enzyme Kinetics

Certain enzymes do not show the normal hyperbola when graphed on a Michaelis-Menten plot ([S] versus V), but rather show sigmoid kinetics owing to cooperativity among substrate binding sites (Figure I-8-10). Cooperative enzymes have multiple subunits and multiple active sites. Enzymes showing cooperative kinetics are often regulatory enzymes in pathways (for example, phosphofructokinase-1 [PFK-1] in glycolysis).

In addition to their active sites, these enzymes often have multiple sites for a variety of activators and inhibitors (e.g., AMP, ATP, citrate, fructose-2,6-bisphosphate [F2,6-BP]). Cooperative enzymes are sometimes referred to as allosteric enzymes because of the shape changes that are induced or stabilized by binding substrates, inhibitors, and activators.

Bridge to Pharmacology

Methanol poisoning (wood alcohol poisoning) is treated with ethanol administration. Both are substrates for alcohol dehydrogenase (ADH), with ethanol having a much lower K_m for the enzyme compared with methanol. This prevents methanol from being converted to formaldehyde, which is toxic and not metabolized further.

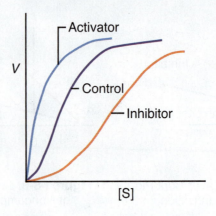

Figure I-8-10. Cooperative Kinetics

Transport Kinetics

The K_m and V_{max} parameters that apply to enzymes are also applicable to transporters in membranes. The kinetics of transport can be derived from the Michaelis-Menten and Lineweaver-Burk equations, where K_m refers to the solute concentration at which the transporter is functioning at half its maximum activity. The importance of K_m values for membrane transporters is exemplified with the variety of glucose transporters (GLUT) and their respective physiologic roles (see Chapter 12).

Chapter Summary

Amino Acids

- Amino acids that have "R-groups" with positive charge at physiologic pH (lysine, arginine).
- Amino acids that have "R-groups" with a negative charge at physiologic pH (aspartic acid, glutamic acid).
- Histidine buffers well in proteins at physiologic pH.

Protein Turnover and Nitrogen Balance

- Essential amino acids: phe, val, trp, thr, ile, met, his, lys, leu, arg (only during positive N-balance)
- Negative nitrogen balance: nitrogen lost > nitrogen gained (illness, protein malnutrition, deficiency of an essential amino acid)
- Positive nitrogen balance: nitrogen lost < nitrogen gained (growth, pregnancy, convalescence)

Enzyme Kinetics

- Enzymes do not affect energy of reaction, ΔG.
- Enzymes lower energy of activation, $\Delta G^{\ddagger}$.
- V_{max} = maximum reaction velocity with a specified amount of enzyme
- K_m = [substrate] required to produce half of the V_{max}
- Inhibitors include:
- (1) competitive (increases K_m)
- (2) noncompetitive (decreases V_{max})
- Rate-limiting enzymes may show cooperative kinetics.

Section I • Biochemistry

Review Questions
Select the ONE best answer.

1. The peptide ala-arg-his-gly-glu is treated with peptidases to release all of the amino acids. The solution is adjusted to pH 7, and electrophoresis is performed. In the electrophoretogram depicted below, the amino acid indicated by the arrow is most likely to be

    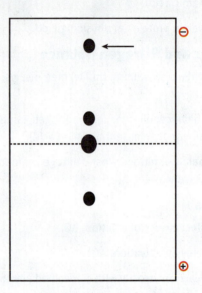

    A. glycine
    B. arginine
    C. glutamate
    D. histidine
    E. alanine

2. The reaction catalyzed by hepatic phosphofructokinase-1 has a ΔG^0 value of -3.5 kcal/mol. This value indicates that under standard conditions this reaction

    A. is reversible
    B. occurs very slowly
    C. produces an activator of pyruvate kinase
    D. is inhibited by ATP
    E. has a low energy of activation
    F. will decrease in activity as the pH decreases
    G. cannot be used for gluconeogenesis
    H. shows cooperative substrate binding
    I. is indirectly inhibited by glucagon
    J. is stimulated by fructose 2,6-bisphosphate

3. The activity of an enzyme is measured at several different substrate concentrations, and the data are shown in the table below.

[S] (mM)	V_0 (mmol/sec)
0.010	2.0
0.050	9.1
0.100	17
0.500	50
1.00	67
5.00	91
10.0	95
50.0	99
100.0	100

   K_m for this enzyme is approximately

   A. 50.0
   B. 10.0
   C. 5.0
   D. 1.0
   E. 0.5

4. Which of the diagrams illustrated below best represents the effect of ATP on hepatic phosphofructokinase-1 (PFK-1)?

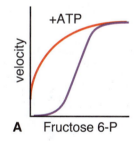 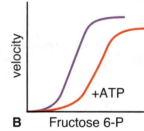 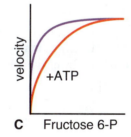 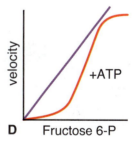 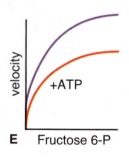

Section I • Biochemistry

5. Several complexes in the mitochondrial electron transport chain contain non-heme iron. The iron in these complexes is bound tightly to the thiol group of which amino acid?

   A. Glutamine
   B. Methionine
   C. Cysteine
   D. Tyrosine
   E. Serine

Items 6–8

Consider a reaction that can be catalyzed by one of two enzymes, A and B, with the following kinetics.

	K_m (M)	Vmax (mmol/min)
A.	5×10^{-6}	20
B.	5×10^{-4}	30

6. At a concentration of 5×10^{-6} M substrate, the velocity of the reaction catalyzed by enzyme A will be

   A. 10
   B. 15
   C. 20
   D. 25
   E. 30

7. At a concentration of 5×10^{-4} M substrate, the velocity of the reaction catalyzed by enzyme B will be

   A. 10
   B. 15
   C. 20
   D. 25
   E. 30

8. At a concentration of 5×10^{-4} M substrate, the velocity of the reaction catalyzed by enzyme A will be

   A. 10
   B. 15
   C. 20
   D. 25
   E. 30

9. A worldwide pandemic of influenza caused by human-adapted strains of avian influenza or bird flu is a serious health concern. One drug for treatment of influenza, Tamiflu (oseltamivir), is an inhibitor of the influenza viral neuraminidase required for release of the mature virus particle from the cell surface. Recent reports have raised concerns regarding viral resistance of Tamiflu compelling the search for alternative inhibitors. Another drug, Relenza (zanamavir), is already FDA approved for use in a prophylactic nasal spray form. The graph below show kinetic data obtained for viral neuraminidase activity (measured as the release of sialic acid from a model substrate) as a function of substrate concentration in the presence and absence of Relenza and Tamiflu.

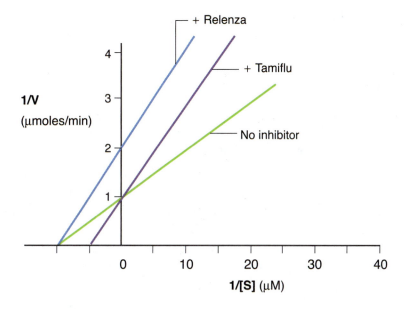

Based on the kinetic data, which of the following statements is correct?

A. Both drugs are competitive inhibitors of the viral neuraminidase.
B. Both drugs are noncompetitive inhibitors of the viral neuraminidase.
C. Tamiflu increases the K_m value for the substrate compared to Relenza.
D. Relenza increases the V_{max} value for the substrate compared to Tamiflu.
E. Relenza is not an inhibitor of neuraminidase, but inhibits another viral enzyme.

Section I • Biochemistry

Answers

1. **Answer: B.** Arginine is the most basic of the amino acids (pI~11) and would have the largest positive charge at pH 7.

2. **Answer: G.** The negative ΔG^0 value indicates the reaction is thermodynamically favorable (irreversible), requiring a different bypass reaction for conversion of F1, 6BP to F6P in the gluconeogenic pathway.

3. **Answer: E.** Because the apparent V_{max} is near 100 mmol/sec, $V_{max}/2$ equals 50 mmol/sec. The substrate concentration giving this rate is 0.50 mM.

4. **Answer: B.** Sigmoidal control curve with ATP inhibiting and shifting curve to the right is needed.

5. **Answer: C.** Cysteine has a sulfhydryl group in its side chain. Although methionine has a sulfur in its side chain, a methyl group is attached to it.

6. **Answer: A.** At the concentration of 5×10^{-6} M, enzyme A is working at one-half of its V_{max} because the concentration is equal to the K_m for the substrate. Therefore, one-half of 20 mmol/min is 10 mmol/min.

7. **Answer: B.** At the concentration of 5×10^{-4} M, enzyme B is working at one-half of its V_{max} because the concentration is equal to the K_m for the substrate. Therefore, one-half of 30 mmol/min is 15 mmol/min.

8. **Answer: C.** At the concentration of 5×10^{-4} M, $100 \times$ the substrate concentration at K_m, enzyme A is working at its V_{max}, which is 20 mmol/min.

9. **Answer: C.** Based on the graph, when the substrate is present, Tamiflu results in the same V_{max} and higher K_m compared to the line when no inhibitor added. These are hallmarks of competitive inhibitors of enzymes, which Tamiflu is. Noncompetitive inhibitors result in decreased V_{max} and the same K_m with no inhibitor added, which is shown by the Relenza line in the graph.

Hormones 9

Learning Objectives

❏ Solve problems concerning hormones and signal transduction

❏ Interpret scenarios about mechanism of water-soluble hormones

❏ Answer questions about G-proteins in signal transduction

❏ Answer questions about lipid-soluble hormones

HORMONES AND SIGNAL TRANSDUCTION

Broadly speaking, a hormone is any compound produced by a cell, which by binding to its cognate receptor alters the metabolism of the cell bearing the hormone–receptor complex. Although a few hormones bind to receptors on the cell that produces them (autoregulation or autocrine function), hormones are more commonly thought of as acting on some other cell, either close by (paracrine) or at a distant site (telecrine). Paracrine hormones are secreted into the interstitial space and generally have a very short half-life. These include the prostaglandins and the neurotransmitters. The paracrine hormones are discussed in the various Lecture Notes, as relevant to the specific topic under consideration. Telecrine hormones are secreted into the bloodstream, generally have a longer half-life, and include the endocrine and gastrointestinal (GI) hormones. The endocrine hormones are the classic ones, and it is sometimes implied that reference is being made to endocrine hormones when the word hormones is used in a general sense. The GI and endocrine hormones are discussed in detail in the GI and endocrinology chapters in the Physiology Lecture Notes. Although there is some overlap, this chapter presents basic mechanistic concepts applicable to all hormones, whereas coverage in the Physiology notes emphasizes the physiologic consequences of hormonal action.

Hormones are divided into two major categories, those that are water soluble (hydrophilic) and those that are lipid soluble (lipophilic, also known as hydrophobic). Important properties of these two classes are shown in Table I-9-1.

Section I • Biochemistry

Table I-9-1. Two Classes of Hormones

Water Soluble	Lipid Soluble
Receptor in cell membrane	Receptor inside cell
Second messengers often involved Protein kinases activated	Hormone–receptor complex binds hormone response elements (HRE) of enhancer regions in DNA
Protein phosphorylation to modify activity of enzymes (requires minutes)	—
Control of gene expression through proteins such as cAMP response element binding (CREB) protein (requires hours)	Control of gene expression (requires hours)
Examples: • Insulin • Glucagon • Catecholamines	Examples: • Steroids • Calcitriol • Thyroxines • Retinoic acid

MECHANISM OF WATER-SOLUBLE HORMONES

Water-soluble hormones must transmit signals to affect metabolism and gene expression without themselves entering the cytoplasm. They often do so via second messenger systems that activate protein kinases.

Protein Kinases

A protein kinase is an enzyme that phosphorylates other proteins, changing their activity (e.g., phosphorylation of acetyl CoA carboxylase inhibits it). Examples of protein kinases are listed in Table I-9-2 along with the second messengers that activate them.

Table I-9-2. Summary of Signal Transduction by Water-Soluble Hormones

Pathway	G Protein	Enzyme	Second Messenger(s)	Protein Kinase	Examples
cAMP	G_s (G_i)	Adenyl cyclase	cAMP	Protein kinase A	Glucagon Epinephrine (β, α-2) Vasopressin (V2, ADH) kidney
PIP_2	G_q	Phospholipase C	DAG, IP_3, Ca^{2+}	Protein kinase C	Vasopressin (V1, V3) vascular smooth muscle Epinephrine ($α_1$)
cGMP	None	Guanyl cyclase	cGMP	Protein kinase G	Atrial natriuretic factor (ANF) Nitric oxide (NO)
Insulin, growth factors	Monomeric $p21^{ras}$	—	—	Tyrosine kinase activity of receptor	Insulin Insulin-like growth factor (IGF) Platelet-derived growth factor (PDGF) Epidermal growth factor (EGF)

Some water-soluble hormones bind to receptors with intrinsic protein kinase activity (often tyrosine kinases). In this case, no second messenger is required for protein kinase activation. The insulin receptor is an example of a tyrosine kinase receptor.

Activation of a protein kinase causes:

- Phosphorylation of enzymes to rapidly increase or decrease their activity.
- Phosphorylation of gene regulatory proteins such as CREB to control gene expression, usually over several hours. The typical result is to add more enzyme to the cell. CREB induces the phosphoenolpyruvate carboxykinase (PEPCK) gene. Kinetically, an increase in the number of enzymes means an increase in V_{max} for that reaction.

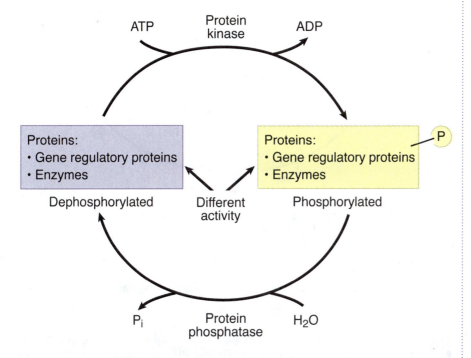

Figure I-9-1. Protein Kinases and Phosphatases

Both represent strategies to control metabolism. The action of protein kinases is reversed by protein phosphatases (Figure I-9-1).

Sequence of Events from Receptor to Protein Kinase

G protein

Receptors in these pathways are coupled through trimetric G proteins in the membrane. The 3 subunits in this type of G protein are α, β, and γ. In its inactive form, the α subunit binds GDP and is in complex with the β and γ subunits. When a hormone binds to its receptor, the receptor becomes activated and, in turn, engages the corresponding G protein (step 1 in Figure I-9-2). The GDP is replaced with GTP, enabling the α subunit to dissociate from the β and γ subunits (step 2 in Figure I-9-2). The activated α subunit alters the activity of adenylate cyclase. If the α subunit is $α_s$, then the enzyme is activated; if the α subunit is $α_i$, then the enzyme is inhibited. The GTP in the activated α subunit will be dephosphorylated to GDP (step 3 in Figure I-9-2) and will rebind to the β and γ subunits (step 4), rendering the G protein inactive.

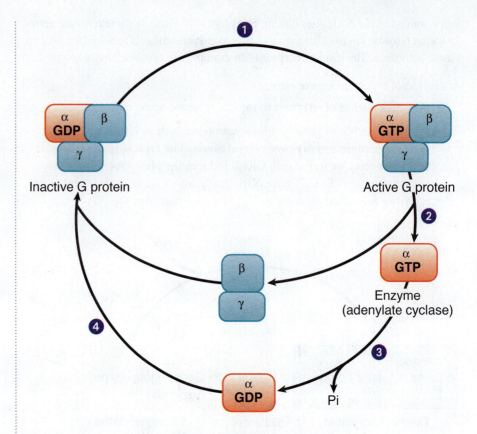

Figure I-9-2. Trimeric G Protein Cycle

Cyclic AMP (cAMP) and phosphatidylinositol bisphosphate (PIP$_2$)

The receptors all have characteristic 7-helix membrane-spanning domains.

The sequence of events (illustrated in Figure I-9-3) leading from receptor to activation of the protein kinase via the cAMP and PIP$_2$ second messenger systems is as follows:

- Hormone binds receptor
- Trimeric G protein in membrane is engaged
- Enzyme (adenylate cyclase or phospholipase) activated
- Second messenger generated
- Protein kinase activated
- Protein phosphorylation (minutes) and gene expression (hours)

An example of inhibition of adenylate cyclase via G$_i$ is epinephrine inhibition (through its binding to α_2 adrenergic receptor) of insulin release from β cells of the pancreas.

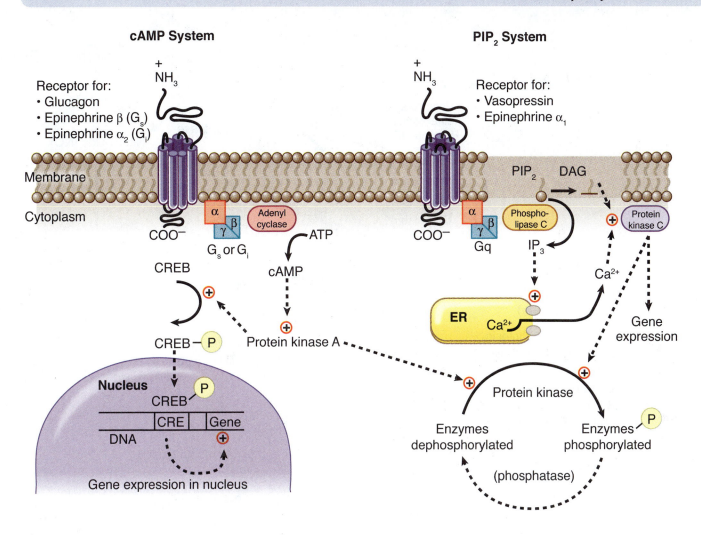

Figure I-9-3. Cyclic AMP and Phosphatidylinositol Bisphosphate (PIP$_2$)

cGMP

Atrial natriuretic factor (ANF), produced by cells in the atrium of the heart in response to distension, binds the ANF receptor in vascular smooth muscle and in the kidney. The ANF receptor spans the membrane and has guanylate cyclase activity associated with the cytoplasmic domain. It causes relaxation of vascular smooth muscle, resulting in vasodilation, and in the kidney it promotes sodium and water excretion.

Nitric oxide (NO) is synthesized by vascular endothelium in response to vasodilators. It diffuses into the surrounding vascular smooth muscle, where it directly binds the heme group of soluble guanylate cyclase, activating the enzyme.

Both the ANF receptor and the soluble guanylate cyclase are associated with the same vascular smooth muscle cells. These cGMP systems are shown in Figure I-9-4.

Note

Once generated, the second messengers cAMP and cGMP are slowly degraded by a class of enzymes called phosphodiesterases (PDEs).

Section I • Biochemistry

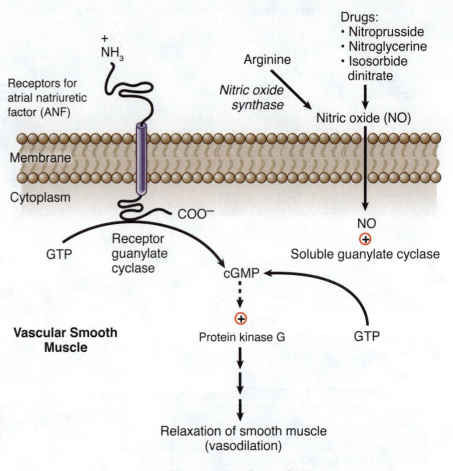

Figure I-9-4. Cyclic GMP

Bridge to Microbiology

***E. coli* heat stable toxin (STa)**

A similar guanylate cyclase receptor in enterocytes is the target of *E. coli* heat-stable toxin (STa). The toxin binds to, and stimulates, the guanylate cyclase increasing cGMP. This causes increased activity of CFTR and diarrhea.

The sequence from receptor to protein kinase is quite similar to the one above for cAMP with two important variations:

- The ANF receptor has intrinsic guanylate cyclase activity. Because no G protein is required in the membrane, the receptor lacks the 7-helix membrane-spanning domain.

- Nitric oxide diffuses into the cell and directly activates a soluble, cytoplasmic guanylate cyclase, so no receptor or G protein is required.

The Insulin Receptor: A Tyrosine Kinase

Insulin binding activates the tyrosine kinase activity associated with the cytoplasmic domain of its receptor as shown in Figure I-9-5. There is no trimeric G protein, enzyme, or second messenger required to activate this protein tyrosine kinase activity:

- Hormone binds receptor
- Receptor tyrosine kinase (protein kinase) is activated
- Protein phosphorylation (autophosphorylation and activation of other proteins)

Once autophosphorylation begins, a complex of other events ensues. An insulin receptor substrate (IRS-1) binds the receptor and is phosphorylated on tyrosine residues, allowing proteins with SH2 (*src* homology) domains to bind to the phosphotyrosine residues on IRS-1 and become active. In this way, the receptor activates several enzyme cascades, which involve:

- Activation of phosphatidylinositol-3 kinase (PI-3 kinase), one of whose effects in adipose and muscle tissues is to increase GLUT-4 in the membrane
- Activation of protein phosphatases. Paradoxically, insulin stimulation via its tyrosine kinase receptor ultimately may lead to dephosphorylating enzymes
- Stimulation of the monomeric G protein (p21^{ras}) encoded by the normal *ras* gene

All these mechanisms can be involved in controlling gene expression, although the pathways by which this occurs have not yet been completely characterized.

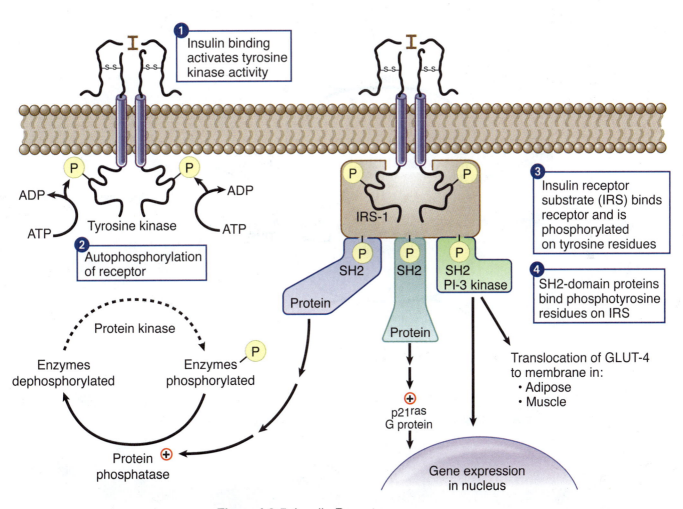

Figure I-9-5. Insulin Receptor

Tyrosine kinase receptors are also involved in signaling by several growth factors, including platelet-derived growth factor (PDGF) and epidermal growth factor (EGF).

Section I • Biochemistry

Functional Relationship of Glucagon and Insulin

Insulin, associated with well-fed, absorptive metabolism, and glucagon, associated with fasting and postabsorptive metabolism, usually oppose each other with respect to pathways of energy metabolism. Glucagon works through the cAMP system to activate protein kinase A favoring phosphorylation of rate-limiting enzymes, whereas insulin often activates protein phosphatases that dephosphorylate many of the same enzymes. An example of this opposition in glycogen metabolism is shown in Figure I-9-6. Glucagon promotes phosphorylation of both rate-limiting enzymes (glycogen phosphorylase for glycogenolysis and glycogen synthase for glycogen synthesis). The result is twofold in that synthesis slows and degradation increases, but both effects contribute to the same physiologic outcome, release of glucose from the liver during hypoglycemia. Insulin reverses this pattern, promoting glucose storage after a meal. The reciprocal relationship between glucagon and insulin is manifested in other metabolic pathways, such as triglyceride synthesis and degradation.

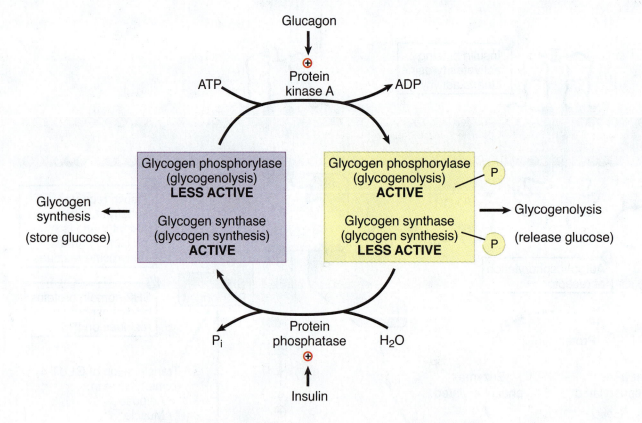

Figure I-9-6. Opposing Activities of Insulin and Glucagon

G PROTEINS IN SIGNAL TRANSDUCTION

Table I-9-2 is a summary of the major components of water-soluble hormone pathways reviewed in this section. There are several different G proteins (GTP-binding) involved. Trimeric G proteins include G_s, G_i, G_q, and in the photoreceptor pathway reviewed in Chapter 10, G_t (transducin). Receptors that engage these all have the seven-helix membrane-spanning structure. Receptor stimulation causes the Gα subunit to bind GTP and become active. The Gα subunit subsequently hydrolyzes the GTP to GDP, terminating the signal. The $p21^{ras}$ G protein is monomeric.

G-protein defects can cause disease in several ways, some of which are summarized in Table I-9-3.

Table I-9-3. Abnormal G Proteins and Disease

Defect	Example	Disease
ADP-ribosylation by:		
• *Cholera* toxin	$G_s\alpha$	Diarrhea of cholera
• *E. coli* toxin	$G_s\alpha$	Traveler's diarrhea
• *Pertussis* toxin	$G_i\alpha$	Pertussis (whooping cough)
Oncogenic mutations	$p21^{ras}$ (*ras*)	Colon, lung, breast, bladder tumors

ADP-Ribosylation by Bacterial Toxins

Certain bacterial exotoxins are enzymes that attach the adenosine diphosphate (ADP)-ribose residue of NAD to Gα subunits, an activity known as ADP-ribosylation. In humans, some ADP-ribosylation is physiological, but it may also be pathological:

- *Vibrio cholerae* exotoxin ADP-ribosylates $G_s\alpha$, leading to an increase in cAMP and subsequently chloride secretion from intestinal mucosal cells, and causing the diarrhea of cholera.

- Certain strains of *Escherichia coli* release toxins (heat labile or LT) similar to cholera toxin, producing traveler's diarrhea.

- *Bordetella pertussis* exotoxin ADP-ribosylates $G_i\alpha$, dramatically reducing its responsiveness to the receptor, thus increasing cAMP. It is not known how this relates to the persistent paroxysmal coughing symptomatic of pertussis (whooping cough).

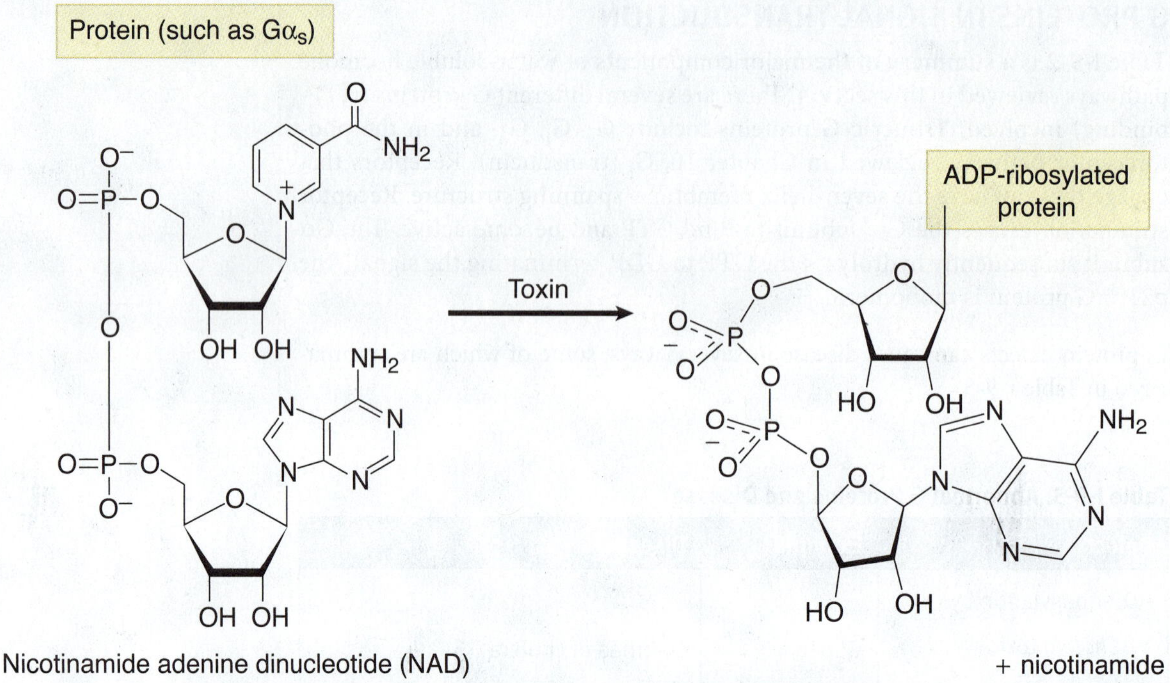

Section I • Biochemistry

Figure I-9-7. ADP-Ribosylation of a Protein

LIPID-SOLUBLE HORMONES

Lipid-soluble hormones diffuse through the cell membrane, where they bind to their respective receptors inside the cell. The receptors have a DNA-binding domain (usually Zn-fingers) and interact with specific response elements in enhancer (or possibly silencer) regions associated with certain genes. For example, the cortisol receptor binds to its response element in the enhancer region of the phosphoenolpyruvate carboxykinase (PEPCK) gene. By increasing the amount of PEPCK in the hepatocyte, cortisol can increase the capacity for gluconeogenesis, one of its mechanisms for responding to chronic stress often associated with injury. The enhancer mechanism was reviewed in Chapter 5.

Review Questions

1. A patient with manic depressive disorder is treated with lithium, which slows the turnover of inositol phosphates and the phosphatidyl inositol derivatives in cells. Which of the following protein kinases is most directly affected by this drug?

   A. Protein kinase C
   B. Receptor tyrosine kinase
   C. Protein kinase G
   D. Protein kinase A
   E. Protein kinase M

Items 2 and 3

Tumor cells from a person with leukemia have been analyzed to determine which oncogene is involved in the transformation. After partial sequencing of the gene, the predicted gene product is identified as a tyrosine kinase.

2. Which of the following proteins would most likely be encoded by an oncogene and exhibit tyrosine kinase activity?

   A. Nuclear transcriptional activator
   B. Epidermal growth factor
   C. Membrane-associated G protein
   D. Platelet-derived growth factor
   E. Growth factor receptor

3. A kinetic analysis of the tyrosine kinase activities in normal and transformed cells is shown below.

   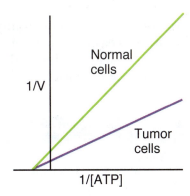

   Which of the following conclusions is best supported by these results?

   A. The tumor cell kinase has a higher-than-normal affinity for ATP
   B. A kinase gene has been deleted from the tumor cell genome
   C. A noncompetitive inhibitor has been synthesized in the tumor cells
   D. A kinase gene has been amplified in the tumor cell genome
   E. The tumor cell kinase has a lower-than-normal affinity for ATP

4. In a DNA sequencing project, an open reading frame (ORF) has been identified. The nucleotide sequence includes a coding region for an SH2 domain in the protein product. This potential protein is most likely to

A. bind to an enhancer region in DNA
B. be a transmembrane hormone receptor
C. transmit signals from a tyrosine kinase receptor
D. bind to an upstream promoter element
E. activate a soluble guanyl cyclase enzyme in vascular smooth muscle

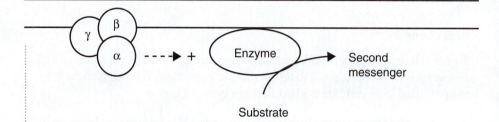

5. The diagram above represents a signal transduction pathway associated with hormone X. The receptor for hormone X is most likely to be characterized as a(n)

A. seven-helix transmembrane domain receptor
B. intracellular receptor with a zinc-finger domain
C. helix-turn-helix transmembrane domain receptor
D. transmembrane receptor with a guanyl cyclase domain
E. tyrosine kinase domain receptor

6. A 58-year-old man with a history of angina for which he occasionally takes isosorbide dinitrate is having erectile dysfunction. He confides in a colleague, who suggests that sildenafil might help and gives him three tablets from his own prescription. The potentially lethal combination of these drugs relates to

	Isosorbide Dinitrate	Sildenafil
A.	Activates nitric oxide synthase in vascular endothelium	Inhibits guanyl cyclase in vascular smooth muscle
B.	Activates nitric oxide synthase in vascular endothelium	Inhibits guanyl cyclase in corpora cavernosa smooth muscle
C.	Releases cyanide as a byproduct	Inhibits cGMP phosphodiesterase in corpora cavernosa smooth muscle
D.	Activates guanyl cyclase in vascular smooth muscle	Inhibits cGMP phosphodiesterase in vascular smooth muscle
E.	Activates the ANF receptor in vascular smooth muscle	Inhibits protein kinase G in vascular smooth muscle

Answers

1. **Answer: A.** The description best fits the PIP_2 system in which protein kinase C is activated.

2. **Answer: E.** Although any of the listed options might be encoded by an oncogene, the "tyrosine kinase" description suggests it is likely to be a growth factor receptor.

3. **Answer: D.** Because the *y*-axis is 1/V, a smaller value for the 1/V means an increase in V_{max}. An increase in V_{max} (with no change in K_m) means an increase in the number of enzymes (a kinase in this problem). Gene amplification (insertion of additional copies of the gene in the chromosome) is a well-known mechanism by which oncogenes are overexpressed and by which resistance to certain drugs is developed. For instance, amplification of the dihydrofolate reductase gene can confer resistance to methotrexate.

4. **Answer: C.** Proteins with SH2 domains might bind to the insulin receptor substrate-1 (IRS-1) to transmit signals from the insulin receptor, a tyrosine kinase type of receptor. PI-3 kinase is an example of an SH2 domain protein. SH2 domains are not involved in DNA binding (**choices A and D**). Examples of protein domains that bind DNA include zinc fingers (steroid receptors), leucine zippers (CREB protein), and helix-turn-helix proteins (homeodomain proteins).

5. **Answer: A.** The diagram indicates that the receptor activates a trimeric G-protein associated with the inner face of the membrane and that the G-protein subsequently signals an enzyme catalyzing a reaction producing a second messenger. Receptors that activate trimeric G-proteins have a characteristic seven-helix transmembrane domain. The other categories of receptors do not transmit signals through trimeric G-proteins.

6. **Answer: D.** Nitrates may be metabolized to nitric oxide (NO) that activates a soluble guanyl cyclase in vascular smooth muscle. The increase in cGMP activates protein kinase G and subsequently leads to vasodilation. Sildenafil inhibits cGMP phosphodiesterase (PDE), potentiating vasodilation that can lead to shock and sudden death. Although sildenafil has much higher potency for the cGMP PDE isozyme in the corpora cavernosa, it can also inhibit the cGMP PDE in vascular smooth muscle. Nitric oxide synthase (**choices A and B**) is the physiologic source of nitric oxide in response to vasodilators such as acetylcholine, bradykinin, histamine, and serotonin.

Vitamins 10

Learning Objectives

❑ Answer questions about vitamin D and calcium homeostasis
❑ Interpret scenarios about vitamin A
❑ Answer questions about vitamin K
❑ Explain information related to vitamin E

OVERVIEW OF VITAMINS

Vitamins have historically been classified as either water soluble or lipid soluble. Water-soluble vitamins are precursors for coenzymes and are reviewed in the context of the reactions for which they are important. A summary of these vitamins is shown in Table I-10-1.

Section I • Biochemistry

Table I-10-1. Water-Soluble Vitamins

Vitamin or Coenzyme	Enzyme	Pathway	Deficiency
Biotin	Pyruvate carboxylase Acetyl CoA carboxylase Propionyl CoA carboxylase	Gluconeogenesis Fatty acid synthesis Odd-carbon fatty acids, Val, Met, Ile, Thr	MCC* (rare): excessive consumption of raw eggs (contain avidin, a biotin-binding protein); also caused by biotinidase deficiency Alopecia (hair loss), bowel inflammation, muscle pain
Thiamine (B_1)	Pyruvate dehydrogenase α-Ketoglutarate dehydrogenase Transketolase Branched chain ketoacid dehydrogenase	PDH TCA cycle HMP shunt Metabolism of valine isoleucine and leucine	MCC: alcoholism (alcohol interferes with absorption) Wernicke (ataxia, nystagmus, ophthalmoplegia) Korsakoff (confabulation, psychosis) Wet beri-beri (high-output cardiac failure, fluid retention, vascular leak) and dry beri-beri (peripheral neuropathy)
Niacin (B_3) NAD(H) NADP(H)	Dehydrogenases	Many	Pellagra: diarrhea, dementia, dermatitis, and, if not treated, death Pellagra may also be related to deficiency of tryptophan (corn is low in triptophan), which supplies a portion of the niacin requirement.
Folic acid THF	Thymidylate synthase Enzymes in purine synthesis need not be memorized	Thymidine (pyrimidine) synthesis Purine synthesis	MCC: alcoholism and pregnancy (body stores depleted in 3 months), hemodialysis Homocystinemia with risk of deep vein thrombosis and atherosclerosis Megaloblastic (macrocytic) anemia Deficiency in early pregnancy causes neural tube defects in fetus
Cyanocobalamin (B_{12})	Homocysteine methyltransferase Methylmalonyl CoA mutase	Methionine, SAM Odd-carbon fatty acids, Val, Met, Ile, Thr	MCC: pernicious anemia. Also in aging, especially with poor nutrition, bacterial overgrowth of terminal ileum, resection of the terminal ileum secondary to Crohn disease, chronic pancreatitis, and, rarely, vegans, or infection with *D. latum* Megaloblastic (macrocytic) anemia Progressive peripheral neuropathy

*MCC, most common cause

(Continued)

Table I-10-1. Water-Soluble Vitamins (*continued*)

Vitamin or Coenzyme	Enzyme	Pathway	Deficiency
Pyridoxine (B$_6$) Pyridoxal-P (PLP)	Aminotransferases (transaminase): AST (GOT), ALT (GPT) δ-Aminolevulinate synthase	Protein catabolism Heme synthesis	MCC: isoniazid therapy Sideroblastic anemia Cheilosis or stomatitis (cracking or scaling of lip borders and corners of the mouth) Convulsions
Riboflavin (B$_2$) FAD(H$_2$)	Dehydrogenases	Many	Corneal neovascularization Cheilosis or stomatitis (cracking or scaling of lip borders and corners of the mouth) Magenta-colored tongue
Ascorbate (C)	Prolyl and lysyl hydroxylases Dopamine hydroxylase	Collagen synthesis Catecholamine synthesis Absorption of iron in GI tract	MCC: diet deficient in citrus fruits and green vegetables Scurvy: poor wound healing, easy bruising (perifollicular hemorrhage), bleeding gums, increased bleeding time, painful glossitis, anemia
Pantothenic acid CoA	Fatty acid synthase Fatty acyl CoA synthetase Pyruvate dehydrogenase α-Ketoglutarate dehydrogenase	Fatty acid metabolism PDH TCA cycle	Rare

Scurvy

A 7-month-old infant presented in a "pithed frog" position, in which he lay on his back and made little attempt to lift the legs and arms because of pain. The infant cried when touched or moved, and there appeared to be numerous areas of swelling and bruising throughout the body. The mother informed the pediatrician that the infant was bottle-fed. However, the mother stated that she always boiled the formula extensively, much longer than the recommended time, to ensure that it was sterile.

Bridge to Pharmacology

High-dose niacin can be used to treat hyperlipidemia.

Section I • Biochemistry

Note
Vitamin Deficiencies

Vitamin D Deficiency

Symptoms
- bone demineralization
- rickets (children)
- osteomalacia (adults)

Causes
- insufficient sunlight
- inadequate fortified foods (milk)
- end-stage renal disease (renal osteodystrophy)

Vitamin A Deficiency

Symptoms
- night blindness
- keratinized squamous epithelia
- xerophthalmia, Bitot spots
- keratomalacia, blindness
- follicular hyperkeratosis
- alopecia

Causes
- fat malabsorption
- fat-free diets

Vitamin E Deficiency

Symptoms
- hemolytic anemia
- acanthocytosis
- peripheral neuropathy
- ataxia
- retinitis pigmentosum

Causes
- fat malabsorption
- premature infants

The patient has infantile scurvy, which often occurs in infants 2–10 months of age who are bottle-fed with formula that is overheated for pasteurization and not supplemented with vitamin C. Vitamin C is destroyed by excessive heat. Although bleeding in an infant with scurvy might occur similarly as in an adult, gum bleeding does not unless there are erupted teeth. Biochemically, vitamin C is necessary as a cofactor by proline and lysine hydroxylases in collagen synthesis. In scurvy, because proline and lysine residues are not hydroxylated, hydrogen bonding within the triple helices does not take place. Consequently, collagen fibers are significantly less stable than normal. Vitamin C also has roles as *1)* an antioxidant, *2)* in reducing iron in the intestine to enable the absorption of iron, and *3)* in hepatic synthesis of bile acids.

There are 4 important lipid-soluble vitamins, D, A, K, and E. Two of these vitamins, A and D, work through enhancer mechanisms similar to those for lipid-soluble hormones. In addition, all 4 lipid-soluble vitamins have more specialized mechanisms through which they act. Table I-10-2 lists their major functions.

Table I-10-2. Lipid-Soluble Vitamins

Vitamin	Important Functions
D (cholecalciferol)	In response to hypocalcemia, helps normalize serum calcium levels
A (carotene)	Retinoic acid and retinol act as growth regulators, especially in epithelium Retinal is important in rod and cone cells for vision
K (menaquinone, bacteria; phytoquinone, plants)	Carboxylation of glutamic acid residues in many Ca^{2+}-binding proteins, importantly coagulation factors II, VII, IX, and X, as well as protein C and protein S
E (α-tocopherol)	Antioxidant in the lipid phase. Protects membrane lipids from peroxidation

VITAMIN D AND CALCIUM HOMEOSTASIS

Hypocalcemia (below-normal blood calcium) stimulates release of parathyroid hormone (PTH), which in turn binds to receptors on cells of the renal proximal tubules. The receptors are coupled through cAMP to activation of a 1α-hydroxylase important for the final, rate-limiting step in the conversion of vitamin D to 1,25-DHCC (dihydroxycholecalciferol or calcitriol).

Once formed, 1,25-DHCC acts on duodenal epithelial cells as a lipid-soluble hormone. Its intracellular receptor (a Zn-finger protein) binds to response elements in enhancer regions of DNA to induce the synthesis of calcium-binding proteins thought to play a role in stimulating calcium uptake from the GI tract.

1,25-DHCC also facilitates calcium reabsorption in the kidney and mobilizes calcium from bone when PTH is also present. All these actions help bring blood calcium levels back within the normal range.

The relation of vitamin D to calcium homeostasis and its *in vivo* activation are shown in Figure I-10-1.

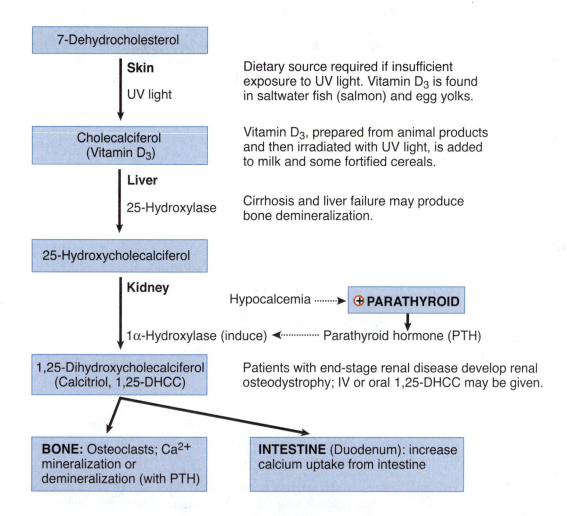

Figure I-10-1. Synthesis and Activation of Vitamin D

Synthesis of 1,25-Dihydroxycholecalciferol (Calcitriol)

Humans can synthesize calcitriol from 7-dehydrocholesterol derived from cholesterol in the liver. Three steps are involved, each occurring in a different tissue:

1. Activation of 7-dehydrocholesterol by UV light in the skin produces cholecalciferol (vitamin D_3) This step is insufficient in many people in cold, cloudy climates, and vitamin D_3 supplementation is necessary.
2. 25-Hydroxylation in the liver (patients with severe liver disease may need to be given 25-DHCC or 1,25-DHCC).
3. 1α-Hydroxylation in the proximal renal tubule cells in response to PTH. Genetic deficiencies or patients with end-stage renal disease develop renal osteodystrophy because of insufficiency of 1,25-DHCC and must be given 1,25-DHCC or a drug analog that does not require metabolism in the kidney. Such patients include those with:
   - End-stage renal disease secondary to diabetes mellitus
   - Fanconi renal syndrome (renal proximal tubule defect)
   - Genetic deficiency of the 1α-hydroxylase (vitamin D-resistant rickets)

Bridge to Pharmacology

Bisphosphonates are a class of drugs used in the treatment of osteoporosis. They function by inhibiting osteoclast action and resorption of bone. This process results in a modest increase in bone mineral density (BMD), leading to strengthening of bone and decrease in fractures. Commonly used bisphosphates are Boniva (ibandronate), Actonel (risedronate), and Fosamax (alendronate).

Vitamin D Toxicity

A 45-year-old man had a 3-week history of weakness, excessive urination, intense thirst, and staggering walk. For most of his adult life, he took excessive amounts of vitamin C because he was told it would help prevent the common cold. The past month, he took excessive amounts of vitamin D and calcium every day because he learned that he was developing osteoporosis. Recent laboratory tests revealed that his serum calcium was greatly elevated, and vitamin D toxicity was the diagnosis.

Vitamin D is highly toxic at consumption levels that continuously exceed 10× RDA, resulting in hypercalcemia. Unlike water-soluble vitamins, which are excreted in excess amounts, vitamin D can be stored in the liver as 25-hydroxycholecalciferol. The excess vitamin D can promote intestinal absorption of calcium and phosphate.

The direct effect of excessive vitamin D on bone is resorption similar to that seen in vitamin D deficiency. Therefore, the increased intestinal absorption of calcium in vitamin D toxicity contributes to hypercalcemia. Rather than helping the man's osteoporosis, a large amount of vitamin D can contribute to it. Hypercalcemia can impair renal function, and early signs include polyuria, polydipsia, and nocturia. Prolonged hypercalcemia can result in calcium deposition in soft tissues, notably the kidney, producing irreversible kidney damage.

Clinical Correlate

Isotretinoin, a form of retinoic acid, is used in the treatment of acne. It is teratogenic (malformations of the craniofacial, cardiac, thymic, and CNS structures) and is therefore absolutely contraindicated in pregnant women and used with caution in women of childbearing age.

Vitamin D Deficiency

Deficiency of vitamin D in childhood produces rickets, a constellation of skeletal abnormalities most strikingly seen as deformities of the legs, but many other developing bones are affected. Muscle weakness is common.

Vitamin D deficiency after epiphyseal fusion causes osteomalacia, which produces less deformity than rickets. Osteomalacia may present as bone pain and muscle weakness.

VITAMIN A

Vitamin A (carotene) is converted to several active forms in the body associated with two important functions, maintenance of healthy epithelium and vision. Biochemically, there are three vitamin A structures that differ on the basis of the functional group on C-1: hydroxyl (retinol), carboxyl (retinoic acid), and aldehyde (retinal).

Maintenance of Epithelium

Retinol and retinoic acid are required for the growth, differentiation, and maintenance of epithelial cells. In this capacity they bind intracellular receptors, which are in the family of Zn-finger proteins, and they regulate transcription through specific response elements.

Vision

When first formed, all the double bonds in the conjugated double bond system in retinal are in the *trans* configuration. This form, all-*trans* retinal is not active. The conversion of all-*trans* retinal to the active form *cis*-retinal takes place in the pigmented epithelial cells. *Cis*-retinal is then transferred to opsin in the rod cells forming the light receptor rhodopsin. It functions similarly in rod and cone cells. When exposed to light, *cis*-retinal is converted all-*trans* retinal. A diagram of the signal transduction pathway for light-activated rhodopsin in the rod cell is shown in Figure I-10-2, along with the relationship of this pathway to rod cell anatomy and changes in the membrane potential. Note the following points:

- Rhodopsin is a 7-pass receptor coupled to the trimeric G protein transducin (G_t).

- When light is present, the pathway activates cGMP phosphodiesterase, which lowers cGMP.

- Rhodopsin and transducin are embedded in the disk membranes in the outer rod segment.

- cGMP-gated Na^+ channels in the cell membrane of the outer rod segment respond to the decrease in cGMP by closing and hyperpolarizing the membrane.

- The rod cell is unusual for an excitable cell in that the membrane is partially depolarized (~ –30 mV) at rest (in darkness) and hyperpolarizes on stimulation.

Because the membrane is partially depolarized in the dark, its neurotransmitter glutamate is continuously released. Glutamate inhibits the optic nerve bipolar cells with which the rod cells synapse. By hyperpolarizing the rod cell membrane, light stops the release of glutamate, relieving inhibition of the optic nerve bipolar cell and thus initiating a signal into the brain.

Section I • Biochemistry

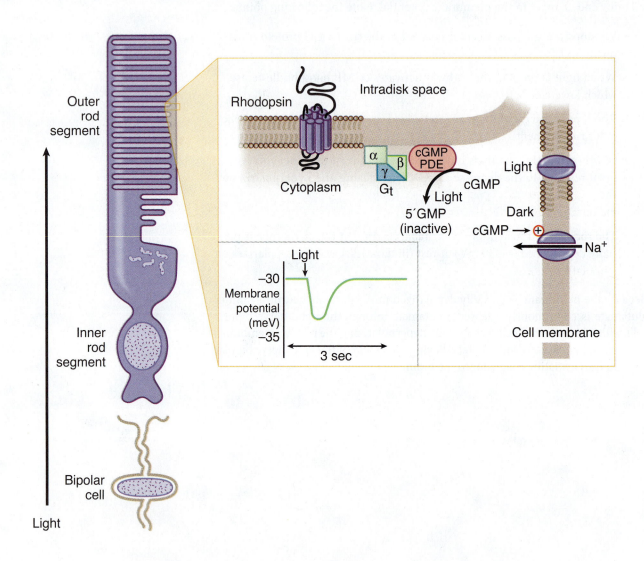

Figure I-10-2. Light-Activated Signal Transduction in the Retinal Rod Cell

> ### Vitamin A Deficiency
>
> A severe drought in portions of Kenya wiped out a family's yam crop, their primary food staple. Within several months, a 3-year-old child in the family began to complain of being unable to see very well, especially at dusk or at night. Also, the child's eyes were red due to constant rubbing because of dryness.
>
> Due to the ability of the liver to store vitamin A, deficiencies that are severe enough to result in clinical manifestations are unlikely to be observed, unless there is an extreme lack of dietary vitamin A over several months. Vitamin A deficiency is the most common cause of blindness and is a serious problem in developing countries. It has a peak incidence at 3–5 years of age. In the U.S., vitamin A deficiency is most often due to fat malabsorption or liver cirrhosis.
>
> Vitamin A deficiency results in night blindness (rod cells are responsible for vision in low light), metaplasia of the corneal epithelium, xerophthalmia (dry eyes), bronchitis, pneumonia, and follicular hyperkeratosis. The spots or patches noted in the eyes of patients with vitamin A deficiency are known as Bitot spots. Because vitamin A is important for differentiation of immune cells, deficiencies can result in frequent infections.
>
> β-carotene is the orange pigment in yams, sweet potatoes, carrots, and yellow squash. Upon ingestion, it can be cleaved relatively slowly to two molecules of retinal by an intestinal enzyme, and each retinal molecule is then converted to all-*trans*-retinol and then absorbed by interstitial cells. Therefore, it is an excellent source of vitamin A.

Note

If vitamin A is continuously ingested at levels greater than 15× RDA, toxicity develops; symptoms include excessive sweeting, brittle nails, diarrhea, hypercalcemia, hepatotoxicity, vertigo, nausea, and vomiting. Unlike vitamin A, β-carotene is not toxic at high levels.

VITAMIN K

Vitamin K is required to introduce Ca^{2+} binding sites on several calcium-dependent proteins. The modification that introduces the Ca^{2+} binding site is a γ-carboxylation of glutamyl residue(s) in these proteins, often identified simply as the γ-carboxylation of glutamic acid. Nevertheless, this vitamin K-dependent carboxylation (Figure I-10-3) is a cotranslational modification occurring as the proteins are synthesized on ribosomes associated with the rough endoplasmic reticulum (RER) during translation.

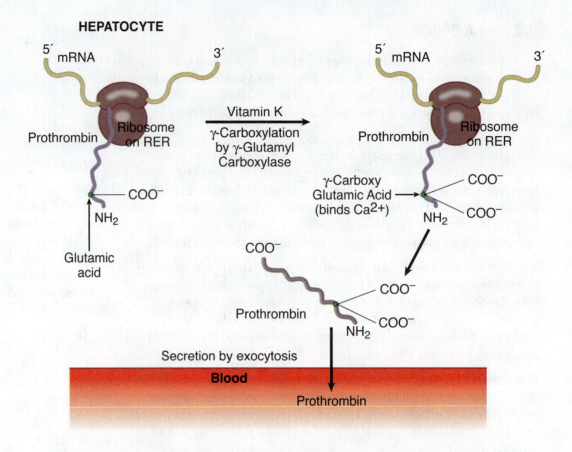

Figure I-10-3. Vitamin K–Dependent γ-Carboxylation of Prothrombin during Translation on the Rough Endoplasmic Reticulum (RER)

Examples of proteins undergoing this vitamin K–dependent carboxylation include the coagulation factors II (prothrombin), VII, IX, and X, as well as the anticoagulant proteins C and S. All these proteins require Ca^{2+} for their function. Vitamin K deficiencies produce prolonged bleeding, easy bruising, and potentially fatal hemorrhagic disease. Conditions predisposing to a vitamin K deficiency include:

- Fat malabsorption (bile duct occlusion)
- Prolonged treatment with broad-spectrum antibiotics (eliminate intestinal bacteria that supply vitamin K)
- Breast-fed newborns (little intestinal flora, breast milk very low in vitamin K), especially in a home-birth where a postnatal injection of vitamin K may not be given
- Infants whose mothers have been treated with certain anticonvulsants during pregnancy such as phenytoin (Dilantin)

Vitamin K Deficiency

A 79-year-old man living alone called his 72-year-old sister and then arrived at the hospital by ambulance complaining of weakness and having a rapid heartbeat. His sister said that he takes no medications and has a history of poor nutrition and poor hygiene. Physical examination confirmed malnourishment and dehydration. A stool specimen was positive for occult blood. He had a prolonged prothrombin time (PT), but his liver function tests (LFTs) were within normal range. He was given an injection of a vitamin that corrected his PT in 2 days.

Poor nutrition and malnourishment, lack of medications, occult blood in the stool specimen, prolonged PT, and normal LFTs are all consistent with vitamin K deficiency. Without vitamin K, several blood clotting factors (prothrombin, X, IX, VII) are not γ-carboxylated on glutamate residues by the γ-glutamyl carboxylase during their synthesis (cotranslational modification) in hepatocytes. The PT returned to normal 2 days after a vitamin K injection.

Vitamin K deficiency should be distinguished from vitamin C deficiency. Table I-10-3 summarizes some of these differences.

Table I-10-3. Comparison of Vitamin K and Vitamin C Deficiencies

Vitamin K Deficiency	Vitamin C Deficiency
Easy bruising, bleeding	Easy bruising, bleeding
Normal bleeding time	Increased bleeding time
Increased PT	Normal PT
Hemorrhagic disease with no connective tissue problems	• Gum hyperplasia, inflammation, loss of teeth • Skeletal deformity in children • Poor wound healing • Anemia
Associated with: • Fat malabsorption • Long-term antibiotic therapy • Breast-fed newborns • Infant whose mother was taking anticonvulsant therapy during pregnancy	Associated with: • Diet deficient in citrus fruit, green vegetables

Section I • Biochemistry

Anticoagulant Therapy

Warfarin and dicumarol antagonize the γ-carboxylation activity of vitamin K and thus act as anticoagulants. They interfere with the cotranslational modification during synthesis of the precoagulation factors. Once these proteins have been released into the bloodstream, vitamin K is no longer important for their subsequent activation and function. Related to this are 2 important points:

- Warfarin and dicumarol prevent coagulation only *in vivo* and cannot prevent coagulation of blood *in vitro* (drawn from a patient into a test tube).

- When warfarin and dicumarol are given to a patient, 2–3 days are required to see their full anticoagulant activity. Heparin or low-molecular- weight heparin is often given to provide short-term anticoagulant activity. Heparin is an activator of antithrombin III.

VITAMIN E

Vitamin E (α-tocopherol) is an antioxidant. As a lipid-soluble compound, it is especially important for protecting other lipids from oxidative damage.

It prevents peroxidation of fatty acids in cell membranes, helping to maintain their normal fluidity. Deficiency can lead to hemolysis, neurologic problems, and retinitis pigmentosa.

High blood levels of Vitamin E can cause hemorrhage in patients given warfarin.

Clinical Correlate

Relative to the other proteins that undergo γ-carboxylation, protein C has a short half-life. Thus, initiation of warfarin therapy may cause a transient hypercoagulable state.

Clinical Correlate

Vitamin K (SC, IM, oral, or IV) is used to reverse bleeding from hypothrombinemia caused by excess warfarin.

Review Questions

Select the ONE best answer.

1. Retinitis pigmentosa (RP) is a genetically heterogeneous disease characterized by progressive photoreceptor degeneration and ultimately blindness. Mutations in more than 20 different genes have been identified in clinically affected patients. Recent studies have mapped an RP locus to the chromosomal location of a new candidate gene at 5q31. One might expect this gene to encode a polypeptide required for the activity of a(n)

   A. receptor tyrosine kinase
   B. cGMP phosphodiesterase
   C. phospholipase C
   D. adenyl cyclase
   E. protein kinase C

2. A 27-year-old woman with epilepsy has been taking phenytoin to control her seizures. She is now pregnant, and her physician is considering changing her medication to prevent potential bleeding episodes in the infant. What biochemical activity might be deficient in the infant if her medication is continued?

   A. Hydroxylation of proline
   B. Glucuronidation of bilirubin
   C. Reduction of glutathione
   D. γ-Carboxylation of glutamate
   E. Oxidation of lysine

3. A 75-year-old woman is seen in the emergency room with a fractured arm. Physical examination revealed multiple bruises and perifollicular hemorrhages, periodontitis, and painful gums. Her diet consists predominately of weak coffee, bouillon, rolls, and plain pasta. Lab results indicated mild microcytic anemia. Which of the following enzymes should be less active than normal in this patient?

   A. Homocysteine methyltransferase
   B. γ-Glutamyl carboxylase
   C. Dihydrofolate reductase
   D. ALA synthase
   E. Prolyl hydroxylase

Answers

1. **Answer: B.** Only phosphodiesterase participates as a signaling molecule in the visual cycle of photoreceptor cells.

2. **Answer: D.** Phenyl hydantoins decrease the activity of vitamin K, which is required for the γ-carboxylation of coagulation factors (II, VII, IX, X), as well as proteins C and S.

3. **Answer: E.** The patient has many signs of scurvy from a vitamin C deficiency. The diet, which contains no fruits or vegetables, provides little vitamin C. Prolyl hydroxylase requires vitamin C, and in the absence of hydroxylation, the collagen α-chains do not form stable, mature collagen. The anemia may be due to poor iron absorption in the absence of ascorbate.

Overview of Energy Metabolism 11

Learning Objectives

❏ Explain information related to metabolic sources of energy

❏ Interpret scenarios about metabolic energy storage

❏ Interpret scenarios about regulation of fuel metabolism

❏ Answer questions about patterns of fuel metabolism in tissues

METABOLIC SOURCES OF ENERGY

Energy is extracted from food via oxidation, resulting in the end products carbon dioxide and water. This process occurs in 4 stages, shown in Figure I-11-1.

In stage 1, metabolic fuels are hydrolyzed in the gastrointestinal tract to a diverse set of monomeric building blocks (glucose, amino acids, and fatty acids) and absorbed.

In stage 2, the building blocks are degraded by various pathways in tissues to a common metabolic intermediate, acetyl-CoA. Most of the energy contained in metabolic fuels is conserved in the chemical bonds (electrons) of acetyl-CoA. A smaller portion is conserved in reducing nicotinamide adenine dinucleotide (NAD) to NADH or flavin adenine dinucleotide (FAD) to $FADH_2$. Reduction indicates the addition of electrons that may be free, part of a hydrogen atom (H), or a hydride ion (H^-).

In stage 3, the citric acid (Krebs, or tricarboxylic acid [TCA]) cycle oxidizes acetyl-CoA to CO_2. The energy released in this process is primarily conserved by reducing NAD to NADH or FAD to $FADH_2$.

The final stage is oxidative phosphorylation, in which the energy of NADH and $FADH_2$ is released via the electron transport chain (ETC) and used by an ATP synthase to produce ATP. This process requires O_2.

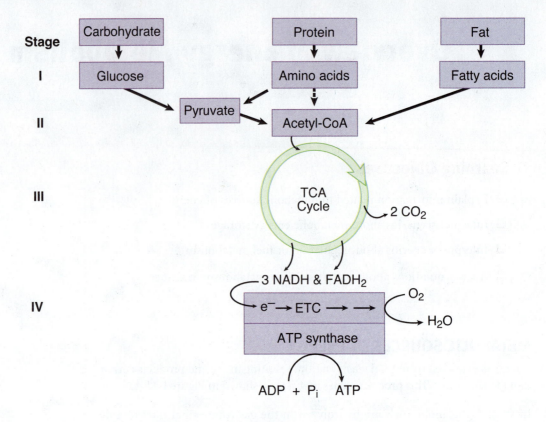

Figure I-11-1. Energy from Metabolic Fuels

METABOLIC ENERGY STORAGE

ATP is a form of circulating energy currency in cells. It is formed in catabolic pathways by phosphorylation of ADP and may provide energy for biosynthesis (anabolic pathways). There is a limited amount of ATP in circulation. Most of the excess energy from the diet is stored as fatty acids (a reduced polymer of acetyl CoA) and glycogen (a polymer of glucose). Although proteins can be mobilized for energy in a prolonged fast, they are normally more important for other functions (contractile elements in muscle, enzymes, intracellular matrix, etc.).

In addition to energy reserves, many other types of biochemicals are required to maintain an organism. Cholesterol is required for cell membrane structure, proteins for muscle contraction, and polysaccharides for the intracellular matrix, to name just a few examples. These substances may be produced from transformed dietary components.

REGULATION OF FUEL METABOLISM

The pathways that are operational in fuel metabolism depend on the nutritional status of the organism. Shifts between storage and mobilization of a particular fuel, as well as shifts among the types of fuel being used, are very pronounced in going from the well-fed state to an overnight fast, and finally to a prolonged state of starvation. The shifting metabolic patterns are regulated mainly by the insulin/glucagon ratio. Insulin is an anabolic hormone that promotes fuel storage. Its action is opposed by a number of hormones, including glucagon, epinephrine, cortisol, and growth hormone. The major function of glucagon is to respond rapidly to decreased blood glucose levels by promoting the synthesis and release of glucose into the circulation. Anabolic and catabolic pathways are controlled at three important levels:

- Allosteric inhibitors and activators of rate-limiting enzymes
- Control of gene expression by insulin and glucagon
- Phosphorylation (glucagon) and dephosphorylation (insulin) of rate-limiting enzymes

Well-Fed (Absorptive) State

Immediately after a meal, the blood glucose level rises and stimulates the release of insulin. The three major target tissues for insulin are liver, muscle, and adipose tissue (Figure I-11-2). Insulin promotes glycogen synthesis in liver and muscle. After the glycogen stores are filled, the liver converts excess glucose to fatty acids and triglycerides. Insulin promotes triglyceride synthesis in adipose tissue and protein synthesis in muscle, as well as glucose entry into both tissues. After a meal, most of the energy needs of the liver are met by the oxidation of excess amino acids.

Two tissues, brain and red blood cells (Figure I-11-2), are insensitive to insulin (are insulin independent). The brain and other nerves derive energy from oxidizing glucose to CO_2 and water in both the well-fed and normal fasting states. Only in prolonged fasting does this situation change. Under all conditions, red blood cells use glucose anaerobically for all their energy needs.

Postabsorptive State

Glucagon and epinephrine levels rise during an overnight fast. These hormones exert their effects on skeletal muscle, adipose tissue, and liver. In liver, glycogen degradation and the release of glucose into the blood are stimulated (Figure I-11-3). Hepatic gluconeogenesis is also stimulated by glucagon, but the response is slower than that of glycogenolysis. The release of amino acids from skeletal muscle and fatty acids from adipose tissue are both stimulated by the decrease in insulin and by an increase in epinephrine. The amino acids and fatty acids are taken up by the liver, where the amino acids provide the carbon skeletons and the oxidation of fatty acids provides the ATP necessary for gluconeogenesis.

Section I • Biochemistry

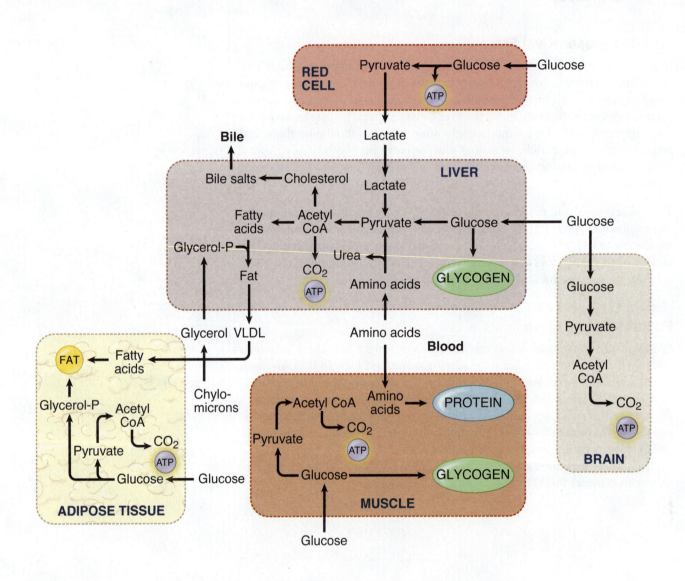

Figure I-11-2. Metabolic Profile of the Well-Fed (Absorptive) State

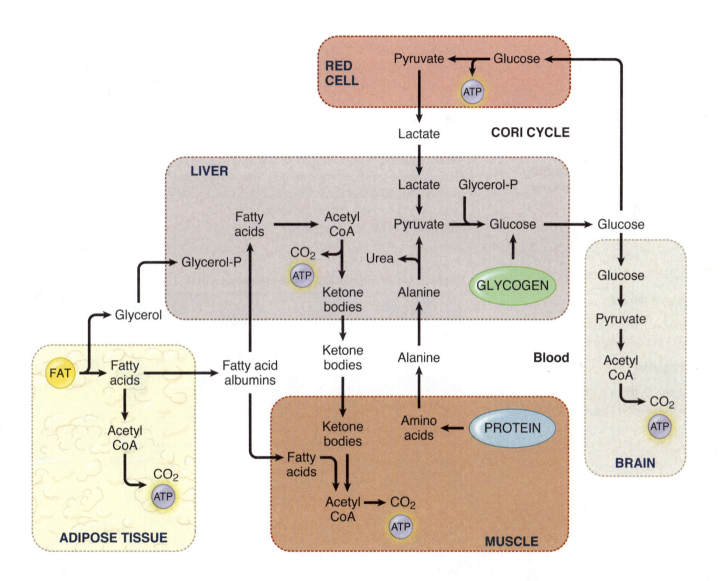

Figure I-11-3. Metabolic Profile of the Postabsorptive State

Section I • Biochemistry

Note

Carbohydrate (4 kcal/gm)

Protein (4 kcal/gm)

Fat (9 kcal/gm)

Alcohol (7 kcal/gm)

Note

Diet

A recommended 2,100-kcal diet consisting of 58% carbohydrate, 12% protein, and 30% fat content:

305 g of carbohydrate

0.58 × 2,100 kcal = 1,218 kcal
1,218 kcal/4 kcal/g = 305 g

63 g of protein

0.12 × 2,100 = 252 kcal
252 kcal/4 kcal/g = 63 g

70 g of fat

0.30 × 2,100 = 630 kcal
630 kcal/9 kcal/g = 70 g

Prolonged Fast (Starvation)

Levels of glucagon and epinephrine are markedly elevated during starvation. Lipolysis is rapid, resulting in excess acetyl-CoA that is used for ketone synthesis. Levels of both lipids and ketones are therefore increased in the blood. Muscle uses fatty acids as the major fuel, and the brain adapts to using ketones for some of its energy. After several weeks of fasting, the brain derives approximately two thirds of its energy from ketones and one third from glucose. The shift from glucose to ketones as the major fuel diminishes the amount of protein that must be degraded to support gluconeogenesis. There is no "energy-storage form" for protein because each protein has a specific function in the cell. Therefore, the shift from using glucose to ketones during starvation spares protein, which is essential for these other functions. Red blood cells (and renal medullary cells) that have few, if any, mitochondria continue to be dependent on glucose for their energy.

PATTERNS OF FUEL METABOLISM IN TISSUES

Fats are much more energy-rich than carbohydrates, proteins, or ketones. Complete combustion of fat results in 9 kcal/g compared with 4 kcal/g derived from carbohydrate, protein, and ketones. The storage capacity and pathways for utilization of fuels varies with different organs and with the nutritional status of the organism as a whole. The organ-specific patterns of fuel utilization in the well-fed and fasting states are summarized in Table I-11-1.

Table I-11-1. Preferred Fuels in the Well-Fed and Fasting States

Organ	Well-Fed	Fasting
Liver	Glucose and amino acids	Fatty acids
Resting skeletal muscle	Glucose	Fatty acids, ketones
Cardiac muscle	Fatty acids	Fatty acids, ketones
Adipose tissue	Glucose	Fatty acids
Brain	Glucose	Glucose (ketones in prolonged fast)
Red blood cells	Glucose	Glucose

Liver

Two major roles of liver in fuel metabolism are to maintain a constant level of blood glucose under a wide range of conditions and to synthesize ketones when excess fatty acids are being oxidized. After a meal, the glucose concentration in the portal blood is elevated. The liver extracts excess glucose and uses it to replenish its glycogen stores. Any glucose remaining in the liver is then converted to acetyl CoA and used for fatty acid synthesis. The increase in insulin after a meal stimulates both glycogen synthesis and fatty acid synthesis in liver. The fatty acids are converted to triglycerides and released into the blood as very low-density lipoproteins (VLDLs). In the well-fed state, the liver derives most of its energy from the oxidation of excess amino acids.

Between meals and during prolonged fasts, the liver releases glucose into the blood. The increase in glucagon during fasting promotes both glycogen degradation and gluconeogenesis. Lactate, glycerol, and amino acids provide carbon skeletons for glucose synthesis.

Adipose Tissue

After a meal, the elevated insulin stimulates glucose uptake by adipose tissue. Insulin also stimulates fatty acid release from VLDL and chylomicron triglyceride (triglyceride is also known as triacylglycerol). Lipoprotein lipase, an enzyme found in the capillary bed of adipose tissue, is induced by insulin. The fatty acids that are released from lipoproteins are taken up by adipose tissue and re-esterified to triglyceride for storage. The glycerol phosphate required for triglyceride synthesis comes from glucose metabolized in the adipocyte. Insulin is also very effective in suppressing the release of fatty acids from adipose tissue.

During the fasting state, the decrease in insulin and the increase in epinephrine activate hormone-sensitive lipase in fat cells, allowing fatty acids to be released into the circulation.

Skeletal Muscle

Resting muscle

The major fuels of skeletal muscle are glucose and fatty acids. Because of the enormous bulk, skeletal muscle is the body's major consumer of fuel. After a meal, under the influence of insulin, skeletal muscle takes up glucose to replenish glycogen stores and amino acids that are used for protein synthesis. Both excess glucose and amino acids can also be oxidized for energy.

In the fasting state, resting muscle uses fatty acids derived from free fatty acids in the blood. Ketones may be used if the fasting state is prolonged. In exercise, skeletal muscle may convert some pyruvate to lactate, which is transported by blood to be converted to glucose in the liver.

Active muscle

The primary fuel used to support muscle contraction depends on the magnitude and duration of exercise as well as the major fibers involved. Skeletal muscle has stores of both glycogen and some triglycerides. Blood glucose and free fatty acids also may be used.

Fast-twitch muscle fibers have a high capacity for anaerobic glycolysis but are quick to fatigue. They are involved primarily in short-term, high-intensity exercise. Slow-twitch muscle fibers in arm and leg muscles are well vascularized and primarily oxidative. They are used during prolonged, low-to-moderate intensity exercise and resist fatigue. Slow-twitch fibers and the number of their mitochondria increase dramatically in trained endurance athletes.

Short bursts of high-intensity exercise are supported by anaerobic glycolysis drawing on stored muscle glycogen.

During moderately high, continuous exercise, oxidation of glucose and fatty acids are both important, but after 1 to 3 hours of continuous exercise at this level, muscle glycogen stores become depleted, and the intensity of exercise declines to a rate that can be supported by oxidation of fatty acids.

Clinical Correlate

Because insulin is necessary for adipose cells to take up fatty acids from triglycerides, high triglyceride levels in the blood may be an indicator of untreated diabetes.

Section I • Biochemistry

Cardiac Muscle

During fetal life cardiac muscle primarily uses glucose as an energy source, but in the postnatal period there is a major switch to β-oxidation of fatty acids. Thus, in humans fatty acids serve as the major fuel for cardiac myocytes. When ketones are present during prolonged fasting, they are also used. Thus, not surprisingly, cardiac myocytes most closely parallel the skeletal muscle during extended periods of exercise.

In patients with cardiac hypertrophy, this situation reverses to some extent. In the failing heart, glucose oxidation increases, and β-oxidation falls.

Brain

Although the brain represents 2% of total body weight, it obtains 15% of the cardiac output, uses 20% of total O_2, and consumes 25% of the total glucose. Therefore, glucose is the primary fuel for the brain. Blood glucose levels are tightly regulated to maintain the concentration levels that enable sufficient glucose uptake into the brain via GLUT 1 and GLUT 3 transporters. Because glycogen levels in the brain are minor, normal function depends upon continuous glucose supply from the bloodstream. In hypoglycemic conditions (<70 mg/dL), centers in the hypothalamus sense a fall in blood glucose level, and the release of glucagon and epinephrine is triggered. Fatty acids cannot cross the blood–brain barrier and are therefore not used at all. Between meals, the brain relies on blood glucose supplied by either hepatic glycogenolysis or gluconeogenesis. Only in prolonged fasts does the brain gain the capacity to use ketones for energy, and even then ketones supply only approximately two thirds of the fuel; the remainder is glucose.

Review Questions

Select the ONE best answer.

1. Two weeks after an episode of the flu, an 8-year-old boy with IDDM is brought to the emergency room in a coma. His breathing is rapid and deep, and his breath has a fruity odor. His blood glucose is 36.5 mM (normal: 4–6 mM [70–110 mg/dL]). The physician administers IV fluids, insulin, and potassium chloride. A rapid effect of insulin in this situation is to stimulate

   A. gluconeogenesis in the liver
   B. fatty acid release from adipose
   C. glucose transport in muscle
   D. ketone utilization in the brain
   E. glycogenolysis in the liver

2. An alcoholic has been on a 2-week drinking binge during which time she has eaten little and has become severely hypoglycemic. Which additional condition may develop in response to chronic, severe hypoglycemia?

   A. Glycogen accumulation in the liver with cirrhosis
   B. Thiamine deficiency
   C. Ketoacidosis
   D. Folate deficiency
   E. Hyperuricemia

3. After a routine physical exam and blood work, a woman with a normal weight for her height was advised that her lipid profile showed an elevation of blood triglycerides. The doctor advises the patient to lower fat consumption which disappoints her since she avidly consumes whole milk. The woman consults a nutritionist, who states that whole milk is 3.5% fat, which corresponds to approximately 11 g of fat in an 8 ounce serving. If she switches to drinking skim milk (nonfat), approximately how much additional grams of carbohydrates should she consume to make up for the loss of fat in the 8 ounce serving?

   A. 5 grams
   B. 11 grams
   C. 15 grams
   D. 25 grams
   E. 35 grams

Answers

1. **Answer: C.** Insulin increases glucose transport in only two tissues, adipose and muscle. The major site of glucose uptake is muscle, which decreases hyperglycemia. Glucose and ketone transport and metabolism are insulin independent in the brain (**choice D**). Insulin would slow gluconeogenesis (**choice A**) and fatty acid release from adipose (**choice B**). Insulin would inhibit glycogenolysis in the liver (**choice E**).

2. **Answer: C.** Severe hypoglycemia lowers the insulin level and increases glucagon. This would favor fatty acid release from the adipose and ketogenesis in the liver.

3. **Answer: D.** It is expected that students know that carbohydrates have 4 Kcal/gram, proteins have 4 Kcal/gram, fat has 9 Kcal/gram, and alcohol has 7 Kcal/gram. In this question, 11 grams of fat times 9 Kcal/gram = 99 Kcal which is rounded to 100 Kcal. Dividing 100 Kcal by 4 Kcal/gram of carbohydrate is 25 grams.

Glycolysis and Pyruvate Dehydrogenase 12

Learning Objectives

❑ Answer questions about carbohydrate digestion

❑ Demonstrate understanding of glucose transport

❑ Solve problems concerning glycolysis

❑ Interpret scenarios about galactose metabolism

❑ Explain information related to fructose metabolism

❑ Answer questions about pyruvate dehydrogenase

OVERVIEW

All cells can carry out glycolysis. In a few tissues, most importantly red blood cells, glycolysis represents the only energy-yielding pathway available. Glucose is the major monosaccharide that enters the pathway, but others such as galactose and fructose can also be used. The first steps in glucose metabolism in any cell are transport across the membrane and phosphorylation by kinase enzymes inside the cell to prevent it from leaving via the transporter.

CARBOHYDRATE DIGESTION

Only a very small amount of the total carbohydrates ingested are monosaccharides. Most of the carbohydrates in foods are in complex forms, such as starch (amylose and amylopectin) and the disaccharides sucrose and lactose. In the mouth, secreted salivary amylase randomly hydrolyzes the starch polymers to dextrins (<8–10 glucoses). Upon entry of food into the stomach, the acid pH destroys the salivary amylase. In the intestine, the dextrins are hydrolyzed to the disaccharides maltose and isomaltose. Disaccharides in the intestinal brush border complete the digestion process:

- Maltase cleaves maltose to 2 glucoses
- Isomaltase cleaves isomaltose to 2 glucoses
- Lactase cleaves lactose to glucose and galactose
- Sucrase cleaves sucrose to glucose and fructose

Uptake of glucose into the mucosal cells is performed by the sodium/glucose transporter, an active transport system.

Section I • Biochemistry

GLUCOSE TRANSPORT

Glucose entry into most cells is concentration driven and independent of sodium. Four glucose transporters (GLUT) are listed in Table I-12-1. They have different affinities for glucose coinciding with their respective physiologic roles. Normal glucose concentration in peripheral blood is 4–6 mM (70–110 mg/dL).

- GLUT 1 and GLUT 3 mediate basal glucose uptake in most tissues, including brain, nerves, and red blood cells. Their high affinities for glucose ensure glucose entry even during periods of relative hypoglycemia. At normal glucose concentration, GLUT 1 and GLUT 3 are at V_{max}.

- GLUT 2, a low-affinity transporter, is in hepatocytes. After a meal, portal blood from the intestine is rich in glucose. GLUT 2 captures the excess glucose primarily for storage. When the glucose concentration drops below the K_m for the transporter, much of the remainder leaves the liver and enters the peripheral circulation. In the β-islet cells of the pancreas. GLUT-2, along with glucokinase, serves as the glucose sensor for insulin release.

- GLUT 4 is in adipose tissue and muscle and responds to the glucose concentration in peripheral blood. The rate of glucose transport in these two tissues is increased by insulin, which stimulates the movement of additional GLUT 4 transporters to the membrane by a mechanism involving exocytosis (Figure I-12-1).

Bridge to Physiology

GLUT 4 translocation to the cell membrane in skeletal muscle is stimulated by exercise. This effect, which is independent of insulin, involves a 5′ AMP-activated kinase.

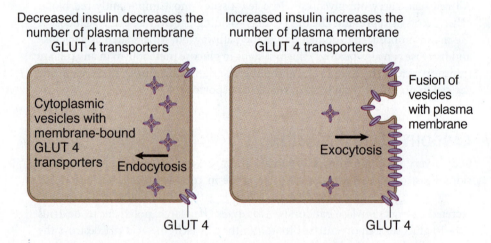

Figure I-12-1. Insulin Regulation of Glucose Transport in Muscle and Adipose Cells

Although basal transport occurs in all cells independently of insulin, the transport rate increases in adipose tissue and muscle when insulin levels rise. Muscle stores excess glucose as glycogen, and adipose tissue requires glucose to form dihydroxyacetone phosphate (DHAP), which is converted to glycerol phosphate used to store incoming fatty acids as triglyceride (TGL, three fatty acids attached to glycerol).

Table I-12-1. Major Glucose Transporters in Human Cells

Name	Tissues	K_m, Glucose	Functions
GLUT 1	Most tissues (brain, red cells)	~1 mM	Basal uptake of glucose
GLUT 2	Liver Pancreatic β-cells	~15 mM	Uptake and release of glucose by the liver β-cell glucose sensor
GLUT 3	Most tissues	~1 mM	Basal uptake
GLUT 4	Skeletal muscle Adipose tissue	~5 mM	Insulin-stimulated glucose uptake; stimulated by exercise in skeletal muscle

Normal blood glucose concentration is 4–6 mM (72–110 mg/dL).

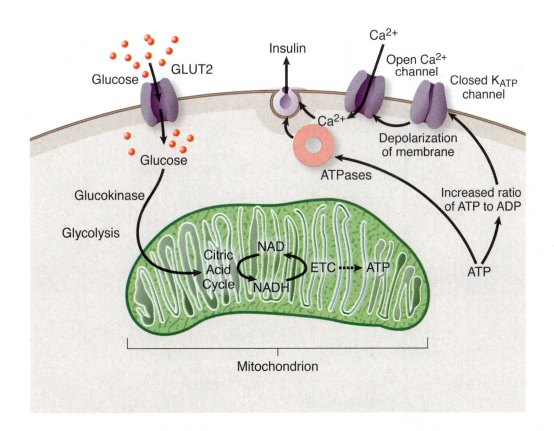

Figure I-12-2. GLUT2 and Glucokinase Together Function as the Glucose Sensor in Pancreatic β-Islet Cells

Note

Glucose induces genetic expression of the insulin gene. Insulin secretion by the pancreatic β-cells is biphasic. Glucose stimulates the first phase (within 15 minutes) with release of preformed insulin. The second phase (several hours) involves insulin synthesis at the gene level.

GLYCOLYSIS

Glycolysis is a cytoplasmic pathway that converts glucose into two pyruvates, releasing a modest amount of energy captured in two substrate-level phosphorylations and one oxidation reaction. If a cell has mitochondria and oxygen, glycolysis is aerobic. If either mitochondria or oxygen is lacking, glycolysis may occur anaerobically (erythrocytes, exercising skeletal muscle), although some of the available energy is lost.

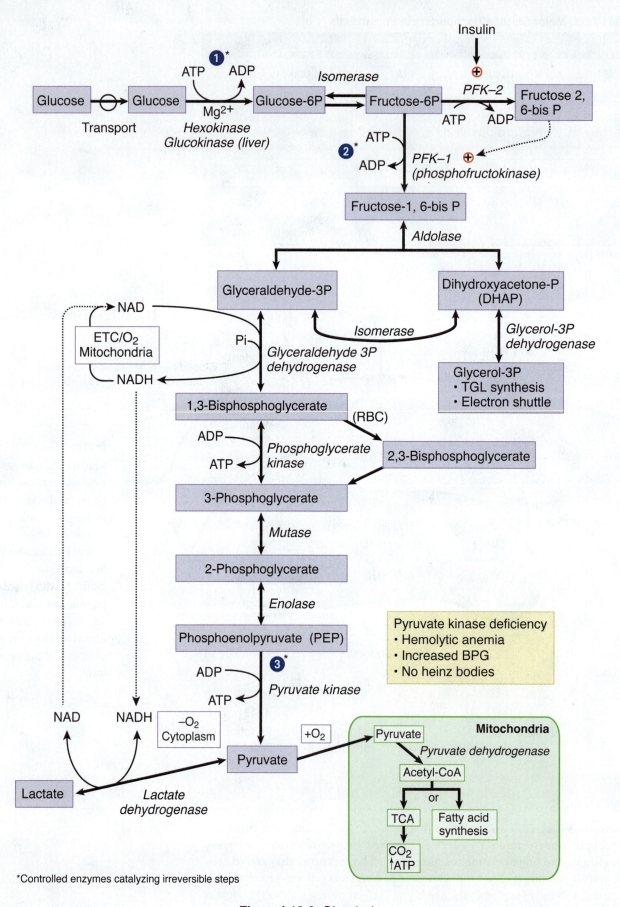

Figure I-12-3. Glycolysis

Glycolysis also provides intermediates for other pathways. In the liver, glycolysis is part of the process by which excess glucose is converted to fatty acids for storage. Glycolysis is shown in Figure I-12-3. Important enzymes in glycolysis include:

1. **Hexokinase/glucokinase:** glucose entering the cell is trapped by phosphorylation using ATP. Hexokinase is widely distributed in tissues, whereas glucokinase is found only in hepatocytes and pancreatic β-islet cells. Table I-12-2 identifies the differences in their respective K_m and V_{max} values. These coincide with the differences in K_m values for the glucose transporters in these tissues listed in Table I-12-1.

Note
Arsenate inhibits the conversion of glyceraldehyde 3-phosphate to 1,3-bisphosphoglycerate by mimicking phosphate in the reaction. The arsenate-containing product is water labile, enabling glycolysis to proceed but resulting in no ATP production.

Table I-12-2. Comparison of Hexokinase and Glucokinase

Hexokinase	Glucokinase
Most tissues	Hepatocytes and pancreatic β-islet cells (along with GLUT-2, acts as the glucose sensor)
Low K_m (0.05 mM in erythrocytes)	High K_m (10 mM)
Inhibited by glucose 6-phosphate	Induced by insulin in hepatocytes

Bridge to Pathology
In ischemic episodes, such as those in myocardial infarction, the lack of oxygen forces cells to rely on anaerobic glycolysis, which increases production of lactic acid. The consequent intracellular acidosis can cause proteins to denature and precipitate, leading to coagulation necrosis.

2. **Phosphofructokinases** (PFK-1 and PFK-2): PFK-1 is the rate-limiting enzyme and main control point in glycolysis. In this reaction, fructose 6-phosphate is phosphorylated to fructose 1,6-bisphosphate using ATP.

   - PFK-1 is inhibited by ATP and citrate, and activated by AMP.
   - Insulin stimulates and glucagon inhibits PFK-1 in hepatocytes by an indirect mechanism involving PFK-2 and fructose 2,6-bisphosphate (Figure I-12-3).

Insulin activates PFK-2 (via the tyrosine kinase receptor and activation of protein phosphatases), which converts a tiny amount of fructose 6-phosphate to fructose 2,6-bisphosphate (F2,6-BP). F2,6-BP activates PFK-1. Glucagon inhibits PFK-2 (via cAMP-dependent protein kinase A), lowering F2,6-BP and thereby inhibiting PFK-1. PFK-1 is a multi-subunit enzyme that demonstrates cooperative kinetics (discussed in Chapter 8).

Section I • Biochemistry

Note

C-peptide is a short polypeptide that connects the A-chain to the B-chain in the proinsulin molecule. It is removed after proinsulin is packaged into vesicles in the Golgi apparatus.

> ### Glucose Sensing in β-Islet Cells
>
> Similar to hepatocytes of the liver, β-islet cells of the pancreas have GLUT 2 on the plasma membrane to transport glucose into the cells, as well as glucokinase to trap the incoming glucose as glucose 6-phosphate. Because both GLUT 2 and glucokinase have high Km values for glucose, glucose is transported and phosphorylated via first-order kinetics (directly proportional to glucose concentration in the bloodstream).
>
> A 1-day-old female infant delivered at 34 weeks' gestation due to intrauterine growth retardation developed progressive respiratory failure that required intermittent mechanical ventilation. Her blood glucose was 13.4 mM and increased to 24.6 mM. Insulin was administered to normalize her glucose. No C-peptide was detectable. Her parents were second cousins. Both had symptoms of mild diabetes controlled by diet alone. Genetic studies revealed a missense mutation (Ala378Val) in the glucokinase gene. The parents were heterozygous, and the infant homozygous, for the mutation. Recombinant mutant glucokinase showed only 0.02% of the wild-type activity.
>
> Near-complete deficiency of glucokinase activity is associated with permanent neonatal type 1 diabetes. Glucokinase deficiency is the problem in this infant. In contrast to the case above, some mutations in the glucokinase gene alter the Km for glucose. Those mutations which decrease the Km (increasing the affinity for glucose) result in hyperinsulinemia and hypoglycemia. Conversely, mutations which increase the Km (decreasing the affinity for glucose) are associated with some cases of maturity-onset diabetes of the young (MODY).

3. **Glyceraldehyde 3-phosphate dehydrogenase**: catalyzes an oxidation and addition of inorganic phosphate (P_i) to its substrate. This results in the production of a high-energy intermediate 1,3-bisphosphoglycerate and the reduction of NAD to NADH. If glycolysis is aerobic, the NADH can be reoxidized (indirectly) by the mitochondrial electron transport chain, providing energy for ATP synthesis by oxidative phosphorylation.

4. **3-Phosphoglycerate kinase**: transfers the high-energy phosphate from 1,3-bisphosphoglycerate to ADP, forming ATP and 3-phosphoglycerate. This type of reaction in which ADP is directly phosphorylated to ATP using a high-energy intermediate is referred to as a substrate-level phosphorylation. In contrast to oxidative phosphorylation in mitochondria, substrate-level phosphorylations are not dependent on oxygen, and are the only means of ATP generation in an anaerobic tissue.

Note

Pyruvate kinase is inactivated by phosphorylation mediated by glucagon.

5. **Pyruvate kinase**: the last enzyme in aerobic glycolysis, it catalyzes a substrate-level phosphorylation of ADP using the high-energy substrate phosphoenolpyruvate (PEP). Pyruvate kinase is activated by fructose 1,6-bisphosphate from the PFK-1 reaction (feed-forward activation).

6. **Lactate dehydrogenase**: is used only in anaerobic glycolysis. It reoxidizes NADH to NAD, replenishing the oxidized coenzyme for glyceraldehyde 3-phosphate dehydrogenase. Without mitochondria and oxygen, glycolysis would stop when all the available NAD had been reduced to NADH. By reducing pyruvate to lactate and oxidizing NADH to NAD, lactate dehydrogenase

prevents this potential problem from developing. In aerobic tissues, lactate does not normally form in significant amounts. However, when oxygenation is poor (skeletal muscle during strenuous exercise, myocardial infarction), most cellular ATP is generated by anaerobic glycolysis, and lactate production increases.

Important Intermediates of Glycolysis

- Dihydroxyacetone phosphate (DHAP) is used in liver and adipose tissue for triglyceride synthesis.
- 1,3-Bisphosphoglycerate and phosphoenolpyruvate (PEP) are high-energy intermediates used to generate ATP by substrate-level phosphorylation.

Glycolysis Is Irreversible

Three enzymes in the pathway catalyze reactions that are irreversible. When the liver produces glucose, different reactions and therefore different enzymes must be used at these three points:

- Glucokinase/hexokinase
- PFK-1
- Pyruvate kinase

ATP Production and Electron Shuttles

Anaerobic glycolysis yields 2 ATP/glucose by substrate-level phosphorylation. Aerobic glycolysis yields these 2 ATP/glucose plus 2 NADH/glucose that can be utilized for ATP production in the mitochondria; however, the inner membrane is impermeable to NADH. Cytoplasmic NADH is reoxidized to NAD and delivers its electrons to one of two electron shuttles in the inner membrane. In the malate shuttle, electrons are passed to mitochondrial NADH and then to the electron transport chain. In the glycerol phosphate shuttle, electrons are passed to mitochondrial $FADH_2$. The two shuttles are diagrammed in Figure I-12-3; important points include:

- Cytoplasmic NADH oxidized using the malate shuttle produces a mitochondrial NADH and yields approximately 3 ATP by oxidative phosphorylation.
- Cytoplasmic NADH oxidized by the glycerol phosphate shuttle produces a mitochondrial $FADH_2$ and yields approximately 2 ATP by oxidative phosphorylation.

Glycolysis in the Erythrocyte

In red blood cells, anaerobic glycolysis represents the only pathway for ATP production, yielding a net 2 ATP/glucose.

Bridge to Physiology

Adaptation to high altitudes (low PO_2) involves:

- Increased respiration
- Respiratory alkalosis
- Lower P_{50} for hemoglobin (initial)
- Increased rate of glycolysis
- Increased [2,3-BPG] in RBC (12–24 hours)
- Normal P_{50} for hemoglobin restored by the increased level of 2,3-BPG
- Increased hemoglobin and hematocrit (days–weeks)

Clinical Correlate

Transfused blood has lower than the expected 2,3-BPG levels, making it less efficient at delivering oxygen to peripheral tissues.

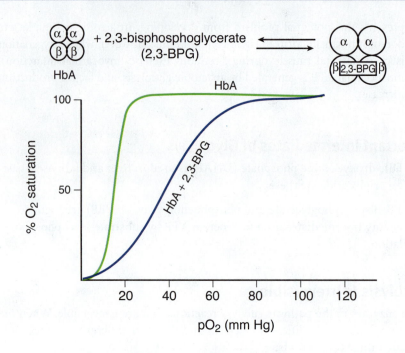

Figure I-12-4. Effect of 2,3-Bisphosphoglycerate on Hemoglobin A

Erythrocytes have bisphosphoglycerate mutase, which produces 2,3-bisphosphoglycerate (BPG) from 1,3-BPG in glycolysis. 2,3-BPG binds to the β-chains of hemoglobin A (HbA) and decreases its affinity for oxygen. This effect of 2,3-BPG is seen in the oxygen dissociation curve for HbA, shown in Figure I-12-4. The rightward shift in the curve is sufficient to allow unloading of oxygen in tissues, but still allows 100% saturation in the lungs. An abnormal increase in erythrocyte 2,3-BPG might shift the curve far enough so HbA is not fully saturated in the lungs.

Although 2,3-BPG binds to HbA, it does not bind well to HbF ($\alpha_2\gamma_2$), with the result that HbF has a higher affinity for oxygen than maternal HbA, allowing transplacental passage of oxygen from mother to fetus.

Pyruvate kinase deficiency

Pyruvate kinase deficiency is the second most common genetic deficiency that causes a hemolytic anemia (glucose 6-phosphate dehydrogenase, G6PDH, is the most common). Characteristics include:

- Chronic hemolysis
- Increased 2,3-BPG and therefore a lower-than-normal oxygen affinity of HbA
- Absence of Heinz bodies (Heinz bodies are more characteristic of G6PDH deficiency)

The red blood cell has no mitochondria and is totally dependent on anaerobic glycolysis for ATP. In pyruvate kinase deficiency, the decrease in ATP causes the erythrocyte to lose its characteristic biconcave shape and signals its destruction in the spleen. In addition, decreased ion pumping by Na^+/K^+-ATPase results in loss of ion balance and causes osmotic fragility, leading to swelling and lysis.

GALACTOSE METABOLISM

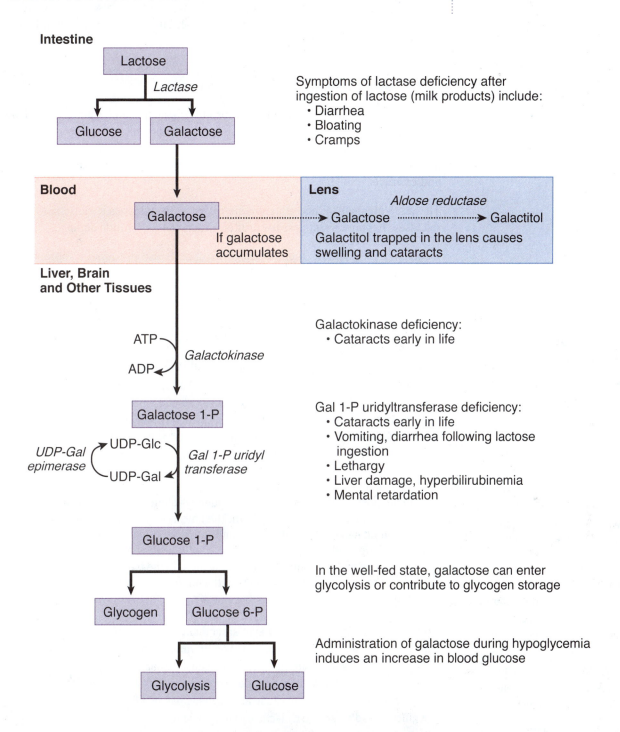

Figure I-12-5. Galactose Metabolism

An important source of galactose in the diet is the disaccharide lactose present in milk. Lactose is hydrolyzed to galactose and glucose by lactase associated with the brush border membrane of the small intestine. Along with other monosaccharides, galactose reaches the liver through the portal blood.

Section I • Biochemistry

Once transported into tissues, galactose is phosphorylated (galactokinase), trapping it in the cell. Galactose 1-phosphate is converted to glucose 1-phosphate by galactose 1-P uridyltransferase and an epimerase. The pathway is shown in Figure I-12-5; important enzymes to remember are:

- Galactokinase
- Galactose 1-phosphate uridyltransferase

Genetic deficiencies of these enzymes produce galactosemia. Cataracts, a characteristic finding in patients with galactosemia, result from conversion of the excess galactose in peripheral blood to galactitol in the lens of the eye, which has aldose reductase. Accumulation of galactitol in the lens causes osmotic damage and cataracts.

The same mechanism accounts for the cataracts in diabetics because aldose reductase also converts glucose to sorbitol, which causes osmotic damage.

Deficiency of galactose 1-phosphate uridyltransferase produces a more severe disease because, in addition to galactosemia, galactose 1-P accumulates in the liver, brain, and other tissues.

Clinical Correlate
Lactose Intolerance

Primary lactose intolerance is caused by a hereditary deficiency of lactase, most commonly found in persons of Asian and African descent. Secondary lactose intolerance can be precipitated at any age by gastrointestinal disturbances such as celiac sprue, colitis, or viral-induced damage to intestinal mucosa, which is why kids with diarrhea should drink clear liquids, and not milk.

Common symptoms of lactose intolerance include vomiting, bloating, explosive and watery diarrhea, cramps, and dehydration. The symptoms can be attributed to bacterial fermentation of lactose to a mixture of CH_4, H_2, and small organic acids. The acids are osmotically active and result in the movement of water into the intestinal lumen.

Diagnosis is based on a positive hydrogen breath test after an oral lactose load. Treatment is by dietary restriction of milk and milk products (except unpasteurized yogurt, which contains active *Lactobacillus*) or by lactase pills.

Galactosemia

Galactosemia is an autosomal recessive trait that results from a defective gene encoding either galactokinase or galactose 1-P uridyltransferase. There are over 100 heritable mutations that can cause galactosemia, and the incidence is approximately 1 in 60,000 births. Galactose will be present in elevated amounts in the blood and urine and can result in decreased glucose synthesis and hypoglycemia.

The parents of a 2-week-old infant who was being breast-fed returned to the hospital because the infant frequently vomited, had a persistent fever, and looked yellow since birth. The physician quickly observed that the infant had early hepatomegaly and cataracts. Blood and urine tests were performed, and it was determined that the infant had elevated sugar (galactose and, to a smaller extent, galactitol) in the blood and urine. The doctor told the parents to bottle-feed the infant with lactose-free formula supplemented with sucrose. Subsequently, the infant improved.

Galactosemia symptoms often begin around day 3 in a newborn and include the hallmark cataracts. Jaundice and hyperbilirubinemia do not resolve if the infant is treated with phototherapy. In the galactosemic infant, the liver, which is the site of bilirubin conjugation, develops cirrhosis. Vomiting and diarrhea occur after milk ingestion because although lactose in milk is hydrolyzed to glucose and galactose by lactase in the intestine, the galactose is not properly metabolized. Severe bacterial infections (*E. coli* sepsis) are common in untreated galactosemic infants. Failure to thrive, lethargy, hypotonia, and mental retardation are other common and apparent features. Many U.S. states have mandatory screening of newborns for galactosemia. If an infant is correctly diagnosed within the first several weeks of life through a newborn screening heel prick test, formulas containing galactose-free carbohydrates are given. The life expectancy will then be normal with an appropriate diet.

Chapter 12 • Glycolysis and Pyruvate Dehydrogenase

FRUCTOSE METABOLISM

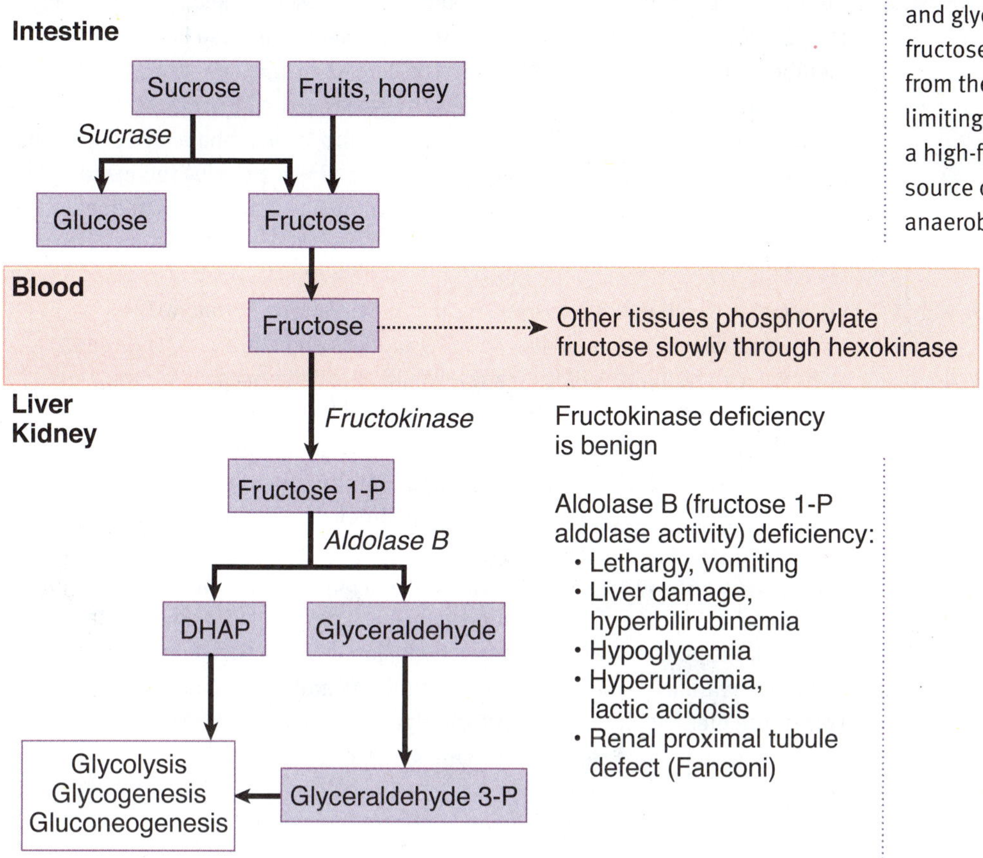

Figure I-12-6. Fructose Metabolism

Pathway summary:
- Intestine: Sucrose → (Sucrase) → Glucose + Fructose; Fruits, honey → Fructose
- Blood: Fructose → Other tissues phosphorylate fructose slowly through hexokinase
- Liver/Kidney: Fructose → (Fructokinase) → Fructose 1-P → (Aldolase B) → DHAP + Glyceraldehyde → Glyceraldehyde 3-P → Glycolysis, Glycogenesis, Gluconeogenesis

Fructokinase deficiency is benign

Aldolase B (fructose 1-P aldolase activity) deficiency:
- Lethargy, vomiting
- Liver damage, hyperbilirubinemia
- Hypoglycemia
- Hyperuricemia, lactic acidosis
- Renal proximal tubule defect (Fanconi)

Note
Because dihydroxyacetone phosphate and glyceraldehyde, the products of fructose metabolism, are downstream from the key regulatory and rate-limiting enzyme of glycolysis (PFK-1), a high-fructose drink supplies a quick source of energy in both aerobic and anaerobic cells.

Fructose is found in honey and fruit and as part of the disaccharide sucrose (common table sugar). Sucrose is hydrolyzed by intestinal brush border sucrase, and the resulting monosaccharides, glucose and fructose, are absorbed into the portal blood. The liver phosphorylates fructose and cleaves it into glyceraldehyde and DHAP. Smaller amounts are metabolized in renal proximal tubules. The pathway is shown in Figure I-12-6; important enzymes to remember are:

- Fructokinase
- Fructose 1-P aldolase (aldolase B)

Genetic deficiency of fructokinase is benign and often detected incidentally when the urine is checked for glucose with a dipstick. Fructose 1-phosphate aldolase deficiency is a severe disease because of accumulation of fructose 1-phosphate in the liver and renal proximal tubules. Symptoms are reversed after removing fructose and sucrose from the diet.

Cataracts are not a feature of this disease because fructose is not an aldose sugar and therefore not a substrate for aldose reductase in the lens.

Section I • Biochemistry

> ### Hereditary Fructose Intolerance
>
> Hereditary fructose intolerance is an autosomal recessive disease (incidence of 1/20,000) due to a defect in the gene that encodes aldolase B in fructose metabolism. In the absence of the enzyme, fructose challenge results in an accumulation of fructose 1-phosphate in hepatocytes and thereby sequestering of inorganic phosphate in this substance. The drop in phosphate levels prevents its use in other pathways, such as glycogen breakdown and gluconeogenesis. Eventually, the liver becomes damaged due to the accumulation of trapped fructose 1-phosphate.
>
> A 4-month-old infant was breast-fed and developing normally. The mother decided to begin the weaning process and started to feed the baby with fruit juices. Within a few weeks, the child became lethargic and yellow-skinned, vomited frequently, and had frequent diarrhea. The mother thought that the child might have had a food allergy and took the child to a clinic for testing. It found that the child had sugar in the urine but did not react with the glucose dipsticks.
>
> If diagnosed early to alleviate complications, a person with fructose intolerance on a diet that excludes fructose and sucrose will develop normally and have a normal lifespan. However, complete exclusion of these sugars is difficult, especially with their widespread use as nutrients and sweeteners. Failure to correct the diet and prolonged fructose ingestion could eventually lead to proximal renal disorder resembling Fanconi syndrome.

PYRUVATE DEHYDROGENASE

Pyruvate from aerobic glycolysis enters mitochondria, where it may be converted to acetyl-CoA for entry into the citric acid cycle if ATP is needed, or for fatty acid synthesis if sufficient ATP is present. The pyruvate dehydrogenase (PDH) reaction (Figure I-12-7) is irreversible and cannot be used to convert acetyl-CoA to pyruvate or to glucose. Pyruvate dehydrogenase in the liver is activated by insulin, whereas in the brain and nerves the enzyme (actually a complex of 5 different enzymatic activities) is not responsive to hormones.

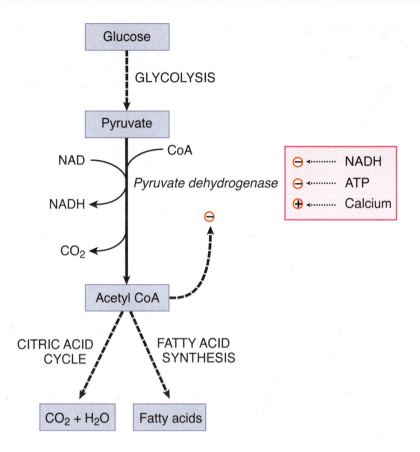

Figure I-12-7. Pyruvate Dehydrogenase

Cofactors and coenzymes used by pyruvate dehydrogenase include:
- Thiamine pyrophosphate (TPP) from the vitamin thiamine
- Lipoic acid
- Coenzyme A (CoA) from pantothenate
- $FAD(H_2)$ from riboflavin
- $NAD(H)$ from niacin (some may be synthesized from tryptophan)

Pyruvate dehydrogenase is inhibited by its product acetyl-CoA. This control is important in several contexts and should be considered along with pyruvate carboxylase, the other mitochondrial enzyme that uses pyruvate (introduced in gluconeogenesis, Chapter 14, Figure I-14-5).

Thiamine Deficiency

Thiamine deficiency is commonly seen in alcoholics, who may develop a complex of symptoms associated with Wernicke peripheral neuropathy and Korsakoff psychosis. Alcohol interferes with thiamine absorption from the intestine. Symptoms include:

- Ataxia
- Ophthalmoplegia, nystagmus
- Memory loss and confabulation
- Cerebral hemorrhage

Congestive heart failure may be a complication (wet beri-beri) owing to inadequate ATP and accumulation of ketoacids in the cardiac muscle.

Two other enzyme complexes similar to pyruvate dehydrogenase that use thiamine are:

- α-Ketoglutarate dehydrogenase (citric acid cycle)
- Branched-chain ketoacid dehydrogenase (metabolism of branched-chain amino acids)

Insufficient thiamine significantly impairs glucose oxidation, causing highly aerobic tissues, such as brain and cardiac muscle, to fail first. In addition, branched-chain amino acids are sources of energy in brain and muscle.

Clinical Correlate

If thiamine deficiency is suspected, patients should be given IV thiamine in the emergency department to prevent lactic acidosis when glucose (dextrose) is administered.

Chapter Summary

Glycolysis

Glucose Transport

- GLUT 2: High K_m; liver (storage) and β-islet (glucose sensor)
- GLUT 4: Lower K_m; insulin-stimulated; adipose and muscle

Important Enzymes

- Glucokinase (induced by insulin in liver), hexokinase (peripheral tissues)
- PFK-1 (rate-limiting)
    - Inhibitors: ATP, citrate
    - Activators: AMP, fructose 2,6-bisphosphate (F2,6-bisP)
- PFK-2 responds to insulin (activated) and glucagon (inhibited).
    - Produces F2,6-bisP that activates PFK-1

Enzymes Catalyzing Irreversible Reactions

- Glucokinase/hexokinase, PFK, pyruvate kinase

Aerobic Glycolysis

- NADH reoxidized by mitochondrial electron transport chain

(Continued)

Chapter Summary (continued)

Anaerobic Glycolysis

- NADH reoxidized by cytoplasmic lactate dehydrogenase
  - Lactate released from tissue
  - RBC, skeletal muscle (short, intense burst of exercise)
  - Any cell deprived of oxygen

ATP Yield

- Anaerobic: 2 ATP/glucose (substrate level phosphorylations)

Genetic Deficiency

- Pyruvate kinase
  - Hemolytic anemia
  - Possible decrease in hemoglobin affinity for oxygen due to increased RBC 2,3-BPG
  - Heinz bodies rarely seen
  - Autosomal recessive

Important Intermediates

- Dihydroxyacetone phosphate (DHAP): forms glycerol 3-P for triglyceride synthesis.

Pyruvate Dehydrogenase (PDH)

  - Mitochondrial
  - Insulin-stimulated

Coenzymes: Thiamine, lipoic acid, CoA, FAD, NAD

Disease Association:

- Wernicke-Korsakoff
  - Most common in alcoholics
  - Thiamine deficiency
  - Neuropathy (ataxia, nystagmus, ophthalmoplegia)
  - Memory loss and confabulation
  - Psychosis
- High-output cardiac failure
  - Chronic, prolonged thiamine deficiency

Section I • Biochemistry

Review Questions

Select the ONE best answer.

1. A 10-month-old child is being evaluated for the underlying cause of a hemolytic anemia. In the diagram shown below, the oxygen dissociation curve for hemoglobin in his erythrocytes is compared with the curve obtained with normal red cells.

   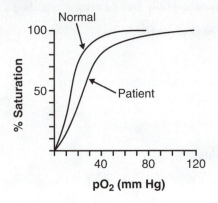

   A deficiency of which enzyme is most likely to account for the hemolytic anemia in this patient?

   A. Glucokinase
   B. Glucose 6-P dehydrogenase
   C. Pyruvate carboxylase
   D. Glutathione reductase
   E. Pyruvate kinase

2. A breast-fed infant begins to vomit frequently and lose weight. Several days later she is jaundiced, her liver is enlarged, and cataracts are noticed in her lenses. These symptoms are most likely caused by a deficiency of

   A. galactose 1-P uridyltransferase
   B. lactase
   C. glucose-6-phosphatase
   D. galactokinase
   E. aldolase B

3. Following an early-morning run, a 29-year-old man consumes an all-American breakfast consisting of cereal, eggs, bacon, sausage, pancakes with maple syrup, doughnuts, and coffee with cream and sugar. Which of the following proteins will most likely be activated in his liver after breakfast?

   A. Cytoplasmic PEP carboxykinase
   B. Plasma membrane GLUT-4 transporter
   C. Cytoplasmic phosphofructokinase-2
   D. Mitochondrial carnitine transporter
   E. Cytoplasmic glycogen phosphorylase

Chapter 12 • Glycolysis and Pyruvate Dehydrogenase

Items 4 and 5

A 55-year-old alcoholic was brought to the emergency department by his friends. During their usual nightly gathering at the local bar, he had passed out and they had been unable to revive him. The physician ordered an injection of thiamine followed by overnight parenteral glucose. The next morning the patient was alert and coherent, serum thiamine was normal, and blood glucose was 73 mg/dL (4 mM). The IV line was removed, and he was taken home.

4. Which of the following enzymes is thiamine-dependent and essential for glucose oxidation in the brain?

   A. Transketolase
   B. Transaldolase
   C. Succinyl-CoA thiokinase
   D. Acetyl-CoA carboxylase
   E. Pyruvate dehydrogenase

5. At the time of discharge from the hospital, which of the following proteins would have no significant physiologic activity in this patient?

   A. Malate dehydrogenase
   B. Glucokinase
   C. α-Ketoglutarate dehydrogenase
   D. GLUT 1 transporter
   E. Phosphofructokinase-1

Answers

1. **Answer: E.** A right-shift in the O_2 binding curve is indicative of abnormally elevated 2,3-BPG secondary to a defect in red cell anaerobic glycolysis. Only pyruvate kinase participates in this pathway.

2. **Answer: A.** Cataracts + liver disease in a milk-fed infant = classic galactosemia.

3. **Answer: C.** Only PFK-2 will be insulin-activated in the postprandial period.

4. **Answer: E.** Most important TPP-dependent enzymes include pyruvate dehydrogenase, α-ketoglutarate dehydrogenase, and transketolase. Transketolase is in the HMP shunt and is not strictly essential for glucose oxidation.

5. **Answer: B.** After an overnight fast (plasma glucose 73 mg/dL), the liver is producing glucose and glucokinase activity would be insignificant (high K_m, low insulin). The other proteins would be needed for aerobic glucose oxidation in the brain or for hepatic gluconeogenesis.

Citric Acid Cycle and Oxidative Phosphorylation 13

Learning Objectives

❏ Solve problems concerning citric acid cycle

❏ Explain information related to electron transport chain

❏ Use knowledge of and oxidative phosphorylation

CITRIC ACID CYCLE

The citric acid cycle, also called the Krebs cycle or the tricarboxylic acid (TCA) cycle, is in the mitochondria. Although oxygen is not directly required in the cycle, the pathway will not occur anaerobically because NADH and $FADH_2$ will accumulate if oxygen is not available for the electron transport chain.

The primary function of the citric acid cycle is oxidation of acetyl-CoA to carbon dioxide. The energy released from this oxidation is saved as NADH, $FADH_2$, and guanosine triphosphate (GTP). The overall result of the cycle is represented by the following reaction:

Acetyl-CoA $\longrightarrow$ 2 CO_2
3 NAD + FAD + GDP + P_i 3 NADH + $FADH_2$ + GTP

Notice that none of the intermediates of the citric acid cycle appear in this reaction, not as reactants or as products. This emphasizes an important (and frequently misunderstood) point about the cycle. It does not represent a pathway for the net conversion of acetyl-CoA to citrate, to malate, or to any other intermediate of the cycle. The only fate of acetyl-CoA in this pathway is its oxidation to CO_2. Therefore, the citric acid cycle does not represent a pathway by which there can be net synthesis of glucose from acetyl-CoA.

The cycle is central to the oxidation of any fuel that yields acetyl-CoA, including glucose, fatty acids, ketone bodies, ketogenic amino acids, and alcohol. There is no hormonal control of the cycle, as activity is necessary irrespective of the fed or fasting state. Control is exerted by the energy status of the cell through allosteric activation or deactivation. Many enzymes are subject to negative feedback.

The citric acid cycle is shown in Figure I-13-1. All the enzymes are in the matrix of the mitochondria except succinate dehydrogenase, which is in the inner membrane.

Section I • Biochemistry

Key points:

1. Isocitrate dehydrogenase, the major control enzyme, is inhibited by NADH and ATP and activated by ADP.

2. α-Ketoglutarate dehydrogenase, like pyruvate dehydrogenase, is a multienzyme complex. It requires thiamine, lipoic acid, CoA, FAD, and NAD. Lack of thiamine slows oxidation of acetyl-CoA in the citric acid cycle.

3. Succinyl-CoA synthetase (succinate thiokinase) catalyzes a substrate-level phosphorylation of GDP to GTP.

4. Succinate dehydrogenase is on the inner mitochondrial membrane, where it also functions as complex II of the electron transport chain.

5. Citrate synthase condenses the incoming acetyl group with oxaloacetate to form citrate.

Note

GTP is energetically equivalent to ATP:

GTP + ADP <----> GDP + ATP

catalyzed by nucleoside diphosphate kinase

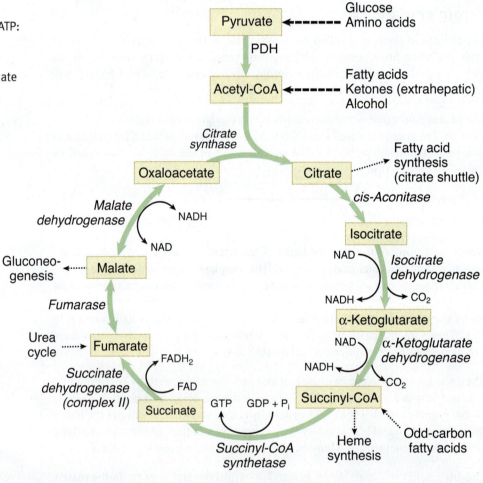

Figure I-13-1. Citric Acid Cycle

Several intermediates of the cycle may serve other functions:
- Citrate may leave the mitochondria (citrate shuttle) to deliver acetyl-CoA into the cytoplasm for fatty acid synthesis.
- Succinyl-CoA is a high-energy intermediate that can be used for heme synthesis and to activate ketone bodies in extrahepatic tissues.
- Malate can leave the mitochondria (malate shuttle) for gluconeogenesis.

When intermediates are drawn out of the citric acid cycle, the cycle slows. Therefore when intermediates leave the cycle they must be replaced to ensure sufficient energy for the cell.

ELECTRON TRANSPORT CHAIN AND OXIDATIVE PHOSPHORYLATION

The mitochondrial electron transport chain (ETC) carries out the following two reactions:

$$NADH + O_2 \longrightarrow NAD + H_2O \quad \Delta G = -56 \text{ kcal/mol}$$
$$FADH_2 + O_2 \longrightarrow FAD + H_2O \quad \Delta G = -42 \text{ kcal/mol}$$

Although the value of ΔG should not be memorized, it does indicate the large amount of energy released by both reactions. The electron transport chain is a device to capture this energy in a form useful for doing work.

Sources of NADH, FADH$_2$, and O$_2$

Many enzymes in the mitochondria, including those of the citric acid cycle and pyruvate dehydrogenase, produce NADH, all of which can be oxidized in the electron transport chain and in the process, capture energy for ATP synthesis by oxidative phosphorylation. If NADH is produced in the cytoplasm, either the malate shuttle or the α-glycerol phosphate shuttle can transfer the electrons into the mitochondria for delivery to the ETC. Once NADH has been oxidized, the NAD can again be used by enzymes that require it.

FADH$_2$ is produced by succinate dehydrogenase in the citric acid cycle and by the α-glycerol phosphate shuttle. Both enzymes are located in the inner membrane and can reoxidize FADH$_2$ directly by transferring electrons into the ETC. Once FADH$_2$ has been oxidized, the FAD can be made available once again for use by the enzyme.

O$_2$ is delivered to tissues by hemoglobin. The majority of oxygen required in a tissue is consumed in the ETC. Its function is to accept electrons at the end of the chain, and the water formed is added to the cellular water. This scheme is shown in Figure I-13-2.

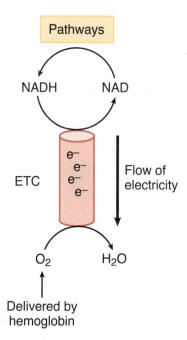

Figure I-13-2. Overview of the Electron Transport Chain

Section I • Biochemistry

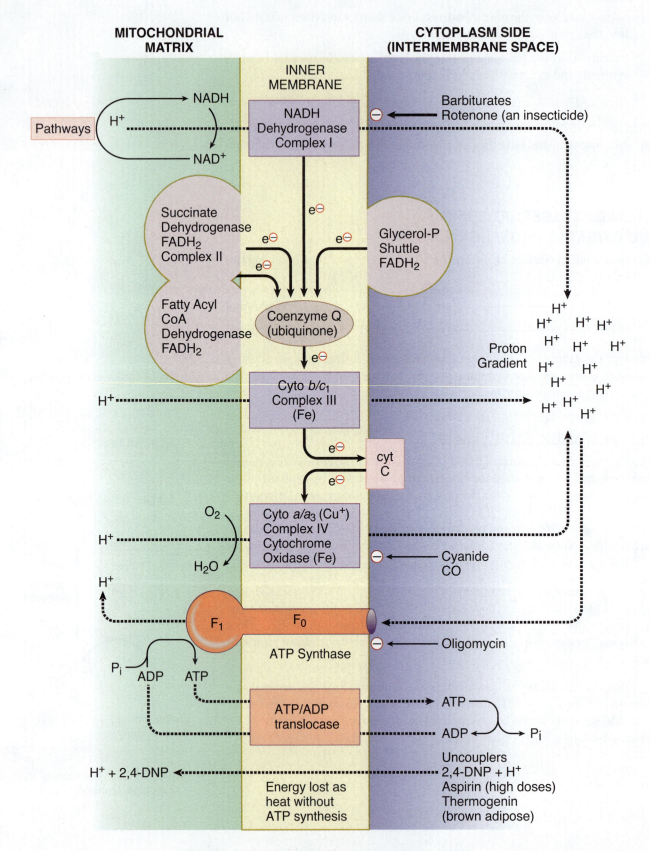

Figure I-13-3. Oxidative Phosphorylation

Capturing Chemical Energy as Electricity

The mitochondrial electron transport chain works like a chemical battery. In one location, an oxidation reaction is poised to release electrons at very high energy; in another location, a potential electron acceptor waits to be reduced. Because the 2 components are physically separated, nothing happens. Once the 2 terminals of the battery are connected by a wire, electrons flow from one compartment to the other through the wire, producing an electrical current or electricity. A light bulb or an electrical pump inserted into the circuit will run on the electricity generated. If no electrical device is in the circuit, all the energy is released as heat. The mitochondrial electron transport chain operates according to the same principle.

Electron Transport Chain

NADH is oxidized by NADH dehydrogenase (complex I), delivering its electrons into the chain and returning as NAD to enzymes that require it. The electrons are passed along a series of protein and lipid carriers that serve as the wire. These include, in order:

- NADH dehydrogenase (complex I) accepts electrons from NADH
- Coenzyme Q (a lipid)
- Cytochrome b/c_1 (an Fe/heme protein; complex III)
- Cytochrome c (an Fe/heme protein)
- Cytochrome a/a_3 (a Cu/heme protein; cytochrome oxidase, complex IV) transfers electrons to oxygen

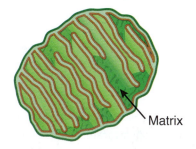

Figure I-13-4. Mitochondrion

All these components are in the inner membrane of the mitochondria as shown in Figure I-13-3. Succinate dehydrogenase and the α-glycerol phosphate shuttle enzymes reoxidize their $FADH_2$ and pass electrons directly to CoQ.

Proton Gradient

The electricity generated by the ETC is used to run proton pumps (translocators), which drive protons from the matrix space across the inner membrane into the intermembrane space, creating a small proton (or pH) gradient. This is similar to pumping any ion, such as Na^+, across a membrane to create a gradient. The three major complexes I, III, and IV (NADH dehydrogenase, cytochrome b/c_1, and cytochrome a/a_3) each translocate protons in this way as the electricity passes through them. The end result is that a proton gradient is normally maintained across the mitochondrial inner membrane. If proton channels open, the protons run back into the matrix. Such proton channels are part of the oxidative phosphorylation complex.

Oxidative Phosphorylation

ATP synthesis by oxidative phosphorylation uses the energy of the proton gradient and is carried out by the F_0F_1 ATP synthase complex, which spans the inner membrane as shown in Figure I-13-3. As protons flow into the mitochondria through the F_0 component, their energy is used by the F_1 component (ATP synthase) to phosphorylate ADP using P_i. On average, when an NADH is oxidized in the ETC, sufficient energy is contributed to the proton gradient for the phosphorylation of 3 ATP by F_0F_1 ATP synthase. $FADH_2$ oxidation provides enough energy for approximately 2 ATP. These figures are referred to as the P/O ratios.

Bridge to Pathology
A genetic defect in oxidative phosphorylation is one cause of Leigh syndrome, a rare neurological disorder.

Section I • Biochemistry

> **Bridge to Pathology**
> **Ischemic Chest Pain**
>
> Patients with chest pain whose symptoms are suggestive of acute myocardial infarction (AMI) are evaluated by electrocardiogram (EKG) and by serial measurements of cardiac enzymes. Although myocardial specific CK-MB has been used as an early indicator of an AMI, measurements of troponin levels are rapidly replacing it.
>
> Troponin I and troponin T are sensitive and specific markers that appear 3 to 6 hours after the onset of symptoms, peak by 16 hours, and remain elevated for nearly a week. In the absence of ST-segment elevation on the EKG, elevated troponin I and troponin T are useful indicators of those patients at high risk for evolving myocardial infarction. LDH isozyme analysis may be helpful if a patient reports chest pain that occurred several days previously because this change ($LDH_1 > LDH_2$) peaks 2 to 3 days following an AMI.

Tissue Hypoxia

Hypoxia deprives the ETC of sufficient oxygen, decreasing the rate of ETC and ATP production. When ATP levels fall, glycolysis increases and, in the absence of oxygen, will produce lactate (lactic acidosis). Anaerobic glycolysis is not able to meet the demand of most tissues for ATP, especially in highly aerobic tissues like nerves and cardiac muscle.

In a myocardial infarction (MI), myocytes swell as the membrane potential collapses and the cell gets leaky. Enzymes are released from the damaged tissue, and lactic acidosis contributes to protein precipitation and coagulation necrosis.

Inhibitors

The ETC is coupled to oxidative phosphorylation so that their activities rise and fall together. Inhibitors of any step effectively inhibit the whole coupled process, resulting in:

- Decreased oxygen consumption
- Increased intracellular NADH/NAD and $FADH_2$/FAD ratios
- Decreased ATP

Important inhibitors include cyanide and carbon monoxide.

Cyanide

Cyanide is a deadly poison because it binds irreversibly to cytochrome a/a_3, preventing electron transfer to oxygen, and producing many of the same changes seen in tissue hypoxia. Sources of cyanide include:

- Burning polyurethane (foam stuffing in furniture and mattresses)
- Byproduct of nitroprusside (released slowly; thiosulfate can be used to destroy the cyanide)

Nitrites may be used as an antidote for cyanide poisoning if given rapidly. They convert hemoglobin to methemoglobin, which binds cyanide in the blood before reaching the tissues. Oxygen is also given, if possible.

Carbon monoxide

Carbon monoxide binds to cytochrome a/a_3 but less tightly than cyanide. It also binds to hemoglobin, displacing oxygen. Symptoms include headache, nausea, tachycardia, and tachypnea. Lips and cheeks turn a cherry-red color. Respiratory depression and coma result in death if not treated by giving oxygen. Sources of carbon monoxide include:

- Propane heaters and gas grills
- Vehicle exhaust
- Tobacco smoke
- House fires
- Methylene chloride–based paint strippers

Other inhibitors include antimycin (cytochrome b/c_1), doxorubicin (CoQ), and oligomycin (F_0).

Uncouplers

Uncouplers are chemicals that decrease the proton gradient, causing:

- Decreased ATP synthesis
- Increased oxygen consumption
- Increased oxidation of NADH

Because the rate of the ETC increases, with no ATP synthesis, energy is released as heat. Important uncouplers include 2,4-dinitrophenol (2,4-DNP) and aspirin (and other salicylates). Brown adipose tissue contains a natural uncoupling protein (UCP, formerly called thermogenin), which allows energy loss as heat to maintain a basal temperature around the kidneys, neck, breastplate, and scapulae in newborns.

Reactive Oxygen Species

When molecular oxygen (O_2) is partially reduced, unstable products called reactive oxygen species (ROS) are formed. These react rapidly with lipids to cause peroxidation, with proteins, and with other substrates, resulting in denaturation and precipitation in tissues. Reactive oxygen species include:

- Superoxide ($O_2^{\cdot-}$)
- Hydrogen peroxide (H_2O_2)
- Hydroxyl radical ($OH^\cdot$)

The polymorphonuclear neutrophil produces these substances to kill bacteria in the protective space of the phagolysosome during the oxidative burst accompanying phagocytosis. Production of these same ROS can occur at a slower rate wherever there is oxygen in high concentration. Small quantities of ROS are inevitable by-products of the electron transport chain in mitochondria. These small quantities are normally destroyed by protective enzymes such as catalase. The rate of ROS production can increase dramatically under certain conditions, such as reperfusion injury in a tissue that has been temporarily deprived of oxygen. ATP levels will be low and NADH levels high in a tissue deprived of oxygen (as in an MI). When oxygen is suddenly introduced, there is a burst of activity in the ETC, generating incompletely reduced ROS.

Defenses against ROS accumulation are particularly important in highly aerobic tissues and include superoxide dismutase and catalase. In the special case of erythrocytes, large amounts of superoxide are generated by the spontaneous dissociation of the oxygen from hemoglobin (occurrence is 0.5–3% of the total hemoglobin per day). The products are methemoglobin and superoxide. The processes that adequately detoxify the superoxide require a variety of enzymes and compounds, including superoxide dismutase, catalase, as well as glutathione peroxidase, vitamin E in membranes, and vitamin C in the cytoplasm. Low levels of any of these detoxifying substances result in hemolysis. For example, inadequate production of NADPH in glucose 6-phosphate dehydrogenase deficiency results in accumulation of the destructive hydrogen peroxide (Chapter 14).

Bridge to Pharmacology

Aspirin in doses used to treat rheumatoid arthritis can result in uncoupling of oxidative phosphorylation, increased oxygen consumption, depletion of hepatic glycogen, and the pyretic effect of toxic doses of salicylate. Depending on the degree of salicylate intoxication, the symptoms can vary from tinnitus to pronounced CNS and acid-base disturbance.

Section I • Biochemistry

Bridge to Medical Genetics
Mitochondrial Diseases

- Leber hereditary optic neuropathy
- MELAS: mitochondrial encephalomyopathy, lactic acidosis, and stroke-like episodes
- Myoclonic epilepsy with ragged red muscle fibers

Mutations in Mitochondrial DNA

The circular mitochondrial chromosome encodes 13 of the more than 80 proteins that comprise the major complexes of oxidative phosphorylation as well as 22 tRNAs and 2 rRNAs. Mutations in these genes affect highly aerobic tissues (nerves, muscle), and the diseases exhibit characteristic mitochondrial pedigrees (maternal inheritance). Key characteristics of most mitochondrial DNA (mtDNA) diseases are lactic acidosis and massive proliferation of mitochondria in muscle, resulting in ragged red fibers. Examples of mtDNA diseases are:

- Mitochondrial encephalomyopathy, lactic acidosis, and stroke-like episodes (MELAS)
- Leber hereditary optic neuropathy
- Ragged red muscle fiber disease

Coordinate Regulation of the Citric Acid Cycle and Oxidative Phosphorylation

The rates of oxidative phosphorylation and the citric acid cycle are closely coordinated, and are dependent mainly on the availability of O_2 and ADP. If O_2 is limited, the rate of oxidative phosphorylation decreases, and the concentrations of NADH and $FADH_2$ increase. The accumulation of NADH, in turn, inhibits the citric acid cycle. The coordinated regulation of these pathways is known as "respiratory control."

In the presence of adequate O_2, the rate of oxidative phosphorylation is dependent on the availability of ADP. The concentrations of ADP and ATP are reciprocally related; an accumulation of ADP is accompanied by a decrease in ATP and the amount of energy available to the cell. Therefore, ADP accumulation signals the need for ATP synthesis. ADP allosterically activates isocitrate dehydrogenase, thereby increasing the rate of the citric acid cycle and the production of NADH and $FADH_2$. The elevated levels of these reduced coenzymes, in turn, increase the rate of electron transport and ATP synthesis.

Chapter Summary

Citric Acid Cycle

- Mitochondria

Function

- Acetyl (CoA) is completely oxidized to carbon dioxide.
  - Energy saved as $FADH_2$, NADH, GTP
  - Cycle functions catalytically; no net synthesis of intermediates from acetyl-CoA

Controlled Step

- Isocitrate dehydrogenase inhibited by NADH (causing the citric acid cycle to stop when the ETC stops in the anaerobic cell).

(Continued)

Chapter Summary (continued)

Other Important Enzymes

- α-Ketoglutarate dehydrogenase (thiamine, lipoic acid, CoA, FAD, NAD)

Links Between Cycle Intermediates and Other Pathways

- Citrate carries acetyl-CoA into cytoplasm for fatty acid synthesis.
- Succinyl-CoA used for heme synthesis
- OAA from pyruvate in gluconeogenesis
- Gluconeogenesis from several amino acids uses the malate shuttle.

Electron Transport and Oxidative Phosphorylation

- Mitochondrial inner membrane (cell membrane in prokaryotes)

Function

- Oxidizes NADH and $FADH_2$
- Generates electrical energy by passing electrons through the ETC to O_2
- Creates a proton gradient across the inner membrane: $[H^+]_{in} < [H^+]_{out}$
- Proton gradient drives phosphorylation of ADP to ATP

Inhibitors

- ATP synthesis decreases, ETC decreases, O_2 consumption decreases
    - Cyanide (complex IV, cytochrome oxidase)
    - Barbiturates and rotenone (complex I, NADH dehydrogenase)
    - Oligomycin (F_0 component of F_0F_1 ATP synthase)

Uncouplers

- ATP synthesis decreases, ETC increases, O_2 consumption increases
    - Destroy the proton gradient
    - Produce heat rather than ATP
    - 2,4-DNP
    - Aspirin in high doses
    - Uncoupling proteins (thermogenin)

Important Patients

- Myocardial (or other) infarction

Genetic Deficiencies

- Mitochondrial pedigrees (neuropathies/myopathies)

Section I • Biochemistry

Review Questions

Select the ONE best answer.

1. During a myocardial infarction, the oxygen supply to an area of the heart is dramatically reduced, forcing the cardiac myocytes to switch to anaerobic metabolism. Under these conditions, which of the following enzymes would be activated by increasing intracellular AMP?

   A. Succinate dehydrogenase
   B. Phosphofructokinase-1
   C. Glucokinase
   D. Pyruvate dehydrogenase
   E. Lactate dehydrogenase

Items 2 and 3

A 40-year-old African American man is seen in the emergency room for a severe headache. His blood pressure is 180/110 mm Hg, and he has evidence of retinal hemorrhage. An infusion of nitroprusside is given.

2. Which of the following enzymes is affected most directly by the active metabolite of this drug?

   A. Phospholipase A2
   B. Cyclic AMP phosphodiesterase
   C. Guanylate cyclase
   D. Cyclic GMP phosphodiesterase
   E. Phospholipase C

3. When nitroprusside is given in higher than usual doses, it may be accompanied by the administration of thiosulfate to reduce potential toxic side effects. Which complex associated with electron transport or oxidative phosphorylation is most sensitive to the toxic byproduct that may accumulate with high doses of nitroprusside?

   A. NADH dehydrogenase
   B. Succinate dehydrogenase
   C. Cytochrome b/c_1
   D. Cytochrome a/a_3
   E. F_0F_1 ATP synthase

4. A patient has been exposed to a toxic compound that increases the permeability of mitochondrial membranes for protons. Which of the following events in liver cells would you expect to occur?

   A. Increased ATP levels
   B. Increased F_1F_0 ATP synthase activity
   C. Increased oxygen utilization
   D. Decreased malate-aspartate shuttle activity
   E. Decreased pyruvate dehydrogenase activity

Items 5 and 6

- A. Citrate shuttle
- B. Glycerolphosphate shuttle
- C. Malate-aspartate shuttle
- D. Carnitine shuttle
- E. Adenine nucleotide shuttle

5. Required for cholesterol and fatty acid synthesis in hepatocytes.

6. Required for the hepatic conversion of pyruvate to glucose.

Answers

1. **Answer: B.** Both PFK-1 and LDH participate in extrahepatic anaerobic glycolysis, but only PFK-1 is regulated by allosteric effectors.

2. **Answer: C.** Nitroprusside is metabolized to produce nitric oxide. NO, normally produced by the vascular endothelium, stimulates the cyclase in vascular smooth muscle to increase cGMP, activate protein kinase G, and cause relaxation.

3. **Answer: D.** In addition to NO, metabolism of nitroprusside also releases small quantities of cyanide, a potent and potentially lethal inhibitor of cyt a/a_3 (complex IV). Thiosulfate is a common antidote for CN poisoning.

4. **Answer: C.** The toxic agent (example, 2,4-dinitrophenol) would uncouple oxidative phosphorylation, leading to a fall in ATP levels, increased respiration, and increased substrate utilization.

5. **Answer: A.** Both fatty acids and cholesterol are synthesized from acetyl-CoA in the cytoplasm. Acetyl-CoA, which is produced in the mitochondria, is delivered to these pathways using the citrate shuttle.

6. **Answer: C.** Oxaloacetate, produced from pyruvate, exits the mitochondrion after conversion to malate.

Glycogen, Gluconeogenesis, and the Hexose Monophosphate Shunt

Learning Objectives

❏ Interpret scenarios about glycogenesis and glycogenolysis
❏ Answer questions about glycogen synthesis
❏ Demonstrate understanding of glycogenolysis
❏ Interpret scenarios about genetic deficiencies of enzymes in glycogen metabolism
❏ Solve problems concerning gluconeogenesis
❏ Use knowledge of hexose monophosphate shunt

GLYCOGENESIS AND GLYCOGENOLYSIS

Glycogen, a branched polymer of glucose, represents a storage form of glucose. Glycogen synthesis and degradation occur primarily in liver and skeletal muscle, although other tissues, including cardiac muscle and the kidney, store smaller quantities.

Glycogen is stored in the cytoplasm as either single granules (skeletal muscle) or as clusters of granules (liver). The granule has a central protein core with polyglucose chains radiating outward to form a sphere (Figure I-14-1). Glycogen granules composed entirely of linear chains have the highest *density* of glucose near the core. If the chains are branched, the glucose *density* is highest at the periphery of the granule, allowing more rapid release of glucose on demand.

Glycogen stored in the liver is a source of glucose mobilized during hypoglycemia. Muscle glycogen is stored as an energy reserve for muscle contraction. In white (fast-twitch) muscle fibers, the glucose is converted primarily to lactate, whereas in red (slow-twitch) muscle fibers, the glucose is completely oxidized.

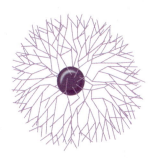

Figure I-14-1.
A glycogen granule

GLYCOGEN SYNTHESIS

Synthesis of glycogen granules begins with a core protein glycogenin. Glucose addition to a granule, shown in Figure I-14-2, begins with glucose 6-phosphate, which is converted to glucose 1-phosphate and activated to UDP-glucose for addition to the glycogen chain by glycogen synthase. Glycogen synthase is the rate-limiting enzyme of glycogen synthesis.

Section I • Biochemistry

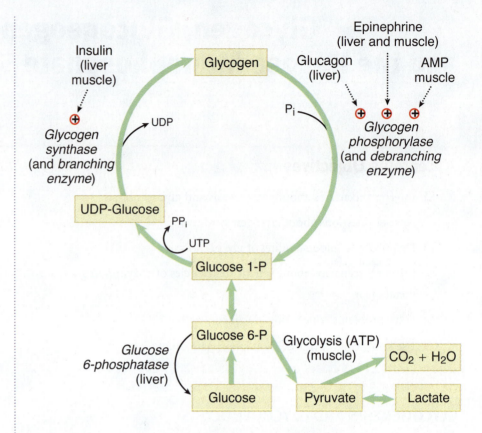

Figure I-14-2. Glycogen Metabolism

Glycogen Synthase

Glycogen synthase forms the α1,4 glycosidic bond found in the linear glucose chains of the granule. Table I-14-1 shows the control of glycogen synthase in liver and skeletal muscle.

Table I-14-1. Comparison of Glycogen Synthase in Liver and Muscle

Glycogen Synthase	Liver	Skeletal Muscle
Activated by	Insulin	Insulin
Inhibited by	Glucagon Epinephrine	Epinephrine

Branching Enzyme (Glycosyl α1,4:α1,6 Transferase)

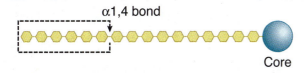

1. Glycogen synthase makes a linear α1,4-linked polyglucose chain (○○○○○).
2. Branching enzyme hydrolyzes an α1,4 bond.

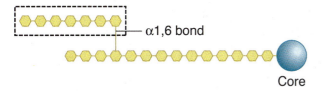

3. Transfers the oligoglucose unit and attaches it with an α1,6 bond to create a branch.
4. Glycogen synthase extends both branches.

Figure I-14-3. Branching Enzyme

Branching enzyme is responsible for introducing α1,6-linked branches into the granule as it grows. The process by which the branch is introduced is shown schematically in Figure I-14-3. Branching enzyme:

- Hydrolyzes one of the α1,4 bonds to release a block of oligoglucose, which is then moved and added in a slightly different location
- Forms an α1,6 bond to create a branch

GLYCOGENOLYSIS

The rate-limiting enzyme of glycogenolysis is glycogen phosphorylase (in contrast to a hydrolase, a phosphorylase breaks bonds using P_i rather than H_2O). The glucose 1-phosphate formed is converted to glucose 6-phosphate by the same mutase used in glycogen synthesis (Figure I-14-2).

Glycogen Phosphorylase

Glycogen phosphorylase breaks α1,4 glycosidic bonds, releasing glucose 1-phosphate from the periphery of the granule. Control of the enzyme in liver and muscle is compared in Table I-14-2.

Section I • Biochemistry

Table I-14-2. Comparison of Glycogen Phosphorylase in Liver and Muscle

Glycogen Phosphorylase	Liver	Skeletal Muscle
Activated by	Epinephrine Glucagon	Epinephrine AMP Ca^{2+} (through calmodulin)
Inhibited by	Insulin	Insulin ATP

Glycogen phosphorylase cannot break α1,6 bonds and therefore stops when it nears the outermost branch points.

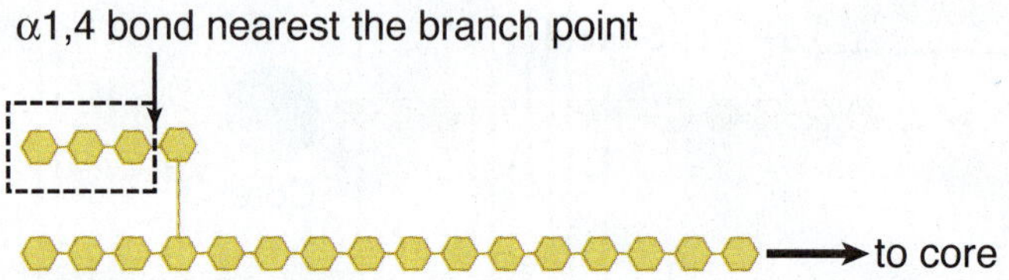

1. Glycogen phosphorylase releases glucose 1-P from the periphery of the granule until it encounters the first branch points.

2. Debranching enzyme hydrolyzes the α1,4 bond nearest the branch point, as shown.

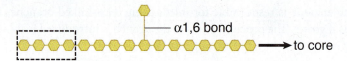

3. Transfers the oligoglucose unit to the end of another chain, then

4. Hydrolyzes the α1,6 bond releasing the single glucose from the former branch.

Figure I-14-4. Debranching Enzyme

Debranching Enzyme (Glucosyl α1,4: α1,4 Transferase and α1,6 Glucosidase)

Debranching enzyme deconstructs the branches in glycogen that have been exposed by glycogen phosphorylase. The two-step process by which this occurs is diagrammed in Figure I-14-4. Debranching enzyme:

- Breaks an α1,4 bond adjacent to the branch point and moves the small oligoglucose chain released to the exposed end of the other chain
- Forms a new α1,4 bond
- Hydrolyzes the α1,6 bond, releasing the single residue at the branch point as free glucose. This represents the only free glucose produced directly in glycogenolysis.

GENETIC DEFICIENCIES OF ENZYMES IN GLYCOGEN METABOLISM

Important genetic deficiencies, listed in Table I-14-3, are classed as glycogen storage diseases because all are characterized by accumulation of glycogen in one or more tissues.

Table I-14-3. Glycogen Storage Diseases

Type	Deficient Enzyme	Cardinal Clinical Features	Glycogen Structure
I: von Gierke	Glucose-6-phosphatase	Severe hypoglycemia, lactic acidosis, hepatomegaly, hyperlipidemia, hyperuricemia, short stature, doll-like facies, protruding abdomen emaciated extremities	Normal
II: Pompe	Lysosomal α1,4-glucosidase	Cardiomegaly, muscle weakness, death by 2 years	Glycogen-like material in inclusion bodies
III: Cori	Glycogen debranching enzyme	Mild hypoglycemia, liver enlargement	Short outer branches Single glucose residue at outer branch
IV: Andersen	Branching enzyme	Infantile hypotonia, cirrhosis, death by 2 years	Very few branches, especially toward periphery
V: McArdle	Muscle glycogen phosphorylase	Muscle cramps and weakness on exercise, myoglobinuria	Normal
VI: Hers	Hepatic glycogen phosphorylase	Mild fasting hypoglycemia, hepatomegaly, cirrhosis	Normal

Glucose-6-Phosphatase Deficiency (von Gierke Disease)

Deficiency of hepatic glucose-6-phosphatase produces a profound fasting hypoglycemia, lactic acidosis, and hepatomegaly. Additional symptoms include:

- Glycogen deposits in the liver (glucose 6-P stimulates glycogen synthesis, and glycogenolysis is inhibited)
- Hyperuricemia predisposing to gout. Decreased P_i causes increased AMP, which is degraded to uric acid. Lactate slows uric acid excretion in the kidney.
- Hyperlipidemia with skin xanthomas; elevation of triglycerides (VLDL)
- Fatty liver

In a person with glucose-6-phosphatase deficiency, ingestion of galactose or fructose causes no increase in blood glucose, nor does administration of glucagon or epinephrine.

Myophosphorylase Deficiency (McArdle Disease)

Myophosphorylase is another name for the muscle glycogen phosphorylase. Symptoms of myophosphorylase deficiency include:

- Exercise intolerance during the initial phase of high-intensity exercise
- Muscle cramping
- Possible myoglobinuria
- Recovery or "second wind" after 10–15 minutes of exercise

A 25-year-old woman had a lifelong history of exercise intolerance that was often accompanied by episodes of cramping. The episodes were somewhat ameliorated by drinking sucrose-rich soft drinks immediately before exercise. The latest episode occurred during her first spin class (stationary bicycling with a resistance load) at her local bicycle shop. She initially had extreme weakness in both legs and muscle cramps and later excreted red-brown urine. In subsequent sessions, in addition to the high-sucrose drink, she reduced the load on the bicycle and was better able to tolerate the initial phase of exercise. After 10–15 minutes, she experienced a "second wind" and was able to continue her exercise successfully.

This woman has myophosphorylase deficiency and is unable to properly break down glycogen to glucose 6-phosphate in her muscles. Without an adequate supply of glucose, sufficient energy via glycolysis for carrying out muscle contraction cannot be obtained, explaining why the muscles are not functioning well (weakness and cramps). The situation is improved by drinking the sucrose-containing drink, which provides dietary glucose for the muscles to use.

Hepatic Glycogen Phosphorylase Deficiency (Hers Disease)

Hepatic glycogen phosphorylase deficiency is usually a relatively mild disease because gluconeogenesis compensates for the lack of glycogenolysis (Figure I-14-5). If present, hypoglycemia, hyperlipidemia, and hyperketosis are mild. Hepatomegaly and growth retardation may be present in early childhood, although hepatomegaly may improve with age.

Lysosomal α1,4 Glucosidase Deficiency (Pompe Disease)

Pompe disease is different from the other diseases in Table I-14-3 because the enzyme missing is not one in the normal process of glycogenolysis described in this chapter. The deficient enzyme normally resides in the lysosome and is responsible for digesting glycogen-like material accumulating in endosomes. In this respect, it is more similar to diseases like Tay-Sachs or even I-cell disease in which indigestible substrates accumulate in inclusion bodies. In Pompe disease, the tissues most severely affected are those that normally have glycogen stores. With infantile onset, massive cardiomegaly is usually the cause of death, which occurs before 2 years of age.

> A 12-month-old girl had slowly progressing muscle weakness involving her arms and legs and developed difficulty breathing. Her liver was enlarged, and a CT scan revealed cardiomegaly. A muscle biopsy showed muscle degeneration with many enlarged, prominent lysosomes filled with clusters of electron-dense granules. Her parents were told that without treatment, the child's symptoms would continue to worsen and likely result in death in 1–2 years. Enzyme replacement therapy was initiated.

This child has a defect of the enzyme lysosomal α1,4 glucosidase (also called acid maltase). Coordinated glycogen breakdown with phosphorylase and debranching enzyme occurs in the cytoplasm. Although the α1,4 glucosidase participates in glycogen breakdown, the purpose of this enzyme and the reason for its location in the lysosome are unknown. Nevertheless, tissues that contain most of the body glycogen (liver and muscle) are severely affected in Pompe disease.

GLUCONEOGENESIS

The liver maintains glucose levels in blood during fasting through either glycogenolysis or gluconeogenesis. These pathways are promoted by glucagon and epinephrine and inhibited by insulin. In fasting, glycogen reserves drop dramatically in the first 12 hours, during which time gluconeogenesis increases. After 24 hours, it represents the sole source of glucose. Important substrates for gluconeogenesis are:

- Glycerol 3-phosphate (from triacylglycerol in adipose)
- Lactate (from anaerobic glycolysis)
- Gluconeogenic amino acids (protein from muscle)

Table I-14-4. Glucogenic and Ketogenic Amino Acids

Ketogenic	Ketogenic and Glucogenic	Glucogenic
Leucine	Phenylalanine	All others
Lysine	Tyrosine	
	Tryptophan	
	Isoleucine	
	Threonine	

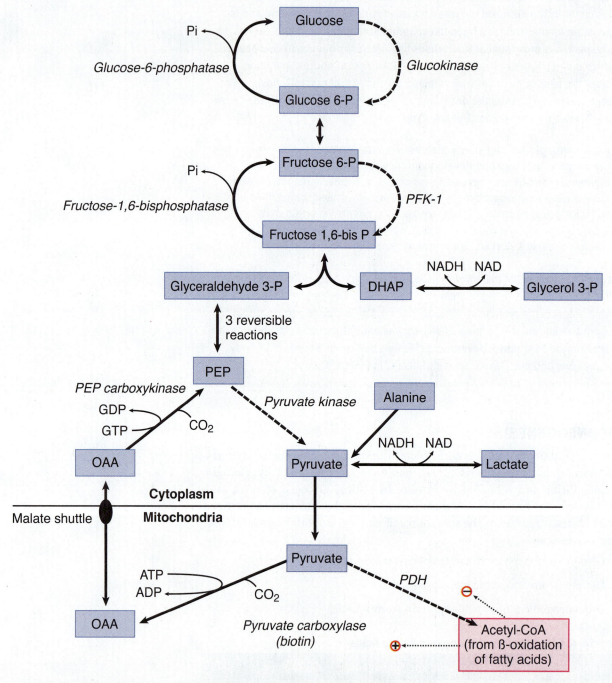

Figure I-14-5. Gluconeogenesis

Dietary fructose and galactose can also be converted to glucose in the liver.

In humans, it is not possible to convert acetyl-CoA to glucose. Inasmuch as most fatty acids are metabolized solely to acetyl-CoA, they are not a major source of glucose either. One minor exception is odd-number carbon fatty acids (e.g., C17), which yield a small amount of propionyl-CoA that is gluconeogenic.

The pathway of gluconeogenesis is diagrammed in Figure I-14-5. Lactate is oxidized to pyruvate by lactate dehydrogenase. The important gluconeogenic amino acid alanine is converted to pyruvate by alanine aminotransferase (ALT or GPT). Glycerol 3-phosphate is oxidized to dihydroxyacetone phosphate (DHAP) by glycerol 3-phosphate dehydrogenase. Most steps represent a reversal of glycolysis, and several of these have been omitted from the diagram. The 4 important enzymes are those required to catalyze reactions that circumvent the irreversible steps:

1. **Pyruvate carboxylase** is a mitochondrial enzyme requiring biotin. It is activated by acetyl-CoA (from β-oxidation). The product oxaloacetate (OAA), a citric acid cycle intermediate, cannot leave the mitochondria but is reduced to malate that can leave via the **malate shuttle**. In the cytoplasm, malate is reoxidized to OAA.

2. **Phosphoenolpyruvate carboxykinase** (PEPCK) in the cytoplasm is induced by glucagon and cortisol. It converts OAA to phosphoenolpyruvate (PEP) in a reaction that requires GTP. PEP continues in the pathway to fructose 1,6-bisphosphate.

3. **Fructose-1,6-bisphosphatase** in the cytoplasm is a key control point of gluconeogenesis. It hydrolyzes phosphate from fructose 1,6-bisphosphate rather than using it to generate ATP from ADP. A common pattern to note is that phosphatases oppose kinases. Fructose- 1,6-bisphosphatase is activated by ATP and inhibited by AMP and fructose 2,6-bisphosphate. Fructose 2,6-bisphosphate, produced by PFK-2, controls both gluconeogenesis and glycolysis (in the liver). Recall from the earlier discussion of this enzyme (see Chapter 12, Figure I-12-3) that PFK-2 is activated by insulin and inhibited by glucagon. Thus, glucagon will lower F 2,6-BP and stimulate gluconeogenesis, whereas insulin will increase F 2,6-BP and inhibit gluconeogenesis.

4. **Glucose-6-phosphatase** is in the lumen of the endoplasmic reticulum. Glucose 6-phosphate is transported into the ER, and free glucose is transported back into the cytoplasm from which it leaves the cell. Glucose-6-phosphatase is only in the liver. The absence of glucose-6-phosphatase in skeletal muscle accounts for the fact that muscle glycogen cannot serve as a source of blood glucose (see Chapter 17, Figure I-17-3).

Although alanine is the major gluconeogenic amino acid, 18 of the 20 (all but leucine and lysine) are also gluconeogenic. Most of these are converted by individual pathways to citric acid cycle intermediates, then to malate, following the same path from there to glucose.

It is important to note that glucose produced by hepatic gluconeogenesis does not represent an energy source for the liver. Gluconeogenesis requires expenditure of ATP that is provided by β-oxidation of fatty acids. Therefore, hepatic gluconeogenesis is always dependent on β-oxidation of fatty acids in the liver. During hypoglycemia, adipose tissue releases these fatty acids by breaking down triglyceride.

Note

Biotin Deficiency

Symptoms

- Alopecia
- Scaly dermatitis
- Waxy pallor
- Acidosis (mild)

Causes

- Raw egg whites (avidin)
- Long-term home TPN

Although the acetyl-CoA from fatty acids cannot be converted to glucose, it can be converted to ketone bodies as an alternative fuel for cells, including the brain. Chronic hypoglycemia is thus often accompanied physiologically by an increase in ketone bodies.

Coordinate Regulation of Pyruvate Carboxylase and Pyruvate Dehydrogenase by Acetyl-CoA

The two major mitochondrial enzymes that use pyruvate, pyruvate carboxylase and pyruvate dehydrogenase, are both regulated by acetyl-CoA. This control is important in these contexts:

- Between meals, when fatty acids are oxidized in the liver for energy, accumulating acetyl-CoA activates pyruvate carboxylase and gluconeogenesis and inhibits PDH, thus preventing conversion of lactate and alanine to acetyl-CoA.

- In the well-fed, absorptive state (insulin), accumulating acetyl-CoA is shuttled into the cytoplasm for fatty acid synthesis. OAA is necessary for this transport, and acetyl-CoA can stimulate its formation from pyruvate (see Chapter 15, Figure I-15-1).

Cori Cycle and Alanine Cycle

During fasting, lactate from red blood cells (and possibly exercising skeletal muscle) is converted in the liver to glucose that can be returned to the red blood cell or muscle. This is called the Cori cycle. The alanine cycle is a slightly different version of the Cori cycle, in which muscle releases alanine, delivering both a gluconeogenic substrate (pyruvate) and an amino group for urea synthesis.

Alcoholism and Hypoglycemia

Alcoholics are very susceptible to hypoglycemia. In addition to poor nutrition and the fact that alcohol is metabolized to acetate (acetyl-CoA), the high amounts of cytoplasmic NADH formed by alcohol dehydrogenase and acetaldehyde dehydrogenase interfere with gluconeogenesis. High NADH favors the formation of:

- Lactate from pyruvate
- Malate from OAA in the cytoplasm
- Glycerol 3-phosphate from DHAP

The effect is to divert important gluconeogenic substrates from entering the pathway (Figure I-14-6).

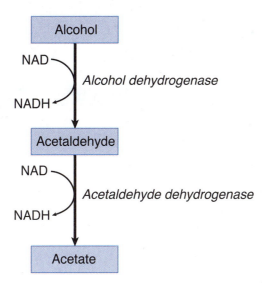

Figure I-14-6. Alcohol Metabolism

Accumulation of cytoplasmic NADH and glycerol 3-P may also contribute to lipid accumulation in alcoholic liver disease. Free fatty acids released from adipose in part enter the liver where β-oxidation is very slow (high NADH). In the presence of high glycerol 3-P, fatty acids are inappropriately stored in the liver as triglyceride.

Extreme Exercise and Alcohol Consumption

Immediately after completing a 26-mile marathon race, a healthy 24-year-old man was extremely dehydrated and thirsty. He quickly consumed a 6-pack of ice-cold beer and shortly thereafter became very weak and light-headed and nearly fainted. He complained of muscle cramping and pain.

Although the effect of alcohol is unrelated to the hormonal control of gluconeogenesis, excessive consumption of alcohol can result in severe hypoglycemia after running a marathon. In exercising muscle, lactic acid builds up in muscle due to anaerobic glycolysis, causing muscle cramping and pain. The lactate spills into blood and is converted to glucose in the liver, as part of the Cori cycle. But to carry out gluconeogenesis, NAD is required by lactate dehydrogenase to oxidize lactate to pyruvate. However, much of the available NAD is being used for ethanol metabolism and is unavailable for lactate oxidation. The result is metabolic acidosis and hypoglycemia.

Clinical Correlate

Alcohol abuse may lead to hepatic steatosis, which is fatty degeneration of liver tissue.

HEXOSE MONOPHOSPHATE SHUNT

The hexose monophosphate (HMP) shunt (pentose phosphate pathway) occurs in the cytoplasm of all cells, where it serves 2 major functions:

- NADPH production
- Source of ribose 5-phosphate for nucleotide synthesis

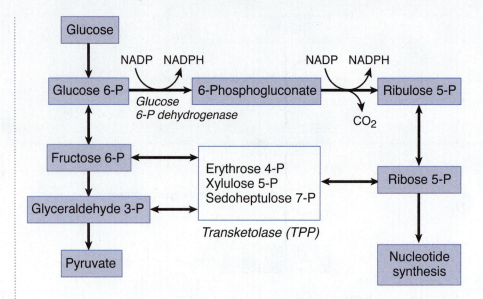

Figure I-14-7. The Hexose Monophosphate Shunt

An abbreviated diagram of the pathway is shown in Figure I-14-7. The first part of the HMP shunt begins with glucose 6-phosphate and ends with ribulose 5-phosphate and is irreversible. This part produces NADPH and involves the important rate-limiting enzyme glucose 6-phosphate dehydrogenase (G6PDH). G6PDH is induced by insulin, inhibited by NADPH, and activated by NADP.

The second part of the pathway, beginning with ribulose 5-phosphate, represents a series of reversible reactions that produce an equilibrated pool of sugars for biosynthesis, including ribose 5-phosphate for nucleotide synthesis. Because fructose 6-phosphate and glyceraldehyde 3-phosphate are among the sugars produced, intermediates can feed back into glycolysis; conversely, pentoses can be made from glycolytic intermediates without going through the G6PDH reaction. Transketolase, a thiamine-requiring enzyme, is important for these interconversions. Transketolase is the only thiamine enzyme in red blood cells.

Functions of NADPH

Cells require NADPH for a variety of functions, including:

- Biosynthesis
- Maintenance of a supply of reduced glutathione to protect against reactive oxygen species (ROS)
- Bactericidal activity in polymorphonuclear leukocytes (PMN)

These important roles are cell specific and shown in Figure I-14-8.

Chapter 14 • Glycogen, Gluconeogenesis, and the Hexose Monophosphate Shunt

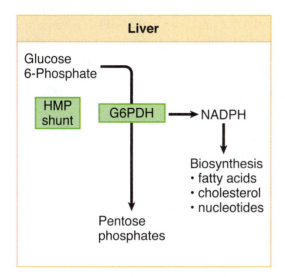
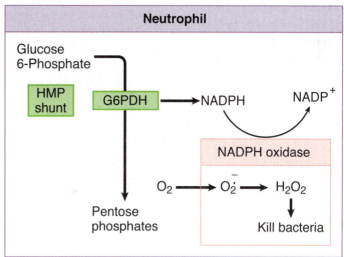
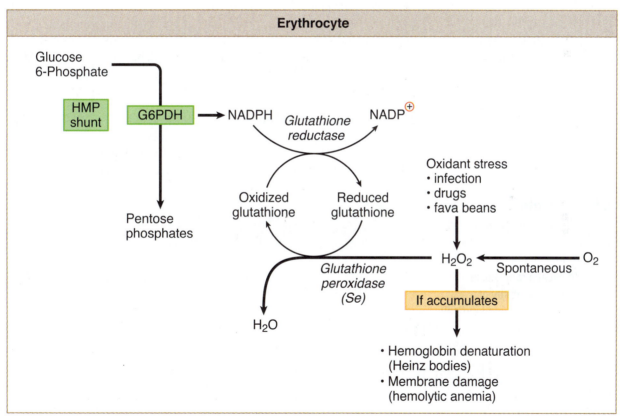

Figure I-14-8. Role of the HMP Shunt in Hepatocytes, Phagocytes, and Erythrocytes

Section I • Biochemistry

Clinical Correlate
Favism

Broad beans, commonly called fava beans, are common to diets in Mediterranean countries (Greece, Italy, Spain, Portugal, and Turkey), in which their ingestion may cause severe hemolysis in G6PDH individuals. Clinically, the condition presents as pallor, hemoglobinuria, jaundice, and severe anemia 24–48 hours after ingestion of the beans.

Clinical Correlate
CGD

Chronic granulomatous disease is most frequently caused by genetic deficiency of NADPH oxidase in the PMN. Patients are susceptible to infection by catalase-positive organisms such as *Staphylococcus aureus*, *Klebsiella*, *Escherichia coli*, *Candida*, and *Aspergillus*. A negative nitroblue tetrazolium test is useful in confirming the diagnosis.

Bridge to Microbiology

Many parasites, such as *Plasmodium*, are deficient in antioxidant mechanisms, making them particularly susceptible to oxygen radicals. In G6PDH deficiency, the ability of erythrocytes to detoxify oxygen radicals is impaired. Ironically, the accumulation of the radicals in erythrocytes in G6PDH deficiency gives protection against malaria.

Glucose 6-Phosphate Dehydrogenase Deficiency

Deficiency of G6PDH may result in hemolytic anemia and, in rare cases, symptoms resembling chronic granulomatous disease (CGD). The disease shows significant allelic heterogeneity (over 400 different mutations in the G6PDH gene are known). The major symptom is either an acute episodic or (rarely) a chronic hemolysis. The disease is X-linked recessive. Female heterozygous for G6PDH deficiency have increased resistance to malaria. Consequently, the deficiency is seen more commonly in families from regions where malaria is endemic.

Because red blood cells contain a large amount of oxygen, they are prone to spontaneously generate ROS that damage protein and lipid in the cell. In the presence of ROS, hemoglobin may precipitate (Heinz bodies) and membrane lipids may undergo peroxidation, weakening the membrane and causing hemolysis. As peroxides form, they are rapidly destroyed by the glutathione peroxidase/glutathione reductase system in the red blood cell, thus avoiding these complications. These enzymes are shown in the red blood cell diagram in Figure I-14-8. NADPH required by glutathione reductase is supplied by the HMP shunt in the erythrocyte.

Persons with mutations that partially destroy G6PDH activity may develop an acute, episodic hemolysis. Certain mutations affect the stability of G6PDH, and, because erythrocytes cannot synthesize proteins, the enzyme is gradually lost over time and older red blood cells lyse. This process is accelerated by certain drugs and, in a subset of patients, ingestion of fava beans. In the United States, the most likely cause of a hemolytic episode in these patients is overwhelming infection, often pneumonia (viral and bacterial) or infectious hepatitis.

In rare instances, a mutation may decrease the activity of G6PDH sufficiently to cause chronic nonspherocytic hemolytic anemia. Symptoms of CGD may also develop if there is insufficient activity of G6PDH (<5% of normal) in the PMN to generate NADPH for the NADPH oxidase bactericidal system.

Chapter Summary

Glycogen Metabolism
- Cytoplasm

Rate-Limiting Enzymes
- Glycogen synthesis: glycogen synthase
  - Activated by insulin in liver and muscle
- Glycogenolysis: glycogen phosphorylase
  - Activated by glucagon in liver (hypoglycemia)
  - Activated by epinephrine and AMP in skeletal muscle (exercise)

Other Enzymes
- Glucose 6-phosphatase releases free glucose; only in liver

Genetic Deficiencies
  - Glucose 6-phosphatase deficiency
  - Hepatic glycogen phosphorylase deficiency
  - Muscle glycogen phosphorylase deficiency
  - Lysosomal α1,4-glucosidase deficiency

Gluconeogenesis
- Cytoplasm and mitochondria; predominantly in liver

Controlled Enzyme
- Fructose 1,6-bisphosphatase
  - Cytoplasm
  - Activated by ATP
  - Inhibited by AMP and fructose 2,6-bisP
  - Insulin (inhibits) glucagon (activates) by their control of PFK-2 (produces fructose 2,6-bisP)

Other Enzymes
- Pyruvate carboxylase
  - Activated by acetyl CoA from β-oxidation
  - Biotin
  - Mitochondria
- Phosphoenolpyruvate carboxykinase (PEPCK)
  - Cytoplasm
  - Induced by glucagon and cortisol
- Glucose 6-phosphatase (endoplasmic reticulum)
  - Only in liver
  - Required to release free glucose from tissue

(Continued)

Section I • Biochemistry

> ### Chapter Summary (continued)
>
> **Important Patients**
>
> - Alcoholic hypoglycemia (high NADH)
> - Glucose 6-phosphatase deficiency
> - Defects in β-oxidation susceptible to hypoglycemic episodes
>
> #### HMP Shunt
> - Cytoplasm of most cells
>
> **Functions**
>
> - Generates NADPH
> - Produces sugars for biosynthesis (ribose 5-P for nucleotides)
>
> **Rate-Limiting Enzymes**
>
> - Glucose 6-phosphate dehydrogenase
>   - Inhibited by NADPH
>   - Induced by insulin in liver
>
> **Genetic Deficiency**
>
> - Glucose 6-phosphate dehydrogenase
>   - Episodic hemolytic anemia (most common) induced by infection and drugs
>   - Chronic hemolysis, CGD-like symptoms (very rare)

Review Questions

Select the ONE best answer.

1. A liver biopsy is done on a child with hepatomegaly and mild fasting hypoglycemia. Hepatocytes show accumulation of glycogen granules with single glucose residues remaining at the branch points near the periphery of the granule. The most likely genetic defect is in the gene encoding a(n):

   A. α-1,4 phosphorylase
   B. α-1,4:α-1,4 transferase
   C. phosphoglucomutase
   D. α-1,6 glucosidase
   E. lysosomal α-1,4 glucosidase

2. When fatty acid β-oxidation predominates in the liver, mitochondrial pyruvate is most likely to be

   A. carboxylated to phosphoenolpyruvate for entry into gluconeogenesis
   B. oxidatively decarboxylated to acetyl CoA for entry into ketogenesis
   C. reduced to lactate for entry into gluconeogenesis
   D. oxidatively decarboxylated to acetyl CoA for oxidation in Krebs cycle
   E. carboxylated to oxaloacetate for entry into gluconeogenesis

Chapter 14 • Glycogen, Gluconeogenesis, and the Hexose Monophosphate Shunt

Items 3 and 4

A 44-year-old man from Limpopo Province in South Africa, living in the United States and receiving antibiotic therapy for a urinary tract infection has a self-limiting episode of hemolysis, back pain, and jaundice. The peripheral blood smear reveals a nonspherocytic, normocytic anemia, and Heinz bodies are seen in some of his erythrocytes.

3. Which of the following genetic deficiencies is most likely related to his hemolytic episode?

    A. Homocysteine methyltransferase
    B. Pyruvate kinase
    C. Dihydrofolate reductase
    D. Ferrochelatase
    E. Glucose 6-phosphate dehydrogenase

4. Which of the following sets of laboratory test results would most likely have been obtained for this patient?

	Direct Bilirubin	Indirect Bilirubin	Urinary Bilirubin
A.	Increased	Increased	Absent
B.	Increased	Increased	Present
C.	Normal	Increased	Absent
D.	Normal	Decreased	Present
E.	Increased	Decreased	Present

Answers

1. **Answer: D.** This activity of the debranching enzyme removes 1,6-linked glucose residues from the branch points during glycogenolysis.

2. **Answer: E.** Hepatic fatty acid oxidation generates energy in the postabsorptive period when pyruvate is being converted to OAA for glucose biosynthesis.

3. **Answer: E.** Only option E is consistent with the constellation of clinical findings presented. Major clue is the positive Heinz body preparation.

4. **Answer: C.** Only option C is characteristic of hemolytic jaundice; indirect hyperbilirubinemia with no spillover of the water-insoluble unconjugated form into the urine.

Lipid Synthesis and Storage 15

Learning Objectives

❑ Answer questions about fatty acid nomenclature
❑ Answer questions about lipid digestion
❑ Answer questions about fatty acid biosynthesis
❑ Demonstrate understanding of triglyceride (triacylglycerol) synthesis
❑ Demonstrate understanding of lipoprotein metabolism
❑ Explain information related to hyperlipidemias
❑ Use knowledge of cholesterol metabolism

FATTY ACID NOMENCLATURE

Fatty acids are long-chain carboxylic acids. The carboxyl carbon is number 1, and carbon number 2 is referred to as the α carbon. When designating a fatty acid, the number of carbons is given along with the number of double bonds (carbons:double bonds). Saturated fatty acids have no double bonds. Palmitic acid (palmitate) is the primary end product of fatty acid synthesis.

$CH_3CH_2CH_2CH_2CH_2CH_2CH_2CH_2CH_2CH_2CH_2CH_2CH_2CH_2CH_2COO^-$
Palmitate   C16:0 or 16:0

Unsaturated fatty acids

Unsaturated fatty acids have one or more double bonds. Humans can synthesize only a few of the unsaturated fatty acids; the rest come from essential fatty acids in the diet that are transported as triglycerides from the intestine in chylomicrons. Two important essential fatty acids are linolenic acid and linoleic acid. These polyunsaturated fatty acids, as well as other acids formed from them, are important in membrane phospholipids to maintain normal fluidity of cell membranes essential for many functions.

The omega (ω) numbering system is also used for unsaturated fatty acids. The ω-family describes the position of the last double bond relative to the end of the chain. The omega designation identifies the major precursor fatty acid, e.g., arachidonic acid is formed from linoleic acid (ω-6 family). Arachidonic acid is itself an important precursor for prostaglandins, thromboxanes, and leukotrienes.

Linoleic	C18:2 (9,12) or $18^{\Delta 9,12}$	ω-6 family (18 − 12 = 6)
Linolenic	C18:3 (9,12,15) or $18^{\Delta 9,12,15}$	ω-3 family
Arachidonic	C20:4 (5,8,11,14) or $20^{\Delta 5,8,11,14}$	ω-6 family

Clinical Correlate
Cardioprotective Effects of Omega-3 Fatty Acids

Omega-3 fatty acids in the diet are correlated with a decreased risk of cardiovascular disease. These appear to replace some of the arachidonic acid (an omega-6 fatty acid) in platelet membranes and may lower the production of thromboxane and the tendency of the platelets to aggregate. A diet high in omega-3 fatty acids has also been associated with a decrease in serum triglycerides. Omega-3 fatty acids are found in cold-water fish, such as salmon, tuna, and herring, as well as in some nuts (walnuts) and seeds (flax seed).

Double bonds in fatty acids are in the *cis-* configuration. *Trans-* double bonds are unnatural and predominate in fatty acids found in margarine and other foods where partial hydrogenation of vegetable oils is used in their preparation. Compared with liquid oils, these partial hydrogenated fatty acids are conveniently solid at cool temperatures. When incorporated into phospholipids that constitute membranes, *trans-* fatty acids decrease membrane fluidity, similar to saturated fatty acids that are found in butter fat and other foods. *Trans-* fatty acids, as well as saturated fatty acids, are associated with increased risk of atherosclerosis.

Activation of Fatty Acids

When fatty acids are used in metabolism, they are first activated by attaching coenzyme A (CoA); fatty acyl CoA synthetase catalyzes this activation step. The product is generically referred to as a fatty acyl CoA or sometimes just acyl CoA. Specific examples would be acetyl CoA with a 2-carbon acyl group, or palmitoyl CoA with a 16-carbon acyl group.

Fatty acid + CoA + ATP → Fatty acyl CoA + AMP + PP_i

LIPID DIGESTION

Typical high-fat meals contain gram-level amounts of triglycerides and milligram-level amounts of cholesterol and cholesterol esters. Upon entry into the intestinal lumen, bile is secreted by the liver to emulsify the lipid contents. The pancreas secretes pancreatic lipase, colipase, and cholesterol esterase that degrade the lipids to 2-monoglyceride, fatty acids, and cholesterol. These lipids are absorbed and re-esterified to tryglycerides and cholesterol esters and packaged, along with apoprotein B-48 and other lipids (e.g., fat-soluble vitamins), into chylomicrons. Normally, there is very little lipid loss in stools. Defects in lipid digestion result in steatorrhea, in which there is an excessive amount of lipids in stool (fatty stools).

FATTY ACID BIOSYNTHESIS

Excess dietary glucose can be converted to fatty acids in the liver and subsequently sent to the adipose tissue for storage. Adipose tissue synthesizes smaller quantities of fatty acids. The pathway is shown in Figure I-15-1. Insulin promotes many steps in the conversion of glucose to acetyl CoA in the liver:

- Glucokinase (induced)
- PFK-2/PFK-1 (PFK-2 dephosphorylated)
- Pyruvate dehydrogenase (dephosphorylated)

Both of the major enzymes of fatty acid synthesis are also affected by insulin:

- Acetyl CoA carboxylase (dephosphorylated, activated)
- Fatty acid synthase (induced)

Citrate Shuttle and Malic Enzyme

The citrate shuttle transports acetyl CoA groups from the mitochondria to the cytoplasm for fatty acid synthesis. Acetyl CoA combines with oxaloacetate in the mitochondria to form citrate, but rather than continuing in the citric acid cycle, citrate is transported into the cytoplasm. Factors that indirectly promote this process include insulin and high-energy status.

In the cytoplasm, citrate lyase splits citrate back into acetyl CoA and oxaloacetate. The oxaloacetate returns to the mitochondria to transport additional acetyl CoA. This process is shown in Figure I-15-1 and includes the important malic enzyme. This reaction represents an additional source of cytoplasmic NADPH in liver and adipose tissue, supplementing that from the HMP shunt.

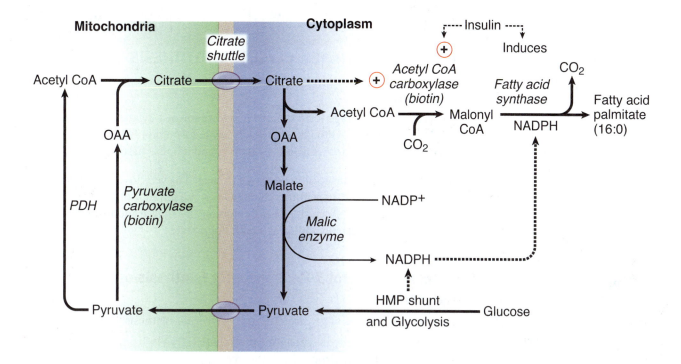

Figure I-15-1. Synthesis of Palmitate from Glucose

Acetyl CoA Carboxylase

Acetyl CoA is activated in the cytoplasm for incorporation into fatty acids by acetyl CoA carboxylase, the rate-limiting enzyme of fatty acid biosynthesis. Acetyl CoA carboxylase requires biotin, ATP, and CO_2. Controls include:

- Activation by insulin (dephosphorylated)
- Activation by citrate

The CO_2 added to form malonyl CoA is never incorporated into the fatty acid because it is removed by fatty acid synthase during the addition of the acetyl group to the fatty acid.

Fatty Acid Synthase

Fatty acid synthase is more appropriately called palmitate synthase because palmitate is the only fatty acid that humans can synthesize *de novo*. This enzyme is a large, multienzyme complex in the cytoplasm that is rapidly induced in the liver after a meal by high carbohydrate and concomitantly rising insulin levels. It contains an acyl carrier protein (ACP) that requires the vitamin pantothenic acid. Although malonyl CoA is the substrate used by fatty acid synthase, only the carbons from the acetyl CoA portion are actually incorporated into the fatty acid produced. Therefore, the fatty acid is derived entirely from acetyl CoA.

NADPH is required to reduce the acetyl groups added to the fatty acid. Eight acetyl CoA groups are required to produce palmitate (16:0).

Fatty acyl CoA may be elongated and desaturated (to a limited extent in humans) using enzymes associated with the smooth endoplasmic reticulum (SER). Cytochrome b_5 is involved in the desaturation reactions. These enzymes cannot introduce double bonds past position 9 in the fatty acid.

TRIGLYCERIDE (TRIACYLGLYCEROL) SYNTHESIS

Triglycerides

Triglycerides, the storage form of fatty acids, are formed by attaching three fatty acids (as fatty acyl CoA) to glycerol. Triglyceride formation from fatty acids and glycerol 3-phosphate occurs primarily in liver and adipose tissue.

Liver sends triglycerides to adipose tissue packaged as very low-density lipoproteins (VLDL; reviewed later in this chapter). A small amount of triglyceride may be stored in the liver. Accumulation of significant triglyceride in tissues other than adipose tissue usually indicates a pathologic state.

Sources of Glycerol 3-Phosphate for Synthesis of Triglycerides

There are two sources of glycerol 3-P for triglyceride synthesis:

- Reduction of dihydroxyacetone phosphate (DHAP) from glycolysis by glycerol 3-P dehydrogenase, an enzyme in both adipose tissue and liver
- Phosphorylation of free glycerol by glycerol kinase, an enzyme found in liver but not in adipose tissue

Glycerol kinase allows the liver to recycle the glycerol released during VLDL metabolism (insulin) back into new triglyceride synthesis. During fasting (glucagon), this same enzyme allows the liver to trap glycerol released into the blood from lipolysis in adipose tissue for subsequent conversion to glucose.

Adipose tissue lacks glycerol kinase and is strictly dependent on glucose uptake to produce DHAP for triglyceride synthesis. In adipose tissue, the GLUT 4 transporter is stimulated by insulin, ensuring a good supply of DHAP for triglyceride synthesis. The roles of glycerol kinase and glycerol 3-P dehydrogenase during triglyceride synthesis and storage are shown in Figure I-15-2.

Bridge to Pathology

Chronic alcohol use can interfere with lipid metabolism in the liver, leading to steatosis, or fatty degeneration of the liver parenchyma.

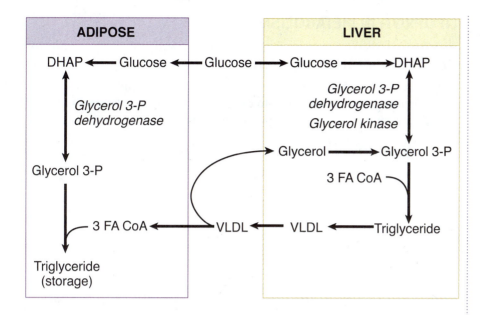

Figure I-15-2. Glycerol 3-P Dehydrogenase and Glycerol Kinase in Triglyceride Synthesis and Storage

Glycerophospholipids

Glycerophospholipids are used for membrane synthesis and for producing a hydrophilic surface layer on lipoproteins such as VLDL. In cell membranes, they also serve as a reservoir of second messengers such as diacylglycerol, inositol 1,4,5-triphosphate, and arachidonic acid. Their structure is similar to triglycerides, except that the last fatty acid is replaced by phosphate and a water-soluble group such as choline (phosphatidylcholine, lecithin) or inositol (phosphatidylinositol).

A comparison of the structures is diagrammed in Figure I-15-3.

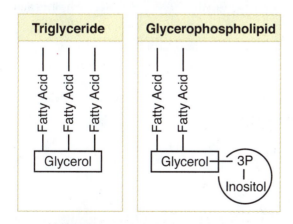

Figure I-15-3. Triglycerides and Glycerophospholipids

Section I • Biochemistry

LIPOPROTEIN METABOLISM

General Concepts: Cholesterol Digestion

Triglycerides and cholesterol are transported in the blood as lipoproteins. Lipoproteins are named according to their density, which increases with the percentage of protein in the particle. From least dense to most dense:

chylomicrons < VLDL < IDL (intermediate-density lipoproteins) < LDL (low-density lipoproteins) < HDL (high-density lipoproteins). An example of a lipoprotein is shown in Figure I-15-4.

The classes of lipoproteins and the important apoproteins associated with their functions are summarized in Table I-15-1 and Figure I-15-5.

Classes of Lipoproteins and Important Apoproteins

Table I-15-1. Classes of Lipoproteins and Important Apoproteins

Lipoprotein	Functions	Apoproteins	Functions
Chylomicrons	Transport dietary triglyceride and cholesterol from intestine to tissues	apoB-48 apoC-II apoE	Secreted by intestine Activates lipoprotein lipase Uptake of remnants by the liver
VLDL	Transports triglyceride from liver to tissues	apoB-100 apoC-II apoE	Secreted by liver Activates lipoprotein lipase Uptake of remnants (IDL) by liver
IDL (VLDL remnants)	Picks up cholesterol from HDL to become LDL Picked up by liver	apoE apoB-100	Uptake by liver
LDL	Delivers cholesterol into cells	apoB-100	Uptake by liver and other tissues via LDL receptor (apoB-100 receptor)
HDL	Picks up cholesterol accumulating in blood vessels Delivers cholesterol to liver and steroidogenic tissues via scavenger receptor (SR-B1) Shuttles apoC-II and apoE in blood	apoA-1	Activates lecithin cholesterol acyltransferase (LCAT) to produce cholesterol esters

Chapter 15 • Lipid Synthesis and Storage

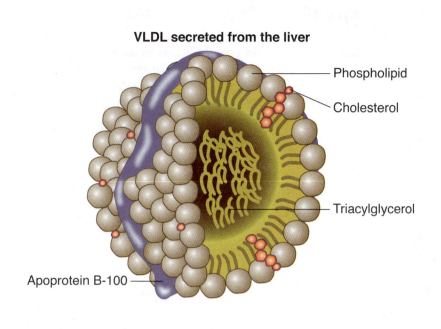

Figure I-15-4. Lipoprotein Structure

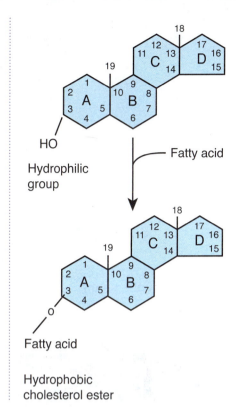

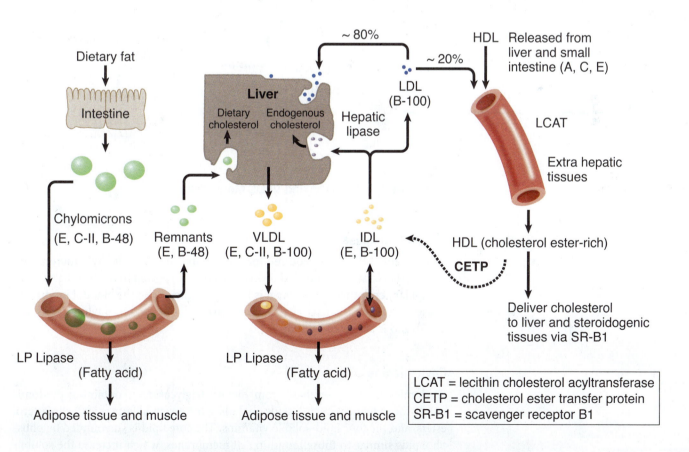

Figure I-15-5. Overview of Lipoprotein Metabolism

Section I • Biochemistry

Chylomicrons, VLDL, and IDL (VLDL Remnants)

Chylomicrons and VLDL are primarily triglyceride particles, although they each have small quantities of cholesterol esters. Chylomicrons transport dietary triglyceride to adipose tissue and muscle, whereas VLDL transport triglyceride synthesized in the liver to these same tissues. Both chylomicrons and VLDL have apoC-II, apoE, and apoB (apoB-48 on chylomicrons and apoB-100 on VLDL). The metabolism of these particles is shown in Figure I-15-6.

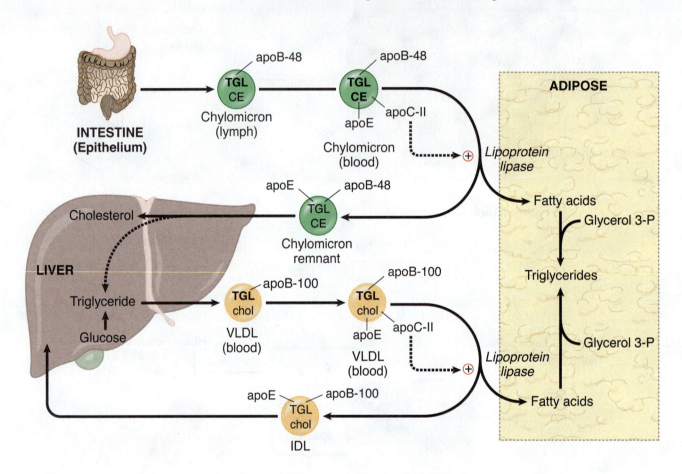

Figure I-15-6. Chylomicron and VLDL Metabolism

Lipoprotein lipase

Lipoprotein (LPLase) is required for the metabolism of both chylomicrons and VLDL. This enzyme is induced by insulin and transported to the luminal surface of capillary endothelium, where it is in direct contact with the blood. Lipoprotein lipase hydrolyzes the fatty acids from triglycerides carried by chylomicrons and VLDL and is activated by apoC-II.

Chylomicrons

Chylomicrons are assembled from dietary triglycerides (containing predominantly the longer chain fatty acids, including the essential fatty acids), cholesterol esters, and the four lipid-soluble vitamins. The core lipid is surrounded by phospholipids similar to those found in cell membranes, which increase the solubility of chylomicrons in lymph and blood. ApoB-48 is attached and required for release from the epithelial cells into the lymphatics.

Chylomicrons leave the lymph and enter the peripheral blood, where the thoracic duct joins the left subclavian vein, thus initially bypassing the liver. After a high-fat meal, chylomicrons cause serum to become turbid or milky. While in the blood, chylomicrons acquire apoC-II and apoE from HDL particles.

In capillaries of adipose tissue (and muscle), apoC-II activates lipoprotein lipase, the fatty acids released enter the tissue for storage, and the glycerol is retrieved by the liver, which has glycerol kinase. The chylomicron remnant is picked up by hepatocytes through the apoE receptor; thus, dietary cholesterol, as well as any remaining triglyceride, is released in the hepatocyte.

VLDL (very low-density lipoprotein)

The metabolism of VLDL is very similar to that of chylomicrons, the major difference being that VLDL are assembled in hepatocytes to transport triglyceride containing fatty acids newly synthesized from excess glucose, or retrieved from the chylomicron remnants, to adipose tissue and muscle. ApoB-100 is added in the hepatocytes to mediate release into the blood. Like chylomicrons, VLDL acquire apoC-II and apoE from HDL in the blood and are metabolized by lipoprotein lipase in adipose tissue and muscle.

VLDL remnants (IDL, intermediate-density lipoprotein)

After triglyceride is removed from the VLDL, the resulting particle is referred to as either a VLDL remnant or as an IDL. A portion of the IDLs is picked up by hepatocytes through their apoE receptor, but some of the IDLs remain in the blood, where they are further metabolized. These IDLs are transition particles between triglyceride and cholesterol transport. In the blood, they can acquire cholesterol esters transferred from HDL particles and thus become converted into LDLs, as shown in Figures I-15-5 and I-15-6.

LDL and HDL

LDL (low-density lipoprotein)

Although both LDL and HDL are primarily cholesterol particles, most of the cholesterol measured in the blood is associated with LDL. The normal role of LDL is to deliver cholesterol to tissues for biosynthesis. When a cell is repairing membrane or dividing, the cholesterol is required for membrane synthesis. Bile acids and salts are made from cholesterol in the liver, and many other tissues require some cholesterol for steroid synthesis. About 80% of LDL are picked up by hepatocytes, the remainder by peripheral tissues. ApoB-100 is the only apoprotein on LDL, and endocytosis of LDL is mediated by apoB-100 receptors (LDL receptors) clustered in areas of cell membranes lined with the protein clathrin.

Regulation of the Cholesterol Level in Hepatocytes

The liver has multiple pathways for acquiring cholesterol, including:

- *De novo* synthesis
- Endocytosis of LDL
- Transfer of cholesterol from HDL via the SR-B1 receptor
- Endocytosis of chylomicron remnants with residual dietary cholesterol

Increased cholesterol in the hepatocytes inhibits further accumulation by repressing the expression of the genes for HMG-CoA reductase, the LDL receptor, and the SR-B1 receptor.

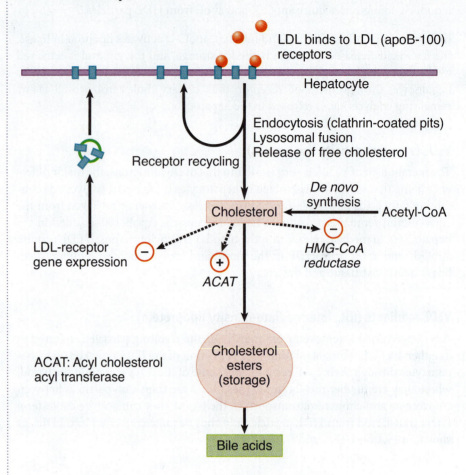

Figure I-15-7. Regulation of Cholesterol Level in Hepatocytes

As shown in Figure I-15-7, endocytosis involves:

- Formation of a coated pit, which further invaginates to become an endosome
- Fusion of the endosome with a lysosome, accompanied by acidification and activation of lysosomal enzymes
- Release of LDL from the LDL receptor

The receptor may recycle to the surface, the LDL is degraded, and cholesterol is released into the cell. Expression of the gene for LDL receptors (apoB-100 receptor) is regulated by the cholesterol level within the cell. High cholesterol decreases expression of this gene as well as the gene for HMG-CoA reductase, the rate limiting enzyme of *de novo* cholesterol synthesis.

HDL (high-density lipoprotein)

HDL is synthesized in the liver and intestines and released as dense, protein-rich particles into the blood. They contain apoA-1 used for cholesterol recovery from fatty streaks in the blood vessels. HDL also carry apoE and apoC-II, but those apoproteins are primarily to donate temporarily to chylomicrons and VLDL.

Lecithin–cholesterol acyltransferase (LCAT)

LCAT (or PCAT, phosphatidylcholine–cholesterol acyltransferase) is an enzyme in the blood that is activated by apoA-1 on HDL. LCAT adds a fatty acid to cholesterol, producing cholesterol esters, which dissolve in the core of the HDL, allowing HDL to transport cholesterol from the periphery to the liver. This process of reverse cholesterol transport is shown in Figure I-15-8.

Cholesterol ester transfer protein (CETP)

HDL cholesterol esters picked up in the periphery can be distributed to other lipoprotein particles such as VLDL remnants (IDL), converting them to LDL. The cholesterol ester transfer protein facilitates this transfer.

Scavenger receptors (SR-B1)

HDL cholesterol picked up in the periphery can also enter cells through a scavenger receptor, SR-B1. This receptor is expressed at high levels in hepatocytes and the steroidogenic tissues, including ovaries, testes, and areas of the adrenal glands. This receptor does not mediate endocytosis of the HDL, but rather transfer of cholesterol into the cell by a mechanism not yet clearly defined.

Atherosclerosis

The metabolism of LDL and HDL intersects in the production and control of fatty streaks and potential plaques in blood vessels. Figure I-15-8 illustrates one model of atherosclerosis involving HDL and LDL at the site of endothelial cell injury. Damage to the endothelium may be related to many factors, including normal turbulence of the blood, elevated LDL, especially modified or oxidized LDL, free radicals from cigarette smoking, homocystinemia (Chapter 17), diabetes (glycation of LDL), and hypertension. The atherosclerotic lesion represents an inflammatory response sharing several characteristics with granuloma formation, and not simple deposition of cholesterol in the blood vessel.

- Endothelial dysfunction increases adhesiveness and permeability of the endothelium for platelets and leukocytes. Infiltrations involve monocytes and T cells. Damaged endothelium has procoagulant rather than anticoagulant properties. In some cases, the endothelial lining may become partially denuded.

- Local inflammation recruits monocytes and macrophages with subsequent production of reactive oxygen species. LDL can become oxidized and then taken up, along with other inflammatory debris, by macrophages, which can become laden with cholesterol (foam cells). Initially the subendothelial accumulation of cholesterol-laden macrophages produces fatty streaks.

- As the fatty streak enlarges over time, necrotic tissue and free lipid accumulates, surrounded by epithelioid cells and eventually smooth muscle cells, an advanced plaque with a fibrous cap. The plaque eventually begins to occlude the blood vessel, causing ischemia and infarction in the heart, brain, or extremities.

Section I • Biochemistry

- Eventually the fibrous cap may thin, and the plaque becomes unstable, leading to rupture and thrombosis.
- HDL may be protective by picking up accumulating cholesterol before the advanced lesion forms. ApoA-1 activates LCAT, which in turn adds a fatty acid to cholesterol to produce a cholesterol ester that dissolves in the core of the HDL.
- The HDL may subsequently be picked up by the liver through the apoE receptor or deliver cholesterol through the scavenger receptor SR-B1 (reverse cholesterol transport from the periphery to the liver). The HDL may also transfer the cholesterol to an IDL, reforming a normal, unoxidized LDL particle.

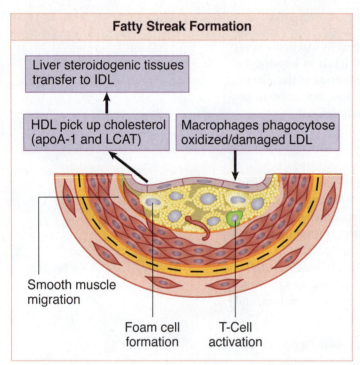
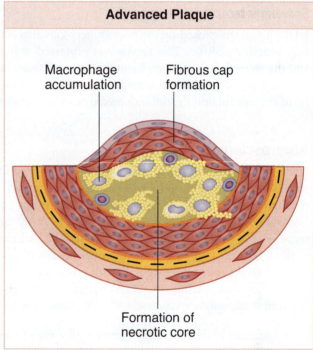

Figure I-15-8. LDL, HDL, and Atherogenesis

Role of Vitamin E

The oxidation of LDL at sites of endothelial damage is thought to be a major stimulus for uptake by macrophages. Some studies have shown a protective role of vitamin E in this process. Vitamin E is a lipid-soluble vitamin that acts as an antioxidant in the lipid phase. In addition to protecting LDL from oxidation, it may also prevent peroxidation of membrane lipids. Vitamins C and A lack this protective effect despite their antioxidant properties.

HYPERLIPIDEMIAS

Excess lipid in the blood can result from primary genetic deficiencies, most of which are rare, or as a secondary consequence of another disease. Two primary hyperlipidemias, type I hypertriglyceridemia and type IIa hypercholesterolemia, are summarized in Table I-15-2.

Table I-15-2. Primary Hyperlipidemias

Type	Deficiency	Lipid Elevated in Blood	Lipoprotein Elevated in Blood	Comments
I	Familial lipoprotein lipase (rare) apoC-II (rare) Autosomal recessive	Triglyceride	Chylomicrons	Red-orange eruptive xanthomas Fatty liver Acute pancreatitis Abdominal pain after fatty meal
IIa	Familial hypercholesterolemia Autosomal dominant (Aa 1/500, AA 1/106) LDL-receptor (LDL-R) deficiency	Cholesterol	LDL	High risk of atherosclerosis and coronary artery disease Homozygous condition, usually death <20 years Xanthomas of the Achilles tendon Tuberous xanthomas on elbows Xanthelasmas Corneal arcus

Type I Hypertriglyceridemia

Rare genetic absence of lipoprotein lipase results in excess triglyceride in the blood and its deposition in several tissues, including liver, skin, and pancreas. Orange-red eruptive xanthomas over the mucous membranes and skin may be seen. Abdominal pain and acute pancreatitis may occur. Fasting chylomicronemia produces a milky turbidity in the serum or plasma.

Diabetes, alcoholism, and glucose-6-phosphatase deficiency all can produce less severe hypertriglyceridemia with an increase in VLDL and chylomicrons. Factors contributing to the hyperlipidemia are:

- Decreased glucose and triglyceride uptake in adipose tissue
- Overactive hormone-sensitive lipase (Chapter 16, Figure I-16-1)
- Underactive lipoprotein lipase

Hyperlipidemia Secondary to Diabetes

A 20-year-old man was studying for his final exams and became hungry. He drove to the nearest fast food restaurant and ordered a double cheeseburger, extra large French fries, and a large soda. About an hour later, he developed serious abdominal distress, became nauseated, and was close to fainting. Upon his arrival at the emergency room, tests showed that he was hyperglycemic, as well as hypertriglyceridemic. His cholesterol levels were only slightly elevated. Additional information revealed that he was diabetic, and he recovered quickly after the administration of insulin.

The most common type of hyperlipidemias is type V, in which patients have elevated serum triglycerides in VLDL and chylomicrons in response to a meal containing carbohydrates and fat, respectively. One of the important regulatory functions of insulin in adipose tissue is promoting lipoprotein lipase activity by increasing transcription of its gene. Therefore, the consequence in diabetes is abnormally low levels of lipoprotein lipase and the inability to adequately degrade the serum triglycerides in lipoproteins to facilitate the uptake of fatty acids into adipocytes.

Type IIa Hypercholesterolemia (LDL Receptor Deficiency)

This is an autosomal dominant genetic disease affecting 1/500 (heterozygous) individuals in the United States. It is characterized by elevated LDL cholesterol and increased risk for atherosclerosis and coronary artery disease. Cholesterol deposits may be seen as:

- Xanthomas of the Achilles tendon
- Subcutaneous tuberous xanthomas over the elbows
- Xanthelasma (lipid in the eyelid)
- Corneal arcus

Homozygous individuals ($1/10^6$) often have myocardial infarctions before 20 years of age.

Abetalipoproteinemia (a Hypolipidemia)

Abetalipoproteinemia and hypobetalipoproteinemia are rare conditions that nevertheless illustrate the importance of lipid absorption and transport. Individuals with these conditions have low to absent serum apoB-100 and apoB-48. Serum triglycerides may be near zero, and cholesterol extremely low.

Because chylomicron levels are very low, fat accumulates in intestinal enterocytes and in hepatocytes. Essential fatty acids and vitamins A and E are not well absorbed. Symptoms in severe cases include:

- Steatorrhea
- Cerebellar ataxia
- Pigmentary degeneration in the retina
- Acanthocytes (thorny appearing erythrocytes)
- Possible loss of night vision

CHOLESTEROL METABOLISM

Cholesterol is required for membrane synthesis, steroid and vitamin D synthesis, and in the liver, bile acid synthesis. Most cells derive their cholesterol from LDL or HDL, but some cholesterol may be synthesized *de novo*. Most *de novo* synthesis occurs in the liver, where cholesterol is synthesized from acetyl-CoA in the cytoplasm. The citrate shuttle carries mitochondrial acetyl-CoA into the cytoplasm, and NADPH is provided by the HMP shunt and malic enzyme. Important points are noted in Figure I-15-9.

Chapter 15 • Lipid Synthesis and Storage

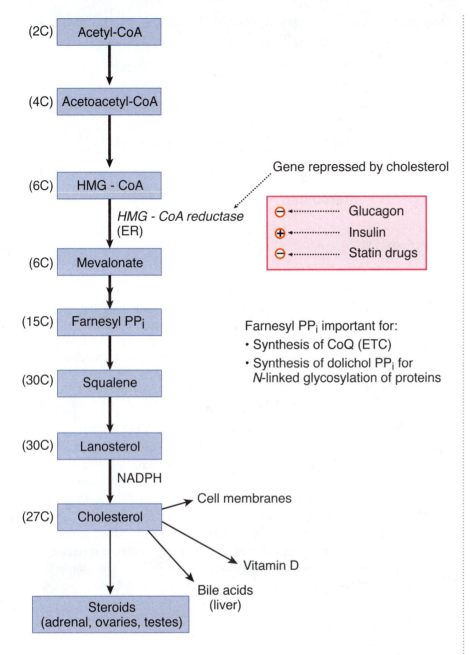

Figure I-15-9. Synthesis of Cholesterol

Bridge to Pharmacology
Treatment of Hypercholesterolemia

Cholestyramine and other drugs which increase elimination of bile salts force the liver to increase their synthesis from cholesterol, thus lowering the internal level of cholesterol in the hepatocytes. Decreased cholesterol within the cell increases LDL receptor expression, allowing the hepatocyte to remove more LDL cholesterol from the blood.

HMG-CoA reductase inhibitors such as atorvastatin and simvastatin inhibit *de novo* cholesterol synthesis in the hepatocyte, which subsequently increases LDL receptor expression.

3-Hydroxy-3-methylglutaryl (HMG)-CoA reductase on the smooth endoplasmic reticulum (SER) is the rate-limiting enzyme. Insulin activates the enzyme (dephosphorylation), and glucagon inhibits it. Mevalonate is the product, and the statin drugs competitively inhibit the enzyme. Cholesterol represses the expression of the HMG-CoA reductase gene and also increases degradation of the enzyme.

Section I • Biochemistry

Farnesyl pyrophosphate, an intermediate in the pathway, may also be used for:

- Synthesis of CoQ for the mitochondrial electron transport chain
- Synthesis of dolichol pyrophosphate, a required cofactor in *N*-linked glycosylation of proteins in the endoplasmic reticulum
- Prenylation of proteins (a posttranslational modification) that need to be held in the cell membrane by a lipid tail. An example is the p21*ras* G protein in the insulin and growth factor pathways.

Hypercholesterolemia

A 55-year-old man went to see his physician for his annual checkup. Over the past 5 years, his bloodwork consistently showed that his total cholesterol was slightly high (205–220 mg/dL), HDL was 45–50 mg/dL, and LDL was approximately 145 mg/dL. His serum C-reactive protein (CRP) value was always within normal range. Despite considerable efforts to lower his total cholesterol and LDL levels (exercise, one glass of wine per day, and carefully controlled diet), his blood cholesterol values did not significantly change. No other problems were evident. He recently heard that the ideal blood level of LDL should be <100 mg/dL. His physician decided to prescribe a statin drug. Within several weeks of taking the statin, he experienced more than usual muscle soreness, pain, and weakness when he exercised. He also noticed that his urine was red-brown.

For a large majority of people, statin drugs work efficiently and without side effects. Maximum lowering of blood cholesterol takes about 4–6 weeks. Because the liver is the site of most cholesterol synthesis, LFTs should be measured 2–3 months after starting the statin regimen. One consequence of statins inhibiting HMG-CoA reductase is the lessening of the downstream synthesis of CoQ, which is needed for the electron transport chain. Without properly functioning mitochondria, muscle would have a decreased ability to generate ATP required for muscle contraction. The red-brown urine is caused by the spillage of myoglobin from damaged muscle cells. CRP is a liver protein that is secreted in inflammation. There is a direct correlation between elevated CRP and atherosclerosis.

Chapter Summary

Fatty Acid Synthesis

- Cytoplasm
- Citrate shuttle
- Acetyl-CoA carboxylase (biotin)
  - Rate-limiting: Citrate activates, insulin activates
- Fatty acid synthase (requires NADPH)
  - Induced by insulin
- Malonyl-CoA is intermediate

Triglyceride Synthesis

- Glycerol 3-P dehydrogenase (liver and adipose)
- Glycerol kinase (liver)

Lipoproteins

- See Table I-15-1.
- Type I: Lipoprotein lipase deficiency (triglycerides)
- Type IIa: LDL (B-100) receptor deficiency (cholesterol)

Cholesterol Synthesis—Rate-Limiting Enzyme

- Most occurs in liver
- HMG-CoA reductase
  - Inhibited by statin drugs
- Precursor for
  - Vitamin D
  - Cell membranes
  - Bile salts/acids
  - Steroid hormones

Section I • Biochemistry

Review Questions

Select the ONE best answer.

1. What is the most positive activator of the process shown below?

   8 Acetyl-CoA + n ATP + 14 NADPH → palmitate + 8 CoASH + nADP + nPi + 14 NADP

   A. Acetyl-CoA
   B. Citrate
   C. Malonyl-CoA
   D. Malate
   E. Oxaloacetate

2. When adipose tissue stores triglyceride arriving from the liver or intestine, glycolysis must also occur in the adipocyte. Which of the following products or intermediates of glycolysis is required for fat storage?

   A. Glycerol
   B. Glucose 6-phosphate
   C. Pyruvate
   D. Acetyl-CoA
   E. Dihydroxyacetone phosphate

Items 3 and 4

Abetalipoproteinemia is a genetic disorder characterized by malabsorption of dietary lipid, steatorrhea (fatty stools), accumulation of intestinal triglyceride, and hypolipoproteinemia.

3. A deficiency in the production of which apoprotein would most likely account for this clinical presentation?

   A. ApoB-100
   B. ApoB-48
   C. ApoC-II
   D. ApoA-I
   E. ApoE

4. Patients with abetalipoproteinemia exhibit membrane abnormalities in their erythrocytes with production of acanthocytes (thorny-appearing cells). This unusual red cell morphology would most likely result from malabsorption of

   A. palmitic acid
   B. ascorbic acid
   C. arachidonic acid
   D. folic acid
   E. linoleic acid

5. A patient with a history of recurring attacks of pancreatitis, eruptive xanthomas, and increased plasma triglyceride levels (2,000 mg/dL) associated with chylomicrons, most likely has a deficiency in

   A. lipoprotein lipase
   B. LDL receptors
   C. HMG-CoA reductase
   D. apoB-48
   E. apoB-100 receptor

6. Uncontrolled phagocytosis of oxidized LDL particles is a major stimulus for the development of foam cells and fatty streaks in the vascular subendothelium. This process may be inhibited by increased dietary intake of

   A. vitamin E
   B. vitamin B_6
   C. vitamin D
   D. vitamin B_{12}
   E. vitamin K

Items 7–9

A 42-year-old man presents with a chief complaint of intermittent claudication during exercise. His family history is significant for the presence of cardiovascular disease on his father's side, but not on his mother's side. Physical exam reveals xanthelasmas and bilateral tendon xanthomas. A plasma lipid profile reveals a cholesterol level of 340 mg/dL, with a high LDL/HDL ratio. He is given instructions for dietary modifications and a prescription for simvastatin.

7. The clinical findings noted in this patient are most likely caused by deficient production of

   A. lethicin cholesterol acyltransferase
   B. apoB-100 receptors
   C. fatty acyl-CoA synthetase
   D. VLDL from LDL
   E. cholesterol ester transfer protein

8. The anticholesterolemic action of simvastatin is based on its effectiveness as a competitive inhibitor of the rate-limiting enzyme in cholesterol biosynthesis. The reaction product normally produced by this enzyme is

   A. squalene
   B. methylmalonate
   C. lanosterol
   D. mevalonate
   E. acetoacetate

Section I • Biochemistry

9. From a Lineweaver-Burk plot, the K_m and V_{max} of this rate-limiting enzyme were calculated to be 4×10^{-3} M and 8×10^2 mmol/h, respectively. If the above experiment is repeated in the presence of simvastatin, which of the following values would be obtained?

	K_m (M)	V_{max} (mmol/h)
A.	4×10^{-3}	3×10^2
B.	2×10^{-3}	1×10^2
C.	4×10^{-3}	9×10^2
D.	8×10^{-3}	8×10^2
E.	8×10^{-3}	9×10^2

10. A 20-year-old man is taken to the university clinic to determine the cause of recurring hyperlipidemia, proteinuria, and anemia. Fasting blood tests reveal slightly elevated concentrations of unesterified cholesterol and phosphatidylcholine. The patient is given a 100 gram chocolate bar and blood lipid levels are monitored hourly. Results reveal significantly increased levels of unesterified cholesterol and phosphatidylcholine for extended periods. A deficiency of which of the following proteins is most likely to be associated with the observations in this patient?

    A. Acyl-CoA:cholesterol acyltransferase (ACAT)
    B. Apoprotein A-1
    C. Apoprotein B48
    D. Apoprotein B100
    E. Lipoprotein lipase

Answers

1. **Answer: B.** Citrate is a potent activator of acetyl-CoA carboxylase for fatty acid synthesis.

2. **Answer: E.** To reform triglycerides from the incoming fatty acids, glycerol 3-P must be available. The adipose can produce this only from DHAP in glycolysis.

3. **Answer: B.** ApoB-48 is required for intestinal absorption of dietary fat in the form of chylomicrons. ApoB-100 formation is also impaired in these patients, but this would not explain the clinical symptoms described.

4. **Answer: E.** The genetic defect would result in malabsorption of the three fatty acids listed, but only linoleate is strictly essential in the diet. Absorption of water-soluble ascorbate and folate would not be significantly affected.

5. **Answer: A.** These are the clinical features of lipoprotein lipase deficiency (type I lipoproteinemia). LDL receptor defects would result in elevated LDLs. HMG-CoA reductase and ApoB-100 have no direct relationship to chylomicrons. ApoB-48 deficiency would result in decreased production of chylomicrons.

6. **Answer: A.** Only vitamin E is an antioxidant.

7. **Answer: B.** The findings are indicative of heterozygous type IIa familial hypercholesterolemia, an autosomal dominant disease. Deficient CETP, LCAT or fatty acid-CoA synthetase would not elevate LDL cholesterol. VLDL are not produced from LDL.

8. **Answer: D.** Must know that mevalonate precedes squalene and lanosterol in the pathway, and that methylmalonate and acetoacetate are not associated with cholesterolgenesis.

9. **Answer: D.** With a competitive inhibitor, there will be an increase in K_m with no change in V_{max}. Option A would be for a noncompetitive inhibitor (V_{max} decreased, K_m unaltered).

10. **Answer: B.** Apo A-1 is present on the surface of HDL and functions to activate circulating LCAT (lecithin:cholesterol acyltransferase) to esterify cholesterol, using lecithin (phosphatidylcholine) as the fatty acid donor. Esterification of cholesterol in blood occurs to trap the resultant cholesterol esters in HDL where they can subsequently be transferred to other lipoproteins (IDL) or taken up directly by hepatocytes and steroidogenic tissues.

    Deficiencies of apoprotein B100 and apoprotein B48 (**choices D and C**) result in abetalipoproteinemia characterized by decreased blood triglycerides and cholesterol.

    ACAT (**choice A**) is an intracellular enzyme and esterifies cholesterol inside cells, but not in blood.

    Deficiency of LPL (**choice E**) would result in type 1 hyperlipidemia and is characterized by elevated serum triglycerides.

Lipid Mobilization and Catabolism 16

Learning Objectives

❏ Solve problems concerning lipid mobilization
❏ Interpret scenarios about fatty acid oxidation
❏ Demonstrate understanding of ketone body metabolism
❏ Use knowledge of sphingolipids

LIPID MOBILIZATION

In the postabsorptive state, fatty acids can be released from adipose tissue to be used for energy. Although human adipose tissue does not respond directly to glucagon, the fall in insulin activates a hormone-sensitive triacylglycerol lipase (HSL) that hydrolyzes triglycerides, yielding fatty acids and glycerol. Epinephrine and cortisol also activate HSL. These steps are shown in Figure I-16-1.

Glycerol may be picked up by liver and converted to dihydroxyacetone phosphate (DHAP) for gluconeogenesis, and the fatty acids are distributed to tissues that can use them. Free fatty acids are transported through the blood in association with serum albumin.

Bridge to Pharmacology

Niacin is a commonly used antihyperlipidemic drug. In large doses (gram-level quantities that are well above the RDA), it works by inhibiting HSL in adipose tissue. With fewer fatty acids entering the liver, very low-density lipoprotein (VLDL) will not be assembled in normal amounts. Both VLDL (carrying triglycerides and cholesterol) and its product, LDL, will be lower in serum.

Section I • Biochemistry

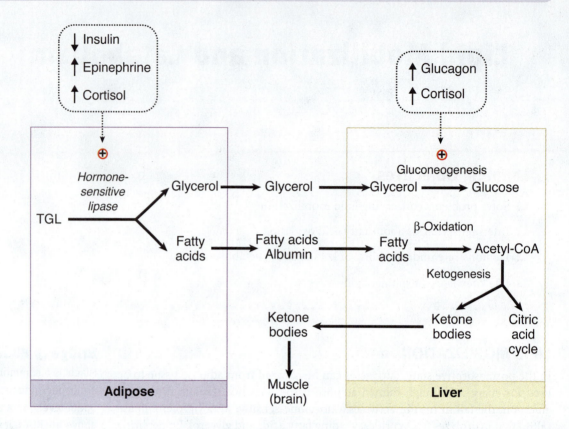

Figure I-16-1. Lipolysis of Triglyceride in Response to Hypoglycemia and Stress

FATTY ACID OXIDATION

Fatty acids are oxidized in several tissues, including liver, muscle, and adipose tissue, by the pathway of β-oxidation. Neither erythrocytes nor brain can use fatty acids and so continue to rely on glucose during normal periods of fasting. Erythrocytes lack mitochondria, and fatty acids do not cross the blood–brain barrier efficiently.

Short-chain fatty acids (2–4 carbons) and medium-chain fatty acids (6–12 carbons) diffuse freely into mitochondria to be oxidized. Long-chain fatty acids (14–20 carbons) are transported into the mitochondrion by a carnitine shuttle (Figure I-16-2) to be oxidized. Very long-chain fatty acids (>20 carbons) enter peroxisomes via an unknown mechanism for oxidation.

Fatty Acid Entry into Mitochondria

Long-chain fatty acids must be activated and transported into the mitochondria. Fatty acyl-CoA synthetase, on the outer mitochondrial membrane, activates the fatty acids by attaching CoA. The fatty acyl portion is then transferred onto carnitine by carnitine acyltransferase-1 for transport into the mitochondria. The sequence of events is shown in Figure I-16-2 and includes the following steps:

- Fatty acyl synthetase activates the fatty acid (outer mitochondrial membrane).
- Carnitine acyltransferase-1 transfers the fatty acyl group to carnitine (outer mitochondrial membrane).
- Fatty acylcarnitine is shuttled across the inner membrane.
- Carnitine acyltransferase-2 transfers the fatty acyl group back to a CoA (mitochondrial matrix).

Carnitine acyltransferase-1 is inhibited by malonyl-CoA from fatty acid synthesis and thereby prevents newly synthesized fatty acids from entering the mitochondria. Insulin indirectly inhibits β-oxidation by activating acetyl-CoA carboxylase (fatty acid synthesis) and increasing the malonyl-CoA concentration in the cytoplasm. Glucagon reverses this process.

β-Oxidation in Mitochondria

β-oxidation reverses the process of fatty acid synthesis by oxidizing (rather than reducing) and releasing (rather than linking) units of acetyl-CoA. The pathway is a repetition of four steps and is shown in Figure I-16-2. Each four-step cycle releases one acetyl-CoA and reduces NAD and FAD (producing NADH and $FADH_2$).

The $FADH_2$ and NADH are oxidized in the electron transport chain, providing ATP. In muscle and adipose tissue, the acetyl-CoA enters the citric acid cycle. In liver, the ATP may be used for gluconeogenesis, and the acetyl-CoA (which cannot be converted to glucose) stimulates gluconeogenesis by activating pyruvate carboxylase.

In a fasting state, the liver produces more acetyl-CoA from β-oxidation than is used in the citric acid cycle. Much of the acetyl-CoA is used to synthesize ketone bodies (essentially two acetyl-CoA groups linked together) that are released into the blood for other tissues.

In a Nutshell
Carnitine Acyltransferases

Carnitine acyltransferase-1 (CAT-1) and carnitine acyltransferase-2 (CAT-2) are also referred to as carnitine palmitoyl transferase-1 (CPT-1) and carnitine palmitoyl transferase-2 (CPT-2). The carnitine transport system is most important for allowing long-chain fatty acids to enter into the mitochondria.

In a Nutshell
β-oxidation of palmitate (16:0) yields 8 acetyl-CoA.

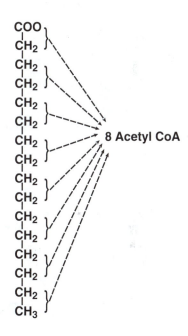

Section I • Biochemistry

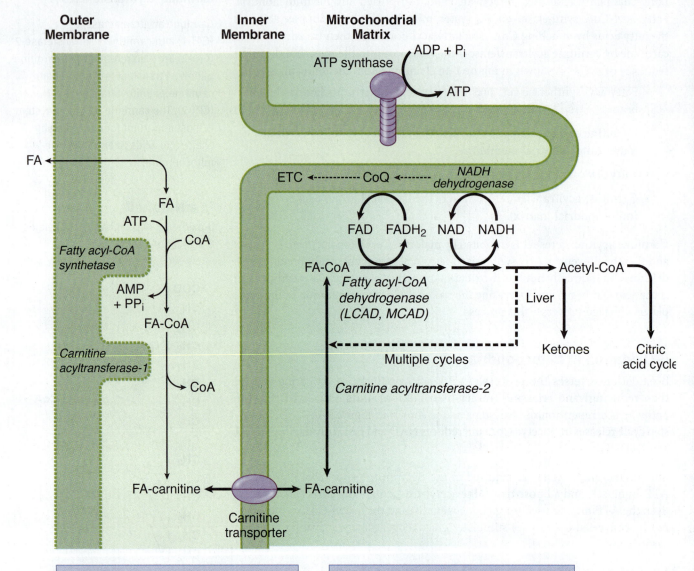

Figure I-16-2. Fatty Acid Activation, Transport, and β-Oxidation

Genetic deficiencies of fatty acid oxidation

Two of the most common genetic deficiencies affecting fatty acid oxidation are:

- Medium chain acyl-CoA dehydrogenase (MCAD) deficiency, primary etiology hepatic
- Myopathic carnitine acyltransferase (CAT/CPT) deficiency, primary etiology myopathic

Medium Chain Acyl-CoA Dehydrogenase (MCAD) Deficiency. Non-ketotic hypoglycemia should be strongly associated with a block in hepatic β-oxidation. During fasting, hypoglycemia can become profound due to lack of ATP to support gluconeogenesis. Decreased acetyl-CoA lowers pyruvate carboxylase activity and also limits ketogenesis. Hallmarks of MCAD deficiency include:

- Profound fasting hypoglycemia
- Low to absent ketones
- Lethargy, coma, death if untreated
- C8–C10 acyl carnitines in blood
- Episode may be provoked by overnight fast in an infant
- In older child, often provoked by illness (flu) that causes loss of appetite and vomiting
- Primary treatment: IV glucose
- Prevention: frequent feeding, high-carbohydrate, low-fat diet

Most individuals affected with MCAD deficiency lead reasonable lives if they take frequent carbohydrate meals to avoid periods of hypoglycemia. Complications arise when fatty meals are ingested and the MCAD enzyme is required to catabolize them. Also, in times of metabolic stress induced by severe fasting, exercise, or infection (conditions with high demands on fatty acid oxidation), symptoms of MCAD deficiency are manifested. It is now believed that some cases of sudden infant death syndrome were due to MCAD deficiency. The incidence of MCAD deficiency is one of the highest of the inborn errors of metabolism (estimated at 1/10,000).

MCAD Deficiency

A 6-year-old suffered gastroenteritis for 3 days that culminated in a brief generalized seizure, which left him semicomatose. Admitting blood glucose was 45 mg/dL (0.25 mM), and his urine was negative for glucose and ketones. Administering intravenous glucose improved his condition within 10 minutes. Subsequent bloodwork revealed elevated C8–C10 acyl carnitines. Following diagnosis of an enzyme deficiency, the boy's parents were cautioned to make sure that he eats meals frequently.

The presence of severe hypoglycemia and absence of ketosis (hypoketosis) is strongly suggestive of a block in β-oxidation. The episode in this case was precipitated by the 3-day gastroenteritis (vomiting/fasting). The elevated C8–C10 acyl carnitines accumulate due to the defective MCAD and they leak into serum. These compounds are detected using sophisticated tandem mass spectrometry.

Clinical Correlate

Ackee, a fruit that grows on the ackee tree found in Jamaica and West Africa, contains hypoglycin, a toxin that acts as an inhibitor of fatty acyl-CoA dehydrogenase. Jamaican vomiting sickness and severe hypoglycemia can result if it is ingested. It is characterized by a sudden onset of vomiting 2–6 hours after ingesting an ackee-containing meal. After a period of prostration that may last as long as 18 hours, more vomiting may occur, followed by convulsions, coma, and death.

Carnitine Acyltransferase-2 CAT-2/CPT-2 (Myopathic Form adolescent or adult onset). Although all tissues with mitochondria contain carnitine acyltransferase, the most common form of this genetic deficiency is myopathic and due to a defect in the muscle-specific CAT/CPT gene. It is an autosomal recessive condition with late onset. Hallmarks of this disease include:

- Muscle aches; mild to severe weakness
- Rhabdomyolysis, myoglobinuria, "red urine"
- Episode provoked by prolonged exercise especially after fasting, cold, or associated stress
- Symptoms may be exacerbated by high-fat, low-carbohydrate diet
- Muscle biopsy shows elevated muscle triglyceride detected as lipid droplets in cytoplasm
- Primary treatment: cease muscle activity and give glucose

A somewhat similar syndrome can be produced by muscle carnitine deficiency secondary to a defect in the transport system for carnitine in muscle.

Propionic Acid Pathway

Fatty acids with an odd number of carbon atoms are oxidized by β-oxidation identically to even-carbon fatty acids. The difference results only from the final cycle, in which even-carbon fatty acids yield two acetyl-CoA (from the 4-carbon fragment remaining) but odd-carbon fatty acids yield one acetyl-CoA and one propionyl-CoA (from the 5-carbon fragment remaining).

Propionyl-CoA is converted to succinyl-CoA, a citric acid cycle intermediate, in the two-step propionic acid pathway. Because this extra succinyl-CoA can form malate and enter the cytoplasm and gluconeogenesis, odd-carbon fatty acids represent an exception to the rule that fatty acids cannot be converted to glucose in humans. The propionic acid pathway is shown in Figure I-16-3 and includes two important enzymes, both in the mitochondria:

- Propionyl-CoA carboxylase requires biotin.
- Methylmalonyl-CoA mutase requires vitamin B_{12}, cobalamin.

Vitamin B_{12} deficiency can cause a megaloblastic anemia of the same type seen in folate deficiency (discussed in Chapter 17). In a patient with megaloblastic anemia, it is important to determine the underlying cause because B_{12} deficiency, if not corrected, produces a peripheral neuropathy owing to aberrant fatty acid incorporation into the myelin sheets associated with inadequate methylmalonyl-CoA mutase activity. Excretion of methylmalonic acid indicates a vitamin B_{12} deficiency rather than folate.

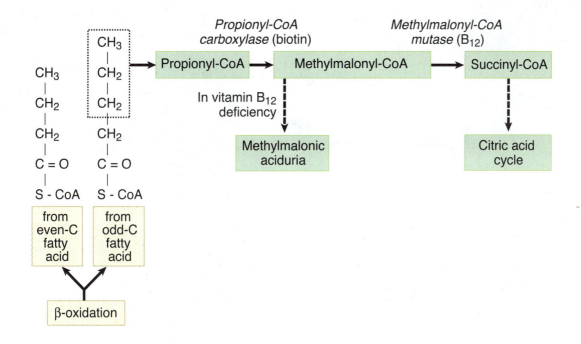

Figure I-16-3. The Propionic Acid Pathway

KETONE BODY METABOLISM

In the fasting state, the liver converts excess acetyl-CoA from β-oxidation of fatty acids into ketone bodies, acetoacetate and 3-hydroxybutyrate (β-hydroxybutyrate), which are used by extrahepatic tissues. Cardiac and skeletal muscles and renal cortex metabolize acetoacetate and 3-hydroxybutyrate to acetyl-CoA. Normally during a fast, muscle metabolizes ketones as rapidly as the liver releases them, preventing their accumulation in blood. After a week of fasting, ketones reach a concentration in blood high enough for the brain to begin metabolizing them. If ketones increase sufficiently in the blood, they can lead to ketoacidosis. Ketogenesis and ketogenolysis are shown in Figure I-16-4.

Section I • Biochemistry

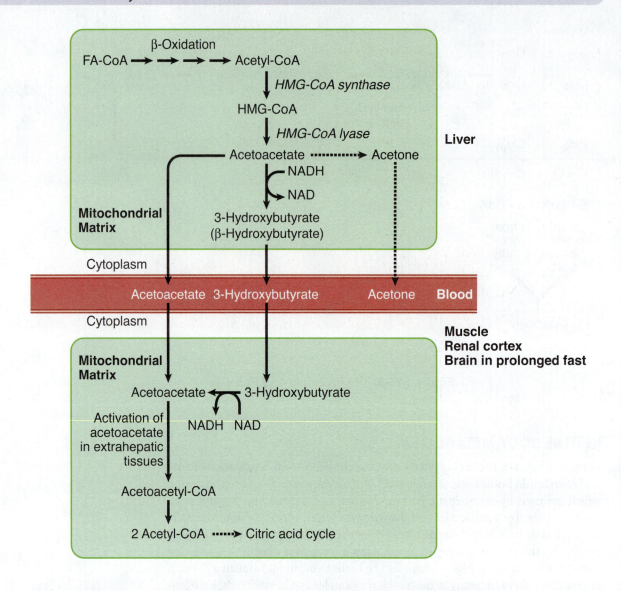

Figure I-16-4. Ketogenesis (Liver) and Ketogenolysis (Extrahepatic)

Clinical Correlate

In untreated type 1 diabetes mellitus, there is no insulin. Although glucose may be high, no insulin is released, HSL is active, b-oxidation is not inhibited, and ketone bodies are generated.

Ketogenesis

Ketogenesis occurs in mitochondria of hepatocytes when excess acetyl-CoA accumulates in the fasting state. HMG-CoA synthase forms HMG-CoA, and HMG-CoA lyase breaks HMG-CoA into acetoacetate, which can subsequently be reduced to 3-hydroxybutyrate. Acetone is a minor side product formed nonenzymatically but is not used as a fuel in tissues. It does, however, impart a strong odor (sweet or fruity) to the breath, which is almost diagnostic for ketoacidosis.

Ketogenolysis

Acetoacetate picked up from the blood is activated in the mitochondria by succinyl-CoA acetoacetyl-CoA transferase (common name thiophorase), an enzyme present only in extrahepatic tissues; 3-hydroxybutyrate is first oxidized to acetoacetate. Because the liver lacks this enzyme, it cannot metabolize the ketone bodies.

Ketogenolysis in brain

Figure I-16-5 shows the major pathways producing fuel for the brain. Note the important times at which the brain switches from:

- Glucose derived from liver glycogenolysis to glucose derived from gluconeogenesis (~12 hours)
- Glucose derived from gluconeogenesis to ketones derived from fatty acids (~1 week)

In the brain, when ketones are metabolized to acetyl-CoA, pyruvate dehydrogenase is inhibited. Glycolysis and subsequently glucose uptake in brain decreases. This important switch spares body protein (which otherwise would be catabolized to form glucose by gluconeogenesis in the liver) by allowing the brain to indirectly metabolize fatty acids as ketone bodies.

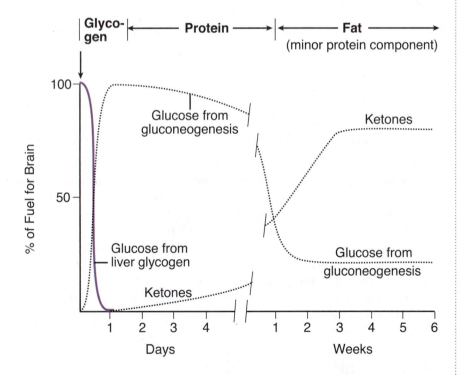

Figure I-16-5. Fuel Use in the Brain During Fasting and Starvation

Ketoacidosis

In patients with type 1 insulin-dependent diabetes mellitus not adequately treated with insulin, fatty acid release from adipose tissue and ketone synthesis in the liver exceed the ability of other tissues to metabolize them, and a profound, life-threatening ketoacidosis may occur. An infection or trauma (causing an increase in cortisol and epinephrine) may precipitate an episode of ketoacidosis by activating HSL. Patients with type 2 non–insulin-dependent diabetes mellitus (NIDDM) are much less likely to show ketoacidosis. The basis for this observation is not completely understood, although type 2 disease has a much slower, insidious onset, and insulin resistance in the periphery is usually not complete. Type 2 diabetics can develop ketoacidosis after an infection or trauma. In certain populations with NIDDM, ketoacidosis is much more common than previously appreciated.

Alcoholics can also develop ketoacidosis. Chronic hypoglycemia, which is often present in chronic alcoholism, favors fat release from adipose. Ketone production increases in the liver, but utilization in muscle may be slower than normal because alcohol is converted to acetate in the liver, diffuses into the blood, and oxidized by muscle as an alternative source of acetyl-CoA.

Associated with ketoacidosis:

- Polyuria, dehydration, and thirst (exacerbated by hyperglycemia and osmotic diuresis)
- CNS depression and coma
- Potential depletion of K^+ (although loss may be masked by a mild hyperkalemia)
- Decreased plasma bicarbonate
- Breath with a sweet or fruity odor, acetone

Laboratory measurement of ketones

In normal ketosis (that accompanies fasting and does not produce an acidosis), acetoacetate and β-hydroxybutyrate are formed in approximately equal quantities. In pathologic conditions, such as diabetes and alcoholism, ketoacidosis may develop with life-threatening consequences. In diabetic and alcoholic ketoacidosis, the ratio between acetoacetate and β-hydroxybutyrate shifts and β-hydroxybutyrate predominates. The urinary nitroprusside test detects only acetoacetate and can dramatically underestimate the extent of ketoacidosis and its resolution during treatment. β-Hydroxybutyrate should be measured in these patients. Home monitors of both blood glucose and β-hydroxybutyrate are available for diabetic patients.

SPHINGOLIPIDS

Sphingolipids are important constituents of cell membranes, as shown in Figure I-16-6. Although sphingolipids contain no glycerol, they are similar in structure to the glycerophospholipids in that they have a hydrophilic region and two fatty acid–derived hydrophobic tails. The various classes of sphingolipids shown in Figure I-16-7 differ primarily in the nature of the hydrophilic region.

Clinical Correlate

Insulin facilitates uptake of potassium by cells, so K^+ levels may be normal before DKA is treated with insulin. Once insulin is administered, however, blood potassium levels need to be monitored.

Chapter 16 • Lipid Mobilization and Catabolism

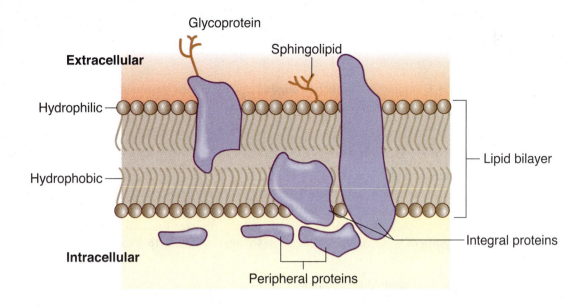

Figure I-16-6. Plasma Membrane

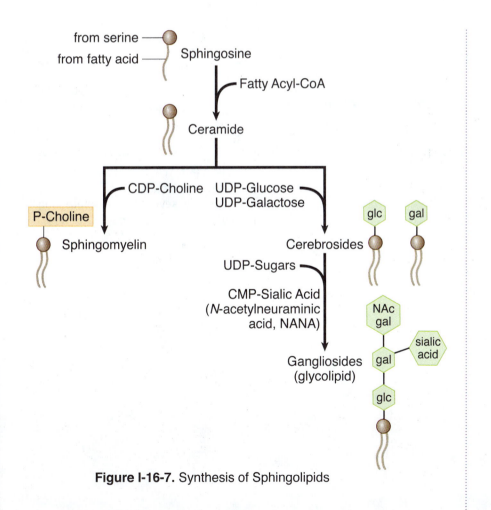

Figure I-16-7. Synthesis of Sphingolipids

Section I • Biochemistry

Classes of sphingolipids and their hydrophilic groups include:
- Sphingomyelin: phosphorylcholine
- Cerebrosides: galactose or glucose
- Gangliosides: branched oligosaccharide chains terminating in the 9-carbon sugar, sialic acid (*N*-acetylneuraminic acid, NANA)

Genetic Deficiencies of Enzymes in Sphingolipid Catabolism

Sphingolipids released when membrane is degraded are digested in endosomes after fusion with lysosomes. Lysosomes contain many enzymes, each of which removes specific groups from individual sphingolipids. Genetic deficiencies of many of these enzymes are known, and the diseases share some of the characteristics of I-cell disease discussed in Chapter 4. Table I-16-1 summarizes these.

Table I-16-1. Genetic Deficiencies of Sphingolipid Catabolism

Disease	Lysosomal Enzyme Missing	Substrate Accumulating in Inclusion Body	Symptoms
Tay-Sachs	Hexosaminidase A	Ganglioside GM_2	Cherry red spots in macula Blindness Psychomotor retardation Death usually <2 years Startle reflex
Gaucher	Glucocerebrosidase	Glucocerebroside	Type 1 (99%): Adult hepatosplenomegaly Erosion of bones, fractures Pancytopenia or thrombocytopenia Characteristic macrophages (crumpled paper inclusions)
Niemann-Pick	Sphingomyelinase	Sphingomyelin	May see cherry red spot in macula Hepatosplenomegaly Microcephaly, severe mental retardation Foamy macrophages with zebra bodies Early death

Gaucher Disease

A 9-year-old boy of Ashkenazic Jewish descent was brought to the university hospital because he was extremely lethargic and bruised easily. The attending physician noted massive hepatomegaly and splenomegaly, marked pallor, and hematologic complications. A histologic examination obtained from bone marrow showed a "wrinkled" appearance of the cytoplasm and that the cytoplasm was highly PAS stain positive. White cells were taken to assay for glucocerebrosidase, and the activity of the enzyme was found to be markedly below normal.

Outside the brain, glucocerebroside arises mainly from the breakdown of old red and white blood cells. In the brain, glucocerebroside arises from the turnover of gangliosides during brain development and formation of the myelin sheath. Without the proper degradation of glucocerebroside due to a lack of glucocerebrosidase, it accumulates in cells and tissues responsible for its turnover. This results in "wrinkled-paper" cytoplasm and carbohydrate positive staining. The easy bruising is due to a low blood platelet count, and the lethargy is due to the anemia.

Highly effective enzyme replacement therapy is available for Gaucher patients. Enzyme replacement therapy results in the reduction of hepatosplenomegaly, skeletal abnormalities, and other Gaucher-associated problems. The major drawback of therapy using intravenously administered recombinant glucocerebrosidase is its prohibitive cost (several hundred thousand dollars per year).

Fabry Disease

In contrast to the other sphingolipidoses (Tay-Sachs, Gaucher, Niemann-Pick) which are all autosomal recessive, Fabry disease is the only one that is X-linked recessive. Fabry is caused by a mutation in the gene that encodes the lysosomal enzyme alpha-galactosidase. Ceramide trihexoside accumulates in the lysosomes. Fabry disease presents during childhood or adolescence:

- Burning sensations in the hands which gets worse with exercise and hot weather
- Small, raised reddish-purple blemishes on the skin (angiokeratomas)
- Eye manifestations, especially cloudiness of the cornea
- Impaired arterial circulation and increased risk of heart attack or stroke
- Enlargement of the heart and kidneys
- Often there is survival into adulthood but with increased risk of cardiovascular disease, stroke.
- Renal failure is often the cause of death.

Enzyme replacement therapy is available and, although expensive, slows the progression of the disease.

Section I • Biochemistry

Chapter Summary

β-Oxidation

Fat Release From Adipose

- Hormone-sensitive lipase
  - Activated by decreased insulin, increased epinephrine
  - Induced by cortisol

Transport of Fatty Acids Into Mitochondria of Target Tissues

- Carnitine shuttle

Rate-Limiting Enzyme

- Carnitine acyltransferase-1 (CAT-1, CPT-1)
  - Inhibited by malonyl-CoA (increases during fatty acid synthesis)

Important Deficiencies

- Medium-chain acyl-CoA dehydrogenase (MCAD)
  - Profound fasting hypoglycemia
  - Hypoketosis
  - C8–C10 Acylcarnitines in blood
- Myopathic CAT-2 (CPT-2) deficiency
  - Extreme muscle weakness associated with endurance exercise and/or exercise after prolonged fasting
  - Rhabdomyolysis and myoglobinuria
- Myopathic carnitine deficiency
  - Similar to CAT-1 deficiency but less severe

Odd-Carbon Fatty Acid Oxidation

- Propionyl-CoA/B_{12} required

Ketone Bodies

- Formed from excess hepatic acetyl-CoA during fasting: acetoacetate, 3-hydroxybutyrate, and acetone (not metabolized further)
- Oxidized in cardiac skeletal muscle, renal cortex, and brain (prolonged fast)

Sphingolipids

- Constituents of lipid bilayer membranes
  - Sphingomyelin (ceramide + P and choline)
  - Cerebrosides (ceramide + glc or gal)
  - Gangliosides/glycolipids (ceramide + oligosaccharides + sialic acid)

Genetic Deficiencies

- Tay-Sachs (hexosaminidase A)
- Niemann-Pick (sphingomyelinase)
- Gaucher (glucocerebrosidase)

Chapter 16 • Lipid Mobilization and Catabolism

Review Questions

Select the ONE best answer.

1. As part of a study to quantify contributors of stress to hyperglycemia and ketosis in diabetes, normal hepatocytes and adipocytes in tissue culture were treated with cortisol and analyzed by Northern blotting using a gene-specific probe. The results of one experiment are shown below.

    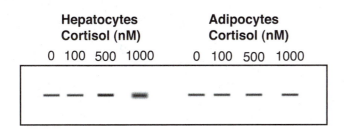

    The ^{32}P-probe used in this experiment most likely binds to a mRNA encoding

    A. phosphoenolpyruvate carboxykinase
    B. lipoprotein lipase
    C. glucokinase
    D. hormone-sensitive lipase
    E. acetyl-CoA carboxylase

2. A child is diagnosed with a congenital deficiency of medium-chain acyl-CoA dehydrogenase activity. Which of the following signs or symptoms would most likely occur upon fasting in this child?

    A. Hypolacticacidemia
    B. Ketoacidosis
    C. Hyperglycemia
    D. Dicarboxylic acidosis
    E. Hyperchylomicronemia

3. A 3-year-old child complains of muscle pain and weakness while in the playground and is admitted to the hospital for examination. Tests reveal slight hepatomegaly and cardiomegaly. A liver biopsy shows extreme but nonspecific fatty changes, and a muscle biopsy contains large amounts of cytoplasmic vacuoles containing neutral lipid. A one-day fast is performed and shows a drop in blood glucose levels without a corresponding production of ketone bodies. The pH of the blood is normal. Which of the following diagnoses might account for this child's problems?

    A. Bilirubin diglucuronide transporter deficiency
    B. Glucose 6-phosphatase deficiency
    C. Mitochondrial 3-hydroxy 3-methylglutaryl-CoA synthase deficiency
    D. Systemic carnitine deficiency
    E. Vitamin D deficiency

Items 4–6

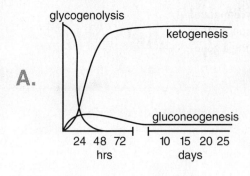

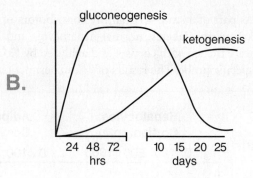

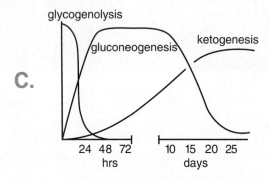

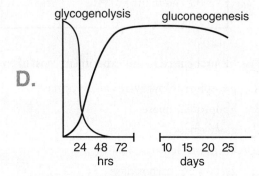

In the options above, each graph depicts the primary source of fuel used by the brain during fasting/starvation. For each condition listed below, select the most closely matched graph.

4. Normal individual

5. Liver phosphorylase deficiency

6. Hepatic fructose-1,6-bisphosphatase deficiency

Items 7–9

A 54-year-old man with type 1 (IDDM) diabetes is referred to an ophthalmologist for evaluation of developing cataracts. Pre-appointment blood work was requested and the results are shown below:

Fasting blood glucose	180 mg/dL
Hemoglobin A	15 gm/dL
Hemoglobin A_{1c}	10% of total Hb
Urine ketones	Positive
Urine glucose	Positive

7. Which of the following enzymes is most strongly associated with cataract formation in this patient?

    A. Galactokinase
    B. Aldose reductase
    C. Glucokinase
    D. Galactose 1-P uridyl transferase
    E. Aldolase B

8. Which of the following best indicates that the blood glucose in this patient has been elevated over a period of weeks?

    A. Presence of ketone bodies
    B. Hyperglycemia
    C. Lipemia
    D. Elevated HbA_{1c}
    E. Lipoprotein lipase

9. Which of the following enzymes would be more active in this patient than in a normal control subject?

    A. Hormone-sensitive lipase
    B. Glucokinase
    C. Fatty acid synthase
    D. Glycogen synthase
    E. Lipoprotein lipase

Section I • Biochemistry

10. A 40-year-old woman with a history of bleeding and pancytopenia now presents with leg pain. She describes a deep, dull pain of increasing severity that required pain medication. Computed tomography examination reveals erosion and thinning of the femoral head. A bone marrow biopsy is performed to confirm a diagnosis of Gaucher disease. What material would be found abnormally accumulating in the lysosomes of her cells?

    A. Mucopolysaccharide
    B. Ganglioside
    C. Ceramide
    D. Cerebroside
    E. Sulfatide

11. An underweight 4-year-old boy presents semicomatose in the emergency room at 10 A.M. Plasma glucose, urea, and glutamine are abnormally low; acetoacetate is elevated; and lactate is normal. He is admitted to the ICU, where an increase in blood glucose was achieved by controlled infusion of glucagon or alanine. Which metabolic pathway is most likely deficient in this child?

    A. Hepatic gluconeogenesis
    B. Skeletal muscle glycogenolysis
    C. Adipose tissue lipolysis
    D. Skeletal muscle proteolysis
    E. Hepatic glycogenolysis

12. After suffering injuries in a motor vehicle accident, a 7-year old boy undergoes open reduction surgery to repair a compound fractured femur. Post-surgically, the boy undergoes severe hemorrhage and requires transfusion of 8 units of blood. Coagulation studies demonstrate the PT time to be normal, but the PTT time is prolonged. Mixing the boy's plasma with normal plasma returns the PTT time to normal. The mode of inheritance of this boy's disease is most similar to which of the following inherited enzyme deficiencies?

    A. Adenosine deaminase deficiency
    B. α-Galactosidase A deficiency
    C. Glucocerebrosidase deficiency
    D. Hexosaminidase A deficiency
    E. Dystrophia myotonica protein kinase deficiency

13. A 15-month-old female infant is brought to the emergency room by her parents. The infant's mother did not receive routine pre-natal care, and limited information is available regarding the infant's pediatric care. The mother does reveal that the infant "doesn't seem like her other children" and has always been very "fussy.'" Physical examination reveals a distressed infant who does not verbalize. Her abdomen is tender and enlargement of both spleen and liver are present. Opthalmoscopic examination fails to reveal cherry-red spots. After a brief hospital course, the infant dies and autopsy is performed. Neural tissue shows parallel striations of electron-dense material within lysosomes. A defect in which of the following was most likely present in this infant?

    A. Golgi-associated phosphate transfer to mannose
    B. Degradation of ganglioside GM2
    C. Degradation of glucocerebrosides
    D. Degradation of sphingomyelin
    E. Synthesis of gangliosides

Items 14–17

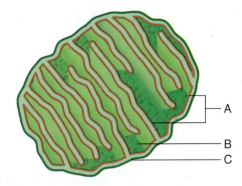

For each item listed below, select the appropriate location from the drawing shown above.

14. Carnitine shuttle

15. F_0F_1 ATP synthase

16. HMG-CoA lyase

17. Carnitine palmitoyltransferase-1

Answers

1. **Answer: A.** Cortisol stimulates transcription of the PEP carboxykinase gene in the liver but not in adipose tissue.

2. **Answer: D.** Fasted MCAD patients typically present with nonketotic hypoglycemia, lactic acidosis, and plasma dicarboxylates.

3. **Answer: D.** Upon entry into the playground to have fun, the child secretes epinephrine, which results in adipose tissue triglyceride (TG) breakdown and entry of fatty acids (FA) into muscle and liver for mitochrondrial

Section I • Biochemistry

β-oxidation. A defect in the carnitine shuttle system in this patient would result in accumulation of TG (re-synthesis from FA) in liver and muscle cytoplasm.

Deficiency of the bilirubin diglucuronide transporter (**choice A**) would result in a liver problem but not the muscle problem that this child has, since the liver processes bilirubin. One would also expect an increase in conjugated bilirubin and clay-colored stools if bilirubin diglucuronide was not entering the bile caniculi.

Glucose 6-phosphatase deficiency (**choice B**) would account for the hepatomegaly and fatty liver, but not for the muscle weakness. These individuals are also prone to lactic acidosis, which would lower the blood pH.

Mitochondrial 3-hydroxy 3-methylglutaryl-CoA (HMG-CoA) synthase deficiency (**choice C**) would present somewhat similarly to a β-oxidation deficiency. Prolonged fasting hypoglycemia would provoke release of fatty acids into the blood and their use by tissues such as the muscle and liver. The deficiency of the mitochondrial HMG-Co synthase prevents ketone formation. There would be no muscle weakness because the muscle can use fatty acids. The brain is unable to do so, and the presence of hypoketotic hypoglycemia would deprive the brain of sufficient energy. Coma and death may result.

Vitamin D deficiency (**choice E**) would not have an effect on organ enlargement and blood glucose levels.

4. **Answer: C.** Glycogen depleted around 18 hours, gluconeogenesis from protein begins to drop gradually, and by 2 weeks, ketones have become the more important fuel for the brain.

5. **Answer: B.** Glycogen would not be mobilized from the liver.

6. **Answer: A.** Gluconeogenesis from proteins would be severely restricted without this enzyme.

7. **Answer: B.** Aldose reductase is rich in lens and nerve tissue (among others) and converts glucose to sorbitol, which causes the osmotic damage. In galactosemia, this same enzyme converts galactose to galactitol, also creating cataracts.

8. **Answer: D.** HbA_{1c} is glycosylated HbA and is produced slowly whenever the glucose in blood is elevated. It persists until the RBC is destroyed and the Hb degraded and so is useful as a long-term indicator of glucose level.

9. **Answer: A.** Because the diabetes is not being well controlled, assume the response to insulin is low and the man would have overstimulated glucagon pathways.

10. **Answer: D.** Glucocerebrosides would accumulate in the cells because the missing enzyme is glucocerebrosidase.

11. **Answer: D.** The patient is hypoglycemic because of deficient release of gluconeogenic amino acid precursors from muscle (low urea and glutamine, alanine and glucagon challenge tests). These results plus normal lactate and hyperketonemia eliminate deficiencies in glycogenolysis, gluconeogenesis, and lipolysis as possibilities; defective muscle glycogenolysis would not produce hypoglycemia.

12. **Answer: B.** The excessive bleeding, increased PTT, and correction of the PTT with addition of normal serum point to hemophilia. The most common types of hemophilia are hemophilia A (deficiency in clotting factor VIII) and hemophilia B (Christmas disease; caused by a deficiency in clotting factor IX). The genes encoding both of these proteins are carried on the X-chromosome, making these X-linked recessive diseases. The only disease listed above which is inherited in an X-linked manner is Fabry disease, caused by a defect in α-galactosidase A involved with degradation of glycosphingolipids.

    (**Choices C and D**) are autosomal recessive inherited disorders of sphingolipid catabolism (Gaucher and Tay-Sachs respectively) classified as lysosomal storage diseases.

    (**Choice E**) is an autosomal dominant inherited disorder (myotonic dystrophy) which displays trinucleotide repeat expansion and anticipation.

13. **Answer: D.** Niemann-Pick (Type A) disease is characterized by hepatosplenomegaly, with or without cherry-red spots in the macular region, neurologic involvement (mental retardation, failure to crawl, sit, or walk independently).

    I-cell disease (**choice A**) is caused by a defect in Golgi-associated phosphotransferase (N-Acetylglucosamine-1-phosphotransferase), which would usually present with cardiomegaly and would not show the Zebra body inclusions typical of Niemann-Pick.

    Tay-Sachs disease (**choice B**) is caused by a defect in hexosaminidase A. In most cases, this will present with the cherry-red spots and would not have Zebra body inclusions inside lysosomes. No hepatosplenomegaly occurs.

    (**Choice C**) describes Gaucher's disease, caused by a defect in glucocerebrosidase and would lead to "crumpled paper inclusions" inside macrophages. The features include bone pain, fractures, and infarctions along with hepatosplenomegaly. Most cases are Type 1 and don't present until late childhood or adolescence.

    (**Choice E**) is a distractor. There are no relevant diseases on Step 1 associated with ganglioside synthesis.

    Note: The patient in this case did not have "cherry-red spots" in the macula of the eye. Both Tay-Sachs and Niemann-Pick disease may present with cherry-red spots, but they are not specific to either disease. Similarly, their absence cannot be used to exclude either disease.

14. **Answer: A.** Needed for transport of fatty acids across the mitochondrial inner membrane.

15. **Answer: A.** Mitochondrial inner membrane.

16. **Answer: B.** Mitochondrial matrix (ketogenesis).

17. **Answer: C.** CAT-1 (CPT-1) and fatty acyl synthetase are among the few enzymes associated with the outer mitochondrial membrane.

Amino Acid Metabolism 17

Learning Objectives

❏ Explain information related to removal and excretion of amino groups
❏ Answer questions about urea cycle
❏ Answer questions about disorders of amino acid metabolism
❏ Explain information related to propionyl-coa carboxylase and methylmalonyl-coa
❏ Use knowledge of mutase deficiencies
❏ Use knowledge of s-adenosylmethionine, folate, and cobalamin
❏ Explain information related to specialized products derived from amino acids
❏ Solve problems concerning heme synthesis
❏ Use knowledge of iron transport and storage
❏ Use knowledge of bilirubin metabolism

OVERVIEW

Protein obtained from the diet or from body protein during prolonged fasting or starvation may be used as an energy source. Body protein is catabolized primarily in muscle and in liver. Amino acids released from proteins usually lose their amino group through transamination or deamination. The carbon skeletons can be converted in the liver to glucose (glucogenic amino acids), acetyl CoA, and ketone bodies (ketogenic), or in a few cases both may be produced (glucogenic and ketogenic).

REMOVAL AND EXCRETION OF AMINO GROUPS

Excess nitrogen is eliminated from the body in the urine. The kidney adds small quantities of ammonium ion to the urine in part to regulate acid-base balance, but nitrogen is also eliminated in this process. Most excess nitrogen is converted to urea in the liver and goes through the blood to the kidney, where it is eliminated in urine.

Amino groups released by deamination reactions form ammonium ion (NH_4^+), which must not escape into the peripheral blood. An elevated concentration of ammonium ion in the blood, hyperammonemia, has toxic effects in the brain (cerebral edema, convulsions, coma, and death). Most tissues add excess nitrogen to the blood as glutamine by attaching ammonia to the γ-carboxyl group of glutamate. Muscle sends nitrogen to the liver as alanine and smaller quantities of other amino acids, in addition to glutamine. Figure I-17-1 summarizes the flow of nitrogen from tissues to either the liver or kidney for excretion.

Bridge to Pharmacology

Lactulose is metabolized to lactic acid in the GI tract by bacteria, which in turn covert ammonia (NH_3) to ammonium (NH_4^+), interfering with absorption and treating hyperammonemia.

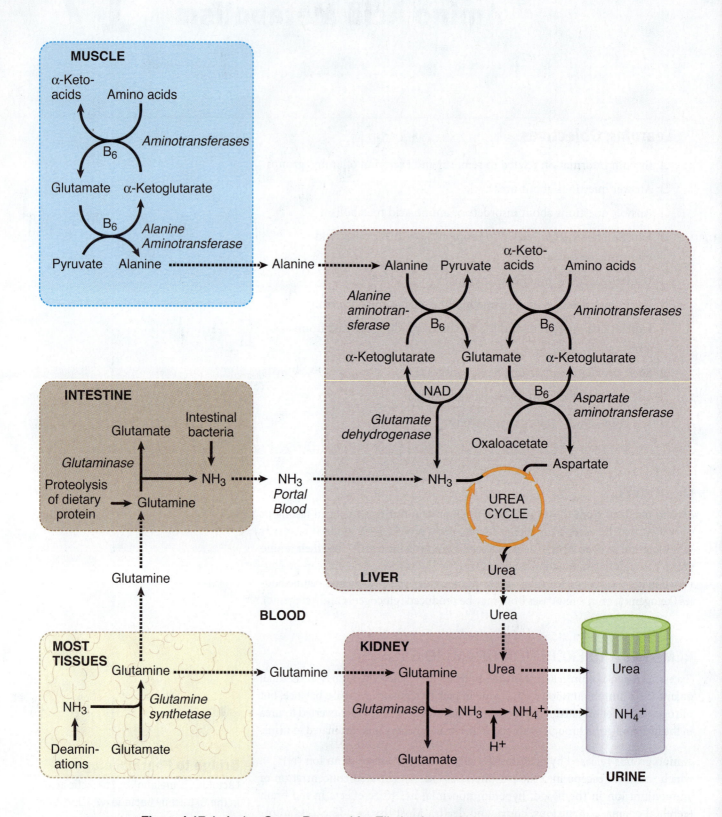

Figure I-17-1. Amino Group Removal for Elimination as Urea and Ammonia

Glutamine Synthetase

Most tissues, including muscle, have glutamine synthetase, which captures excess nitrogen by aminating glutamate to form glutamine. The reaction is irreversible. Glutamine, a relatively nontoxic substance, is the major carrier of excess nitrogen from tissues.

Glutaminase

The kidney contains glutaminase, allowing it to deaminate glutamine arriving in the blood and to eliminate the amino group as ammonium ion in urine. The reaction is irreversible. Kidney glutaminase is induced by chronic acidosis, in which excretion of ammonium may become the major defense mechanism. The liver has only small quantities of glutaminase; however, levels of the enzyme are high in the intestine where the ammonium ion from deamination can be sent directly to the liver via the portal blood and used for urea synthesis. The intestinal bacteria and glutamine from dietary protein contribute to the intestinal ammonia entering the portal blood.

Aminotransferases (Transaminases)

Both muscle and liver have aminotransferases, which, unlike deaminases, do not release the amino groups as free ammonium ion. This class of enzymes transfers the amino group from one carbon skeleton (an amino acid) to another (usually α-ketoglutarate, a citric acid cycle intermediate). Pyridoxal phosphate (PLP) derived from vitamin B_6 is required to mediate the transfer.

Aminotransferases are named according to the amino acid donating the amino group to α-ketoglutarate. Two important examples are alanine aminotransferase (ALT, formerly GPT) and aspartate aminotransferase (AST, formerly GOT). Although the aminotransferases are in liver and muscle, in pathologic conditions these enzymes may leak into the blood, where they are useful clinical indicators of damage to liver or muscle.

The reactions catalyzed by aminotransferases are reversible and play several roles in metabolism:

- During protein catabolism in muscle, they move the amino groups from many of the different amino acids onto glutamate, thus pooling it for transport. A portion of the glutamate may be aminated by glutamine synthetase (as in other tissues) or may transfer the amino group to pyruvate, forming alanine using the aminotransferase ALT.

- In liver, aminotransferases ALT and AST can move the amino group from alanine arriving from muscle into aspartate, a direct donor of nitrogen into the urea cycle.

Glutamate Dehydrogenase

This enzyme is found in many tissues, where it catalyzes the reversible oxidative deamination of the amino acid glutamate. It produces the citric acid cycle intermediate α-ketoglutarate, which serves as an entry point to the cycle for a group of glucogenic amino acids. Its role in urea synthesis and nitrogen removal is still controversial, but has been included in Figure I-17-1.

UREA CYCLE

Urea, which contains two nitrogens, is synthesized in the liver from aspartate and carbamoyl phosphate, which in turn is produced from ammonium ion and carbon dioxide by mitochondrial carbamoyl phosphate synthetase. This enzyme requires N-acetylglutamate as an activator. N-acetylglutamate is produced only when free amino acids are present. The urea cycle and the carbamoyl phosphate synthetase reaction are shown in Figure I-17-2.

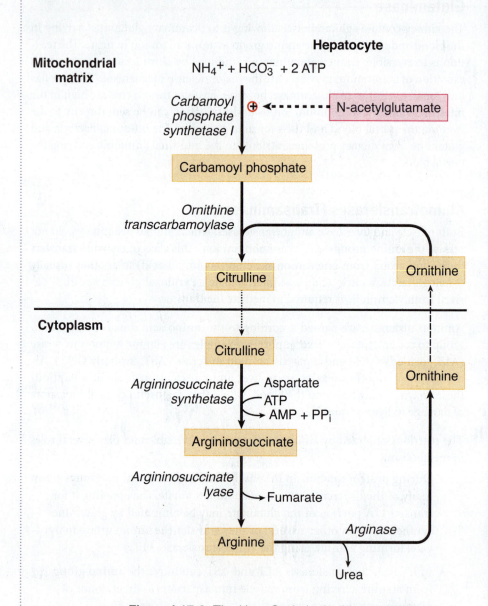

Figure I-17-2. The Urea Cycle in the Liver

The urea cycle, like the citric acid cycle, acts catalytically. Small quantities of the intermediates are sufficient to synthesize large amounts of urea from aspartate and carbamoyl phosphate. The cycle occurs partially in the mitochondria and partially in the cytoplasm.

- Citrulline enters the cytoplasm, and ornithine returns to the mitochondria.
- Carbamoyl phosphate synthetase and ornithine transcarbamoylase are mitochondrial enzymes.

- Aspartate enters the cycle in the cytoplasm and leaves the cycle (minus its amino group) as fumarate. If gluconeogenesis is active, fumarate can be converted to glucose.
- The product urea is formed in the cytoplasm and enters the blood for delivery to the kidney.

Genetic Deficiencies of the Urea Cycle

A combination of hyperammonemia, elevated blood glutamine, and decreased blood urea nitrogen (BUN) suggests a defect in the urea cycle. With neonatal onset, infants typically appear normal for the first 24 hours. Sometime during the 24- to 72-hour postnatal period, symptoms of lethargy, vomiting, and hyperventilation begin and, if not treated, progress to coma, respiratory failure, and death. Table I-17-1 compares the deficiencies of the two mitochondrial enzymes in the urea cycle, carbamoyl phosphate synthetase and ornithine transcarbamoylase.

The two conditions can be distinguished by an increase in orotic acid and uracil, which occurs in ornithine transcarbamoylase deficiency, but not in the deficiency of carbamoyl phosphate synthetase. Orotic acid and uracil are intermediates in pyrimidine synthesis (see Chapter 18). This pathway is stimulated by the accumulation of carbamoyl phosphate, the substrate for ornithine transcarbamoylase in the urea cycle and for aspartate transcarbamoylase in pyrimidine synthesis.

These conditions can be treated with a low protein diet and administration of sodium benzoate or phenylpyruvate to provide an alternative route for capturing and excreting excess nitrogen.

Table I-17-1. Genetic Deficiencies of Urea Synthesis

Carbamoyl Phosphate Synthetase	Ornithine Transcarbamoylase
↑ $[NH_4^+]$; hyperammonemia	↑ $[NH_4^+]$; hyperammonemia
Blood glutamine is increased	Blood glutamine is increased
BUN is decreased	BUN is decreased
No orotic aciduria Autosomal recessive	Orotic aciduria X-linked recessive
Cerebral edema	Cerebral edema
Lethargy, convulsions, coma, death	Lethargy, convulsions, coma, death

DISORDERS OF AMINO ACID METABOLISM

Figure I-17-3 presents a diagram of pathways in which selected amino acids are converted to citric acid cycle intermediates (and glucose) or to acetyl-CoA (and ketones). Important genetic deficiencies are identified on the diagram.

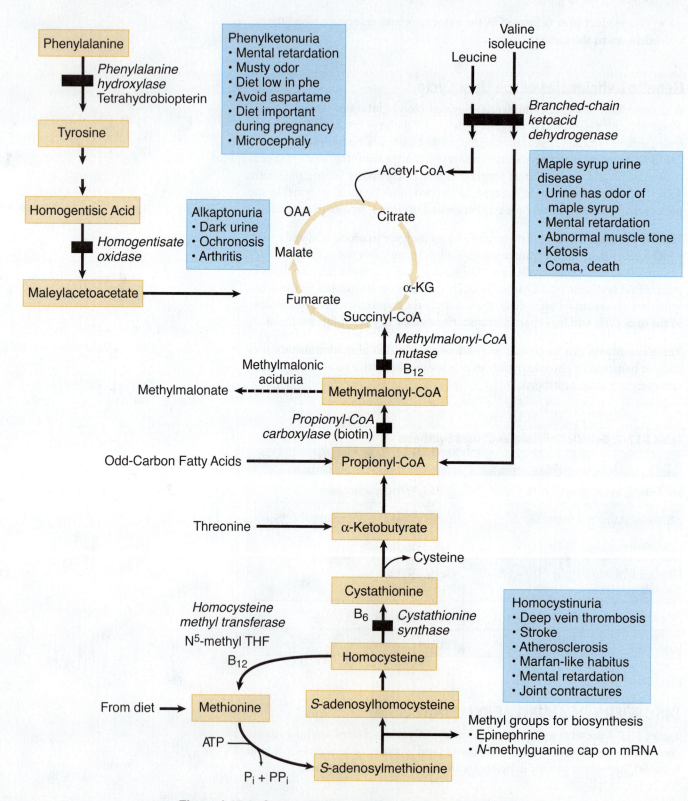

Figure I-17-3. Genetic Deficiencies of Amino Acid Metabolism

Phenylalanine Hydroxylase Deficiency (Phenylketonuria)

Infants with classic phenylketonuria (PKU) are normal at birth but if untreated show slow development, severe mental retardation, autistic symptoms, and loss of motor control. Children may have pale skin and white-blonde hair. The neurotoxic effects relate to high levels of phenylalanine and not to the phenylketones from which the name of the disease derives. Infants are routinely screened a few days after birth for blood phenylalanine level. Treatment consists of a life-long semisynthetic diet restricted in phenylalanine (small quantities are necessary because it is an essential amino acid). Aspartame (*N*-aspartyl-phenylalanine methyl ester), which is widely used as an artificial sweetener, must be strictly avoided by phenylketonurics.

Women with PKU who become pregnant must be especially careful about the phenylalanine level in their blood so as not to adversely affect neurologic development in the fetus. Infants whose phenylketonuric mothers have not maintained adequate metabolic control during pregnancy have a high risk for mental retardation (although less profound than in a child with untreated PKU), microcephaly, and low birth weight.

Bridge to Medical Genetics
There are more than 100 known mutations in the gene for phenylalanine hydroxylase, causing PKU. This is an example of allelic heterogeneity.

Albinism

Albinism (1:15,000) is a group of conditions in which then normal conversion of tyrosine to melanin is altered. The most severe form is a deficiency of tyrosinase, causing an absence of pigment in the skin, hair, and eyes.

Homogentisate Oxidase Deficiency (Alcaptonuria)

Accumulation of homogentisic acid in the blood causes its excretion in urine, after which it gradually darkens upon exposure to air. This sign of alcaptonuria is not present in all patients with the enzyme deficiency. The dark pigment also accumulates over years in the cartilage (ochronosis) and may be seen in the sclera of the eye, in ear cartilage and patients develop arthritis in adulthood, usually beginning in the third decade. Treatment is targeted to managing the symptoms.

Branched-Chain Ketoacid Dehydrogenase Deficiency (Maple Syrup Urine Disease)

Branched-chain ketoacid dehydrogenase, an enzyme similar to α-ketoglutarate dehydrogenase (thiamine, lipoic acid, CoA, FAD, NAD^+), metabolizes branched-chain ketoacids produced from their cognate amino acids, valine, leucine, and isoleucine. In the classic form of the disease, infants are normal for the first few days of life, after which they become progressively lethargic, lose weight, and have alternating episodes of hypertonia and hypotonia, and the urine develops a characteristic odor of maple syrup. Ketosis, coma, and death ensue if not treated. Treatment requires restricting dietary valine, leucine, and isoleucine.

Propionyl-CoA Carboxylase and Methylmalonyl-CoA Mutase Deficiencies

Valine, methionine, isoleucine, and threonine are all metabolized through the propionic acid pathway (also used for odd-carbon fatty acids). Deficiency of either enzyme results in neonatal ketoacidosis from failure to metabolize ketoacids produced from these four amino acids. The deficiencies may be distinguished

Note
Propionyl CoA carboxylase deficiency:

Accumulation of
- propionic acid
- methyl citrate
- hydroxypropionic acid

Methylmalonyl CoA mutase deficiency:

Accumulation of
- methylmalonic acid

based on whether methylmalonic aciduria is present (methylmalonyl CoA mutase deficiency) or by the presence of methyl citrate and hydroxypropionate (propionyl CoA carboxylase deficiency). A diet low in protein or a semisynthetic diet with low amounts of valine, methionine, isoleucine, and threonine is used to treat both deficiencies.

> ### Homocystinemia/Homocystinuria
>
> Accumulation of homocystine in blood is associated with cardiovascular disease; deep vein thrombosis, thromboembolism, and stroke; dislocation of the lens (ectopic lens); and mental retardation. Homocystine is a disulfide dimer of homocysteine. Homocystinemia caused by an enzyme deficiency is a rare, but severe, condition in which atherosclerosis in childhood is a prominent finding. These children often have myocardial infarctions before 20 years of age. All patients excrete high levels of homocystine in the urine. Treatment includes a diet low in methionine. The major enzyme deficiency producing homocystinemia is that of cystathionine synthase:
>
>> A 5-year-old girl was brought to her pediatrician because she had difficulty with her vision and seemed to be slow in her mental and physical development since birth. The physician noted that the girl had abnormally long, "spidery" fingers and a downward dislocation of the right lens of her eye. Further examination revealed a deep vein thrombosis. A laboratory examination of her blood indicated increased methionine. She also had increased urinary excretion of homocystine, indicated by a cyanide-nitroprusside test. The parents were advised to restrict methionine to low levels and supplement folate, vitamin B_{12}, and vitamin B_6 in the girl's diet.
>
> Homocystinuria caused by a genetic defect in the enzyme cystathionine synthase is rare and can present similarly to Marfan syndrome. The latter is a defect in the fibrillin gene, resulting in tall stature, long fingers and toes, lens dislocation, and a tendency toward aortic wall ruptures. In cystathionine synthase deficiency subluxation of the lens is downward and inward. In Marfan syndrome subluxation of the lens is upward and outward. Cystathionine synthase deficiency results in the accumulation of homocysteine and methionine and their spillage into blood and urine. Two molecules of homocysteine can oxidize to the disulfide-crosslinked homocystine. Many patients with homocystinuria who have partial activity of cystathionine synthase respond well to pyridoxine administration. If left untreated, patients will usually succumb to myocardial infarction, stroke, or pulmonary embolism.

Homocystinemia from Vitamin Deficiencies

Vitamin deficiencies may produce a more mild form of homocystinemia. Mild homocystinemia is associated with increased risk for atherosclerosis, deep vein thrombosis, and stroke. The vitamin deficiencies causing homocystinemia include:

- Folate deficiency: The recommended dietary intake of folate has been increased (also protects against neural tube defects in the fetus), and additional folate is now added to flour (bread, pasta, and other products made from flour)
- Vitamin B_{12}
- Vitamin B_6

S-ADENOSYLMETHIONINE, FOLATE, AND COBALAMIN

One-Carbon Units in Biochemical Reactions

One-carbon units in different oxidation states are required in the pathways producing purines, thymidine, and many other compounds. When a biochemical reaction requires a methyl group (methylation), S-adenosylmethionine (SAM) is generally the methyl donor. If a 1-carbon unit in another oxidation state is required (methylene, methenyl, formyl), tetrahydrofolate (THF) typically serves as its donor.

S-Adenosylmethionine

Important pathways requiring SAM include synthesis of epinephrine and of the 7-methylguanine cap on eukaryotic mRNA. Synthesis of SAM from methionine is shown in Figure I-17-3. After donating the methyl group, SAM is converted to homocysteine and remethylated in a reaction catalyzed by N-methyl THF–homocysteine methyltransferase requiring both vitamin B_{12} and N-methyl-THF. The methionine produced is once again used to make SAM.

Note
THB (BH4) is necessary for tyrosine hydroxylase, phenylalanine hydroxylase, and tryptophan hydroxylase (serotonin synthesis) and is regenerated by dihydropteridine reductase.

Clinical Correlate
Parkinson's disease is caused by loss of dopaminergic neurons in the substantia nigra. It is treated with levodopa (L-dopa).

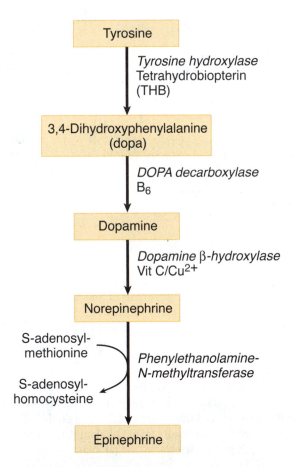

Figure I-17-4. Catecholamine Synthesis

Tetrahydrofolate

THF is formed from the vitamin folate through two reductions involving NADPH and catalyzed by dihydrofolate reductase shown in Figure I-17-5. It picks up a 1-carbon unit from a variety of donors and enters the active 1-carbon pool. Important pathways requiring forms of THF from this pool include the synthesis of all purines and thymidine, which in turn are used for DNA and RNA synthesis during cell growth and division.

Megaloblastic anemia results from insufficient active THF to support cell division in the bone marrow. Methotrexate inhibits DHF reductase, making it a useful antineoplastic drug. Folate deficiencies may be seen during pregnancy and in alcoholism.

Additional folate may be stored as the highly reduced N^5-methyl-THF. This form is referred to as the storage pool as there is only one known enzyme that uses it, and in turn moves it back into the active pool. This enzyme is N-methyl THF-homocysteine methyltransferase, discussed above, which also requires vitamin B_{12} and is involved in regenerating SAM as a methyl donor for reactions.

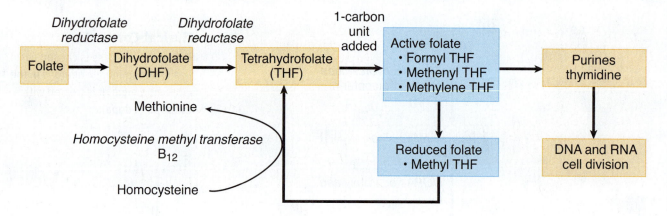

Figure I-17-5. Folate Metabolism

Cobalamin

The vitamin cobalamin (vitamin B_{12}) is reduced and activated in the body to two forms, adenosylcobalamin, used by methylmalonyl-CoA mutase, and methylcobalamin, formed from N^5-methyl-THF in the N-methyl THF-homocysteine methyltransferase reaction. These are the only two enzymes that use vitamin B_{12} (other than the enzymes that reduce and add an adenosyl group to it).

Cobalamin deficiency can create a secondary deficiency of active THF by preventing its release from the storage pool through the N-methyl THF-homocysteine methyltransferase reaction, and thus also result in megaloblastic anemia. Progressive peripheral neuropathy also results from cobalamin deficiency. Treating a cobalamin deficiency with folate corrects the megaloblastic anemia but does not halt the neuropathy.

The most likely reason for cobalamin deficiency is pernicious anemia (failure to absorb vitamin B_{12} in the absence of intrinsic factor from parietal cells). Vitamin B_{12} absorption also decreases with aging and in individuals with chronic pancreatitis. Less common reasons for B_{12} deficiency include a long-term completely vegetarian diet (plants don't contain vitamin B_{12}) and infection with *Diphyllobothrium latum*, a parasite found in raw fish. Excess vitamin B_{12} is stored in the body, so deficiencies develop slowly.

Deficiencies of folate and cobalamin are compared in Table I-17-2.

Table I-17-2. Comparison of Folate and Vitamin B12 Deficiencies

Folate Deficiency	Vitamin B$_{12}$ (Cobalamin) Deficiency
Megaloblastic anemia • Macrocytic • MCV greater than 100 femtolitres (fL) • PMN nucleus more than 5 lobes Homocysteinemia with risk for cardiovascular disease Deficiency develops in 3–4 months Risk factors for deficiency: • Pregnancy (neural tube defects in fetus may result) • Alcoholism • Severe malnutrition • Gastric or terminal ileum resection	Megaloblastic anemia • Macrocytic • MCV greater than 100 femtolitres (fL) • PMN nucleus more than 5 lobes Homocysteinemia with risk for cardiovascular disease Methylmalonic aciduria Progressive peripheral neuropathy Deficiency develops in years Risk factors for deficiency: • Pernicious anemia • Gastric resection • Chronic pancreatitis • Severe malnutrition • Vegan • Infection with *D. latum* • Ageing • Bacterial overgrowth of the terminal ileum • *H. pylori* infection

Bridge to Pathology

Vitamin B$_{12}$ deficiency causes demyelination of the posterior columns and lateral corticospinal tracts in the spinal cord.

SPECIALIZED PRODUCTS DERIVED FROM AMINO ACIDS

Table I-17-3 identifies some important products formed from amino acids.

Table I-17-3. Products of Amino Acids

Amino Acid	Products
Tyrosine	Thyroid hormones T$_3$ and T$_4$ Melanin Catecholamines
Tryptophan	Serotonin NAD, NADP
Arginine	Nitric oxide (NO)
Glutamate	γ-Aminobutyric acid (GABA)
Histidine	Histamine

HEME SYNTHESIS

Heme synthesis occurs in almost all tissues because heme proteins include not only hemoglobin and myoglobin but all the cytochromes (electron transport chain,

Section I • Biochemistry

cytochrome P-450, cytochrome b_5), as well as the enzymes catalase, peroxidase, and the soluble guanylate cyclase stimulated by nitric oxide. The pathway producing heme, shown in Figure I-17-6, is controlled independently in different tissues. In liver, the rate-limiting enzyme δ-aminolevulinate synthase (ALA) is repressed by heme.

Note

Compounds with an "-ogen" suffix, such as urobilinogen, are colorless substances. In the presence of oxygen, they spontaneously oxidize, forming a conjugated double-bond network in the compounds. These oxidized compounds are highly colored substances and have an "-in" suffix (e.g., porphobilin, urobilin).

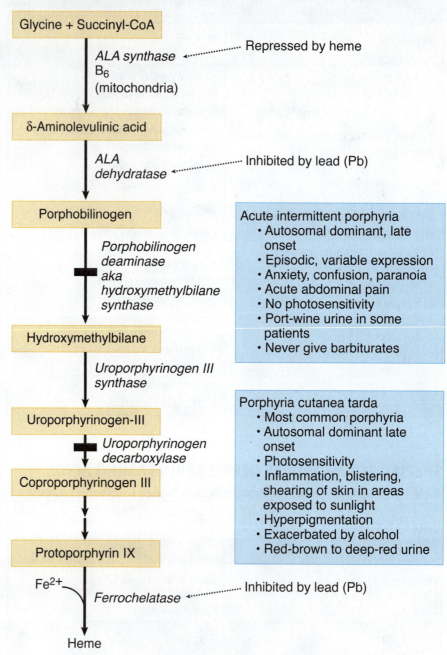

Figure I-17-6. Heme Synthesis

Acute Intermittent Porphyria: Porphobilinogen Deaminase (Hydroxymethylbilane Synthase) Deficiency

This late-onset autosomal dominant disease exhibits variable expression. Many heterozygotes remain symptom-free throughout their lives. Signs and symptoms, when present, include:

- Abdominal pain, often resulting in multiple laparoscopies (scars on abdomen)
- Anxiety, paranoia, and depression
- Paralysis
- Motor, sensory or autonomic neuropathy
- Weakness
- Excretion of ALA (δ-aminolevulinic) and PBG (porphobilinogen) during episodes
- In severe cases, dark port-wine color to urine on standing

Some of these individuals are incorrectly diagnosed and placed in psychiatric institutions. Episodes may be induced by hormonal changes and by many drugs, including barbiturates.

Other Porphyrias

Deficiencies of other enzymes in the heme pathway produce porphyrias in which photosensitivity is a common finding. Chronic inflammation to overt blistering and shearing in exposed areas of the skin characterize these porphyrias. The most common is porphyria cutanea tarda (deficiency of uroporphyrinogen decarboxylase), an autosomal dominant condition with late onset. β-Carotene is often administered to porphryia patients with photosensitivity to reduce the production of reactive oxygen species.

> ### Porphyria cutanea tarda
>
> A 35-year-old man was becoming very sensitive to sunlight and often detected persistent rashes and blisters throughout areas of his body that were exposed to the sun. He also observed that drinking excessive alcohol with his friends after softball games worsened the incidence of the recurrent blisters and sunburns. He became even more concerned after he noticed his urine became a red-brown tint if he did not flush the toilet.
>
> Porphyria cutanea tarda is an adult-onset hepatic porphyria in which hepatocytes are unable to decarboxylate uroporphyrinogen in heme synthesis. The uroporphyrin spills out of the liver and eventually into urine, giving rise to the characteristic red-wine urine if it is allowed to stand, a hallmark of porphyrias. Hepatotoxic substances, such as excessive alcohol or iron deposits, can exacerbate the disease. Skin lesions are related to high circulating levels of porphyrins.

Vitamin B₆ Deficiency

ALA synthase, the rate-limiting enzyme, requires pyridoxine (vitamin B_6). Deficiency of pyridoxine is associated with isoniazid therapy for tuberculosis and may cause sideroblastic anemia with ringed sideroblasts.

Iron Deficiency

The last enzyme in the pathway, heme synthase (ferrochelatase), introduces the Fe^{2+} into the heme ring. Deficiency of iron produces a microcytic hypochromic anemia.

Bridge to Pharmacology

Barbiturates are hydroxylated by the microsomal cytochrome P-450 system in the liver to facilitate their efficient elimination from the body. Administration of the barbiturates results in stimulation of cytochrome P-450 synthesis, which in turn reduces heme levels. The reduction in heme lessens the repression of ALA synthase, causing more porphyrin precursor synthesis. In porphyrias, the indirect production of more precursors by the barbiturates exacerbates the disease.

Section I • Biochemistry

Lead Poisoning

Lead inactivates many enzymes including ALA dehydrase and ferrochelatase (heme synthase), and can produce a microcytic sideroblastic anemia with ringed sideroblasts in the bone marrow. Other symptoms include:

- Coarse basophilic stippling of erythrocytes
- Headache, nausea, memory loss
- Abdominal pain, diarrhea (lead colic)
- Lead lines in gums
- Lead deposits in abdomen and epiphyses of bone seen on radiograph
- Neuropathy (claw hand, wrist-drop)
- Increased urinary ALA
- Increased free erythrocyte protoporphyrin

Vitamin B_6 deficiency, iron deficiency, and lead poisoning all can cause anemia. These three conditions are summarized and compared in Table I-17-4.

Clinical Correlate

The failure of ferrochelatase to insert Fe^{2+} into protoporphyrin IX to form heme, such as in lead poisoning or iron deficiency anemia, results in the nonenzymatic insertion of Zn^{2+} to form zinc-protoporphyrin. This complex is extremely fluorescent and is easily detected.

Table I-17-4. Comparison of Vitamin B6 Deficiency, Iron Deficiency, and Lead Poisoning

Vitamin B_6 (Pyridoxine) Deficiency	Iron Deficiency	Lead Poisoning
Microcytic	Microcytic	Microcytic Coarse basophilic stippling in erythrocytes
Ringed sideroblasts in bone marrow		Ringed sideroblasts in bone marrow
Protoporphyrin: ↓	Protoporphyrin: ↑	Protoporphyrin: ↑
δ-ALA: ↓	δ-ALA: Normal	δ-ALA: ↑
Ferritin: ↑	Ferritin: ↓	Ferritin: ↑
Serum iron: ↑	Serum iron: ↓	Serum iron: ↑
Isoniazid for tuberculosis	Dietary iron insufficient to compensate for normal loss	Lead paint Pottery glaze Batteries (Diagnose by measuring blood lead level)

Bridge to Pathology

Hemochromatosis is an inherited, autosomal recessive disease (prevalence of 1/200) generally seen in men >40 years old and in older women. The disease is characterized by a daily intestinal absorption of 2–3 mg of iron compared with the normal 1 mg. Over a period of 20–30 years, this disease results in levels of 20–30 grams of iron in the body compared with the normal 4 grams. Hemosiderin deposits are found in the liver, pancreas, skin, and joints.

IRON TRANSPORT AND STORAGE

Iron (Fe^{3+}) released from hemoglobin in the histiocytes is bound to ferritin and then transported in the blood by transferrin, which can deliver it to tissues for synthesis of heme. Important proteins in this context are:

- Ferroxidase (also known as ceruloplasmin, a Cu^{2+} protein) oxidizes Fe^{2+} to Fe^{3+} for transport and storage (Figure I-17-7).

- Transferrin carries Fe^{3+} in blood.
- Ferritin itself oxidizes Fe^{2+} to Fe^{3+} for storage of normal amounts of Fe^{3+} in tissues. Loss of iron from the body is accomplished by bleeding and shedding epithelial cells of the mucosa and skin. The body has no mechanism for excreting iron, so controlling its absorption into the mucosal cells is crucial. No other nutrient is regulated in this manner.
- Hemosiderin binds excess Fe^{3+} to prevent escape of free Fe^{3+} into the blood, where it is toxic.

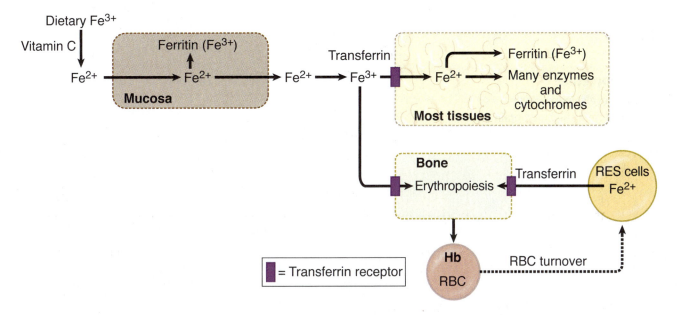

Figure I-17-7. Iron Metabolism

BILIRUBIN METABOLISM

Subsequent to lysis of older erythrocytes in the spleen, heme released from hemoglobin is converted to bilirubin in the histiocytes. This sequence is shown in Figure I-17-8.

- Bilirubin is not water soluble and is therefore transported in the blood attached to serum albumin.
- Hepatocytes conjugate bilirubin with glucuronic acid, increasing its water solubility.
- Conjugated bilirubin is secreted into the bile.
- Intestinal bacteria convert conjugated bilirubin into urobilinogen.
- A portion of the urobilinogen is further converted to bile pigments (stercobilin) and excreted in the feces, producing their characteristic red-brown color. Bile duct obstruction results in clay-colored stools.
- Some of the urobilinogen is converted to urobilin (yellow) and excreted in urine.

Clinical Correlate

Excessive RBC destruction in hemolytic anemia results in excessive conversion of bilirubin to urobilinogen in the intestine. Higher-than-normal absorption of the urobilinogen and its subsequent excretion in the urine results in a deeper-colored urine.

Clinical Correlate

At very high levels, lipid-soluble bilirubin may cross the blood-brain barrier and precipitate in the basal ganglia, causing irreversible brain damage (kernicterus).

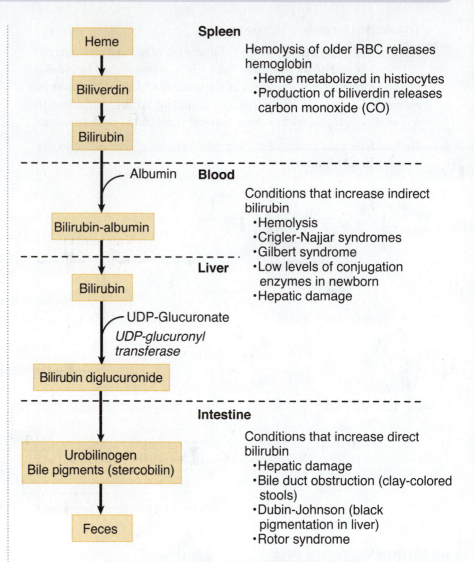

Figure I-17-8. Heme Catabolism and Bilirubin

Bilirubin and Jaundice

Jaundice (yellow color of skin, whites of the eyes) may occur when blood levels of bilirubin exceed normal (icterus). Jaundice may be characterized by an increase in unconjugated (indirect) bilirubin, conjugated (direct) bilirubin, or both. Accumulation of bilirubin (usually unconjugated) in the brain (kernicterus) may result in death. When conjugated bilirubin increases, it may be excreted, giving a deep yellow-red color to the urine. Examples of conditions associated with increased bilirubin and jaundice include hemolytic crisis, UDP-glucuronyl transferase deficiency, hepatic damage, and bile duct occlusion.

Hemolytic crisis

With severe hemolysis, more bilirubin is released into the blood than can be transported on albumin and conjugated in the liver. Unconjugated and total bilirubin increase and may produce jaundice and kernicterus. Examples include:

- Episode of hemolysis in G6PDH deficiency
- Sickle cell crisis
- Rh disease of newborn

Hemolytic crisis may be confirmed by low hemoglobin and elevated reticulocyte counts.

UDP-glucuronyl transferase deficiency

When bilirubin conjugation is low because of genetic or functional deficiency of the glucuronyl transferase system, unconjugated and total bilirubin increase. Examples include:

- Crigler-Najjar syndromes (types I and II)
- Gilbert syndrome
- Physiologic jaundice in the newborn, especially premature infants (enzymes may not be fully induced)

Hepatic damage

Viral hepatitis or cirrhosis produces an increase in both direct and indirect bilirubin. Aminotransferase levels will also be elevated.

- Alcoholic liver disease, AST increases more than ALT
- Viral hepatitis, ALT increases more than AST

Bile duct occlusion

Occlusion of the bile duct (gallstone, primary biliary cirrhosis, pancreatic cancer) prevents conjugated bilirubin from leaving the liver. Conjugated bilirubin increases in blood and may also appear in urine. Feces are light-colored.

Chapter Summary

Amino Acid Metabolism
- Major transport forms of excess nitrogen from tissues
  - Muscle: alanine
  - Other tissues: glutamine

Enzymes
- Glutamine synthetase (most tissues)
- Glutaminase (kidney, intestine)
- Aminotransferases (transaminases)
  - Muscle and liver
  - Require vitamin B_6, pyridoxine
  - AST (GOT), ALT (GPT)

(Continued)

Chapter Summary (Continued)

Urea Cycle

- Liver (mitochondria and cytoplasm)
- Rate-limiting enzyme: carbamoyl phosphate synthetase-1 (activated by N-acetylglutamate)

Urea Cycle Deficiencies

- Most result in hyperammonemia and cerebral edema, decreased BUN, increased blood glutamine
    - Carbamoyl phosphate synthetase (no increase in orotic acid or uracil)
    - Ornithine transcarbamoylase (increase in uracil and orotic acid)

Other Genetic Diseases Associated with Amino Acid Metabolism

- Phenylketonuria (phenylalanine hydroxylase)
- Alcaptonuria (homogentisate oxidase)
- Maple syrup urine disease (branched-chain ketoacid dehydrogenase)
- Homocystinuria (cystathionine synthase or homocysteine methyl transferase)

Vitamin Deficiencies

- Homocystinemia (folate, B_{12}, B_6)
- Megaloblastic anemia (folate, B_{12})

Heme Synthesis

Rate-Limiting Enzyme

- δ-aminolevulinate synthase (B_6)

    Repressed by heme

Anemias

- Differentiate microcytic anemias due to iron deficiency, B_6 deficiency, lead poisoning

Porphyrias

- Acute intermittent porphyria (porphobilinogen deaminase/ hydroxymethylbilane synthase)
    - Neurologic and hepatic
    - May show port-wine urine during episode
- Porphyria cutanea tarda
    - Most common porphyria
    - Photosensitivity
    - Red-brown urine

Review Questions

Select the ONE best answer.

1. Which enzymes are responsible for producing the direct donors of nitrogen into the pathway producing urea?

    A. Arginase and argininosuccinate lyase
    B. Xanthine oxidase and guanine deaminase
    C. Glutamate dehydrogenase and glutaminase
    D. Argininosuccinate synthetase and ornithine transcarbamoylase
    E. Aspartate aminotransferase and carbamoyl phosphate synthetase

2. Two days after a full-term normal delivery, a neonate begins to hyperventilate, develops hypothermia and cerebral edema, and becomes comatose. Urinalysis reveals high levels of glutamine and orotic acid. The BUN is below normal. Which enzyme is most likely to be deficient in this child?

    A. Cytoplasmic glutaminase
    B. Cytoplasmic carbamoyl phosphate synthetase
    C. Cytoplasmic orotidylate decarboxylase
    D. Mitochondrial carbamoyl phosphate synthetase
    E. Mitochondrial ornithine transcarbamoylase

Items 3 and 4

A 49-year-old man with a rare recessive condition is at high risk for deep vein thrombosis and stroke and has had replacement of ectopic lenses. He has a normal hematocrit and no evidence of megaloblastic anemia.

3. A mutation in the gene encoding which of the following is most likely to cause this disease?

    A. Cystathionine synthase
    B. Homocysteine methyltransferase
    C. Fibrillin
    D. Lysyl oxidase
    E. Branched chain α-ketoacid dehydrogenase

4. Amino acid analysis of this patient's plasma would most likely reveal an abnormally elevated level of

    A. lysine
    B. leucine
    C. methionine
    D. ornithine
    E. cysteine

5. A 56-year-old man with a history of genetic disease undergoes hip replacement surgery for arthritis. During the operation the surgeon notes a dark pigmentation (ochronosis) in the man's cartilage. His ochronotic arthritis is most likely caused by oxidation and polymerization of excess tissue

   A. homogentisic acid
   B. orotic acid
   C. methylmalonic acid
   D. uric acid
   E. ascorbic acid

Items 6–8

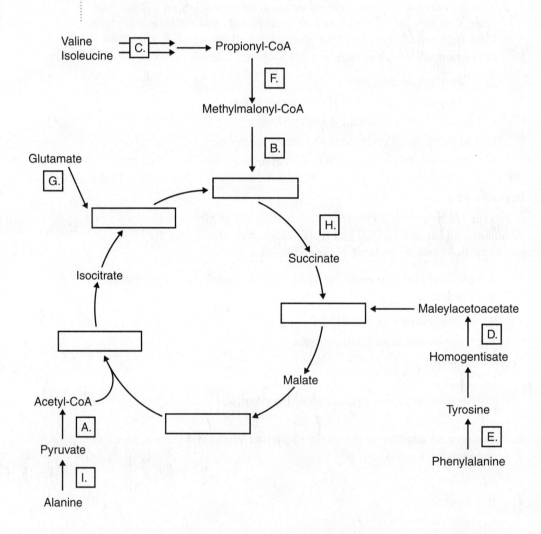

For each of the conditions below, link the missing substrate or enzyme.

6. A 9-week-old boy, healthy at birth, begins to develop symptoms of ketoacidosis, vomiting, lethargy, seizures and hypertonia. Urine has characteristic odor of maple syrup.

7. A child with white-blond hair, blue eyes, and pale complexion is on a special diet in which one of the essential amino acids is severely restricted. He has been told to avoid foods artificially sweetened with aspartame.

8. A chronically ill patient on long-term (home) parenteral nutrition develops metabolic acidosis, a grayish pallor, scaly dermatitis, and alopecia (hair loss). These symptoms subside upon addition of the B vitamin biotin to the alimentation fluid.

9. A woman 7 months pregnant with her first child develops anemia. Laboratory evaluation indicates an increased mean cell volume (MVC), hypersegmented neutrophils, and altered morphology of several other cell types. The most likely underlying cause of this woman's anemia is

    A. folate deficiency
    B. iron deficiency
    C. glucose 6-phosphate dehydrogenase deficiency
    D. cyanocobalamin (B_{12}) deficiency
    E. lead poisoning

Items 10 and 11

A 64-year-old woman is seen by a hematologist for evaluation of a macrocytic anemia. The woman was severely malnourished. Both homocysteine and methylmalonate were elevated in her blood and urine, and the transketolase level in her erythrocytes was below normal.

10. What is the best evidence cited that the anemia is due to a primary deficiency of cyanocobalamin (B_{12})?

    A. Macrocytic anemia
    B. Elevated methylmalonate
    C. Low transketolase activity
    D. Elevated homocysteine
    E. Severe malnutrition

11. In response to a B_{12} deficiency, which of the additional conditions may develop in this patient if she is not treated?

    A. Progressive peripheral neuropathy
    B. Gout
    C. Wernicke-Korsakoff
    D. Destruction of parietal cells
    E. Bleeding gums and loose teeth

Section I • Biochemistry

Items 12–15

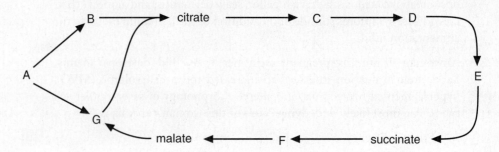

Link the following to the letters in the cycle.

12. Obligate activator of hepatic pyruvate carboxylase in the postabsorptive state.

13. Product formed by argininosuccinate lyase during urea synthesis.

14. Substrate and energy source for synthesis of δ-aminolevulinate in the heme pathway.

15. Converted to glutamate in a reaction requiring the coenzyme form of pyridoxine (B_6)

16. A 62-year-old man being treated for tuberculosis develops a microcytic, hypochromic anemia. Ferritin levels are increased, and marked sideroblastosis is present. A decrease in which of the following enzyme activities is most directly responsible for the anemia in this man?

    A. Cytochrome oxidase
    B. Cytochrome P_{450} oxidase
    C. Pyruvate kinase
    D. δ-Aminolevulinate synthase
    E. Lysyl oxidase

17. A 48-year-old man developed abdominal colic, muscle pain, and fatigue. Following a 3-week hospitalization, acute intermittent porphyria was initially diagnosed based on a high level of urinary δ-aminolevulinic acid. Subsequent analysis of the patient's circulating red blood cells revealed that 70% contained elevated levels of zinc protoporphyrin, and the diagnosis was corrected. The correct diagnosis is most likely to be

    A. protoporphyria
    B. congenital erythropoietic porphyria
    C. lead poisoning
    D. barbiturate addiction
    E. iron deficiency

18. A 3-week-old infant has been having intermittent vomiting and convulsions. She also has had episodes of screaming and hyperventilation. The infant has been lethargic between episodes. Tests reveal an expanded abdomen, and blood values show decreased citrulline amounts as well as a decreased BUN. What other clinical outcomes would be expected in this infant?

    A. Decreased blood pH and uric acid crystals in urine
    B. Decreased blood pH and increased lactic acid in blood
    C. Increased blood glutamine and increased orotic acid in urine
    D. Increased blood ammonia and increased urea in urine
    E. Megaloblastic anemia and increased methylmalonic acid in blood

19. A 69-year-old male presents to his family physician with a complaint of recent onset difficulty in performing activities of daily living. He is a retired factory worker who last worked 4 years ago. Upon questioning, his spouse reveals that he "hasn't been able to get around the way he used to." Physical examination reveals a well-nourished 69-year-old man who walks with an exaggerated kyphosis. His gait appears to be quite slow and wide-based. He also appears to have a resting tremor. The appropriate management of his case would target which of the following?

    A. Amino acid degradation
    B. Catecholamine synthesis
    C. Ganglioside degradation
    D. Prostaglandin synthesis
    E. Sphingolipid degradation

Section I • Biochemistry

Answers

1. **Answer: E.** Aspartate is produced by AST and carbamoyl phosphate by CPS-I.

2. **Answer: E.** Given these symptoms, the defect is in the urea cycle and the elevated orotate suggests deficiency of ornithine transcarbamoylase.

3. **Answer: A.** Homocysteine, the substrate for the enzyme, accumulates increasing the risk of deep vein thrombosis and disrupting the normal crosslinking of fibrillin. Deficiency of homocysteine methyltransferase would cause homocystinuria, but would also predispose to megaloblastic anemia.

4. **Answer: C.** Only methionine is degraded via the homocysteine/cystathionine pathway and would be elevated in the plasma of a cystathionine synthase–deficient patient via activation of homocysteine methyltransferase by excess substrate.

5. **Answer: A.** Adults with alcaptonuria show a high prevalence of ochronotic arthritis due to deficiency of homogentisate oxidase.

6. **Answer: C.** Maple syrup urine disease; substrates are branched chain α-ketoacids derived from the branched chain amino acids.

7. **Answer: E.** The child has PKU; aspartame contains phenylalanine. These children may be blond, blue-eyed, and pale complected because of deficient melanin production from tyrosine.

8. **Answer: F.** The only biotin-dependent reaction in the diagram. The enzyme is propionyl- CoA carboxylase.

9. **Answer: A.** Pregnant woman with megaloblastic anemia and elevated serum homocysteine strongly suggests folate deficiency. Iron deficiency presents as microcytic, hypochromic anemia and would not elevate homocysteine. B_{12} deficiency is not most likely in this presentation.

10. **Answer: B.** Methylmalonyl-CoA mutase requires B_{12} but not folate for activity. Macrocytic anemia, elevated homocysteine, and macrocytic anemia can be caused by either B_{12} or folate deficiency.

11. **Answer: A.** Progressive peripheral neuropathy. A distractor may be D, but this would be the cause of a B_{12} deficiency, not a result of it.

12. **Answer: B.** Acetyl-CoA activates pyruvate carboxylase and gluconeogenesis during fasting.

13. **Answer: F.** Fumarate.

14. **Answer: E.** Succinyl-CoA.

15. **Answer: D.** Glutamate is produced by B_6-dependent transamination of α-ketoglutarate.

16. **Answer: D.** Sideroblastic anemia in a person being treated for tuberculosis (with isoniazid) is most likely due to vitamin B_6 deficiency. δ-Aminolevulinate synthase, the first enzyme in heme synthesis, requires vitamin B_6 (pyridoxine).

17. **Answer: C.** Lead inhibits both ferrochelatase (increasing the zinc protoporphyrin) and ALA dehydrase (increasing δ-ALA).

18. **Answer: C.** The infant has a defect in the urea cycle, resulting from ornithine transcarbamylase (OTC) deficiency. OTC deficiency would result in decreased intermediates of the urea cycle, including decreased urea formation as indicated by the decreased BUN. OTC can be diagnosed by elevated orotic acid since carbamyl phosphate accumulates in the liver mitochondria and spills into the cytoplasm entering the pyrimidine-synthesis pathway.

    Methylmalonic acid in blood (**choice E**) is seen in vitamin B12 disorders.

    A decreased BUN would result in *elevated ammonia* in blood, raising the pH (**choices A and B**).

    Decreased BUN means decreased blood urea, hence, decreased urea in urine (**choice D**).

19. **Answer: B.** The above case describes a patient with Parkinson's disease, which is caused by degeneration of the substantia nigra. This leads to dopamine deficiency in the brain and results in resting tremors, bradykinesia, cog-wheeling of the hand joints, and rigidity of musculature. In addition, patients are often described as having "mask-like facies." Dopamine is one of the catecholamines synthesized in a common pathway with norepinephrine and epinephrine.

    The diseases involving amino acid degradation (**choice A**), ganglioside degradation (**choice C**), and sphingolipid degradation (**choice E**) do not match the presentation seen in the case.

Purine and Pyrimidine Metabolism 18

Learning Objectives

❑ Explain information related to pyrimidine synthesis
❑ Use knowledge of pyrimidine catabolism
❑ Explain information related to purine synthesis
❑ Demonstrate understanding of purine catabolism and the salvage enzyme HGPRT

OVERVIEW

Nucleotides are needed for DNA and RNA synthesis (DNA replication and transcription) and for energy transfer. Nucleoside triphosphates (ATP and GTP) provide energy for reactions that would otherwise be extremely unfavorable in the cell.

Ribose 5-phosphate for nucleotide synthesis is derived from the hexose monophosphate shunt and is activated by the addition of pyrophosphate from ATP, forming phosphoribosyl pyrophosphate (PRPP) using PRPP synthetase (Figure I-18-1). Cells synthesize nucleotides in two ways, *de novo* synthesis and salvage pathways (Figure I-18-1). In *de novo* synthesis, which occurs predominantly in the liver, purines and pyrimidines are synthesized from smaller precursors, and PRPP is added to the pathway at some point. In the salvage pathways, preformed purine and pyrimidine bases can be converted into nucleotides by salvage enzymes distinct from those of *de novo* synthesis. Purine and pyrimidine bases for salvage enzymes may arise from:

- Synthesis in the liver and transport to other tissues
- Digestion of endogenous nucleic acids (cell death, RNA turnover)

In many cells, the capacity for *de novo* synthesis to supply purines and pyrimidines is insufficient, and the salvage pathway is essential for adequate nucleotide synthesis. In patients with Lesch-Nyhan disease, an enzyme for purine salvage (hypoxanthine guanine phosphoribosyl pyrophosphate transferase, HPRT) is absent or deficient. People with this genetic deficiency have CNS deterioration, mental retardation, and spastic cerebral palsy associated with compulsive self-mutilation. Cells in the basal ganglia of the brain (fine motor control) normally have very high HPRT activity. These patients also all have hyperuricemia because purines cannot be salvaged, causing gout.

Section I • Biochemistry

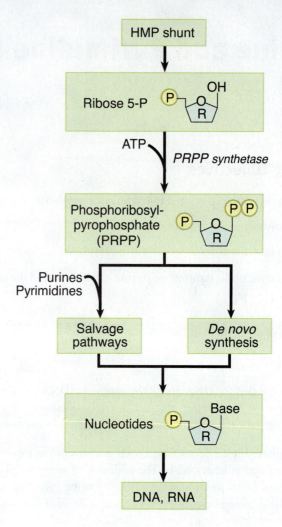

Figure I-18-1. Nucleotide Synthesis by Salvage and De Novo Pathways

PYRIMIDINE SYNTHESIS

Pyrimidines are synthesized *de novo* in the cytoplasm from aspartate, CO_2, and glutamine, as shown in Figure I-18-2. Synthesis involves a cytoplasmic carbamoyl phosphate synthetase that differs from the mitochondrial enzyme with the same name used in the urea cycle.

Orotic Aciduria

Several days after birth, an infant was observed to have severe anemia, which was found to be megaloblastic. There was no evidence of hepatomegaly or splenomegaly. The pediatrician started the newborn on a bottle-fed regimen containing folate, vitamin B_{12}, vitamin B_6, and iron. One week later, the infant's condition did not improve. The pediatrician noted that the infant's urine contained a crystalline residue, which was analyzed and determined to be orotic acid. Laboratory tests indicated no evidence of hyperammonemia. The infant was given a formula that contained uridine. Shortly thereafter, the infant's condition improved significantly.

Orotic aciduria is an autosomal recessive disorder caused by a defect in uridine monophosphate (UMP) synthase. This enzyme contains two activities, orotate phosphoribosyltransferase and orotidine decarboxylase. The lack of pyrimidines impairs nucleic acid synthesis needed for hematopoiesis, explaining the megaloblastic anemia in this infant. Orotic acid accumulates and spills into the urine, resulting in orotic acid crystals and orotic acid urinary obstruction. The presence of orotic acid in urine might suggest that the defect could be ornithine transcarbamylase (OTC) deficiency, but the lack of hyperammonemia rules out a defect in the urea cycle. Uridine administration relieves the symptoms by bypassing the defect in the pyrimidine pathway. Uridine is salvaged to UMP, which feedback-inhibits carbamoyl phosphate synthase-2, preventing orotic acid formation.

Note
Two Orotic Acidurias

1. Hyperammonemia

    No megaloblastic anemia
    - Pathway: Urea cycle
    - Enzyme deficient: OTC

2. Megaloblastic anemia

    No hyperammonemia
    - Pathway: Pyrimidine synthesis
    - Enzyme deficient: UMP synthase

Folate and vitamin B_{12} deficiency: megaloblastic anemia, but no orotic aciduria

Section I • Molecular Biology and Biochemistry

Bridge to Pharmacology
Cotrimoxazole

Cotrimoxazole contains the synergistic antibiotics sulfamethoxazole and trimethoprim, which inhibit different steps in the prokaryotic synthesis of tetrahydrofolate.

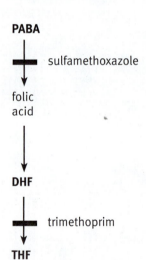

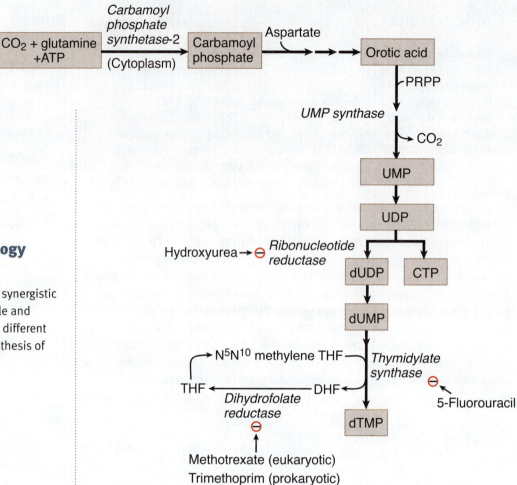

Figure I-18-2. *De Novo* Pyrimidine Synthesis

The primary end product of pyrimidine synthesis is UMP. In the conversion of UMP to dTMP, three important enzymes are ribonucleotide reductase, thymidylate synthase, and dihydrofolate reductase. All three enzymes are targets of antineoplastic drugs and are summarized in Table I-18-1.

Table I-18-1. Important Enzymes of Pyrimidine Synthesis

Enzyme	Function	Drug
Ribonucleotide reductase	Reduces all NDPs to dNDPs for DNA synthesis	Hydroxyurea (S phase)
Thymidylate synthase	Methylates dUMP to dTMP Requires THF	5-Fluorouracil (S phase)
Dihydrofolate reductase (DHFR)	Converts DHF to THF Without DHFR, thymidylate synthesis will eventually stop	Methotrexate (eukaryotic) (S phase) Trimethoprim (prokaryotic) Pyrimethamine (protozoal)

Ribonucleotide Reductase

Ribonucleotide reductase is required for the formation of the deoxyribonucleotides for DNA synthesis. Figure I-18-2 shows its role in dTMP synthesis, and Figure I-18-3 shows all four nucleotide substrates:

- All four nucleotide substrates must be diphosphates.
- dADP and dATP strongly inhibit ribonucleotide reductase.
- Hydroxyurea, an anticancer drug, blocks DNA synthesis indirectly by inhibiting ribonucleotide reductase.

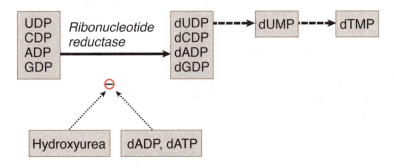

Figure I-18-3. Ribonucleotide Reductase

PYRIMIDINE CATABOLISM

Pyrimidines may be completely catabolized (NH_4^+ is produced) or recycled by pyrimidine salvage enzymes.

PURINE SYNTHESIS

Purines are synthesized *de novo* beginning with PRPP as shown in Figure I-18-4. The most important enzyme is PRPP amidotransferase, which catalyzes the first and rate-limiting reaction of the pathway. It is inhibited by the three purine nucleotide end products AMP, GMP, and IMP.

Section I • Biochemistry

The drugs allopurinol (used for gout) and 6-mercaptopurine (antineoplastic) also inhibit PRPP amidotransferase. These drugs are purine analogs that must be converted to their respective nucleotides by HGPRT within cells. Also note that:

- The amino acids glycine, aspartate, and glutamine are used in purine synthesis.
- Tetrahydrofolate is required for synthesis of all the purines.
- Inosine monophosphate (contains the purine base hypoxanthine) is the precursor for AMP and GMP.

Bridge to Microbiology

Protozoan and multicellular parasites and many obligate parasites, such as *Chlamydia*, cannot synthesize purines *de novo* because they lack the necessary genes in the purine pathway. However, they have elaborate salvage mechanisms for acquiring purines from the host to synthesize their own nucleic acids to grow.

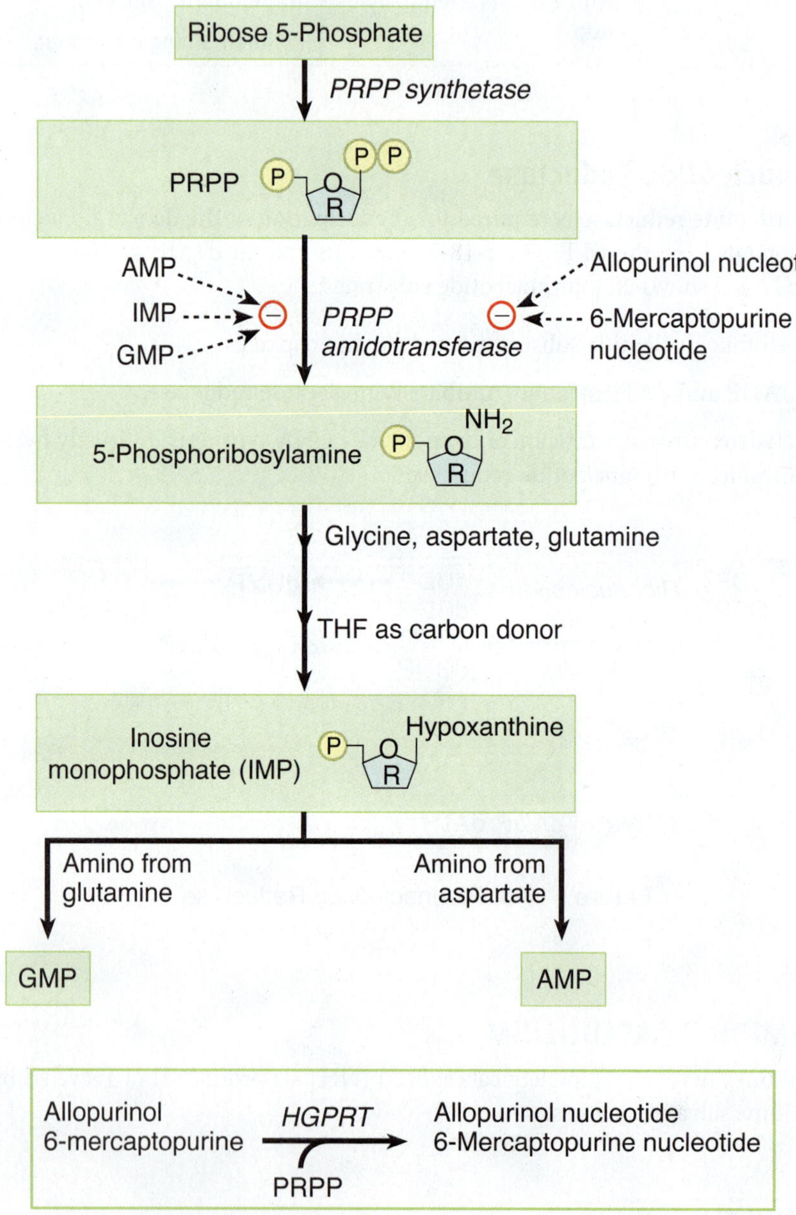

Figure I-18-4. *De Novo* Purine Synthesis

PURINE CATABOLISM AND THE SALVAGE ENZYME HGPRT

Excess purine nucleotides or those released from DNA and RNA by nucleases are catabolized first to nucleosides (loss of P_i) and then to free purine bases (release of ribose or deoxyribose). Excess nucleoside monophosphates may accumulate when:

- RNA is normally digested by nucleases (mRNAs and other types of RNAs are continuously turned over in normal cells).
- Dying cells release DNA and RNA, which is digested by nucleases.
- The concentration of free P_i decreases as it may in galactosemia, hereditary fructose intolerance, and glucose-6-phosphatase deficiency.

Salvage enzymes recycle normally about 90% of these purines, and 10% are converted to uric acid and excreted in urine. When purine catabolism is increased significantly, a person is at risk for developing hyperuricemia and potentially gout.

Purine catabolism to uric acid and salvage of the purine bases hypoxanthine (derived from adenosine) and guanine are shown in Figure I-18-5.

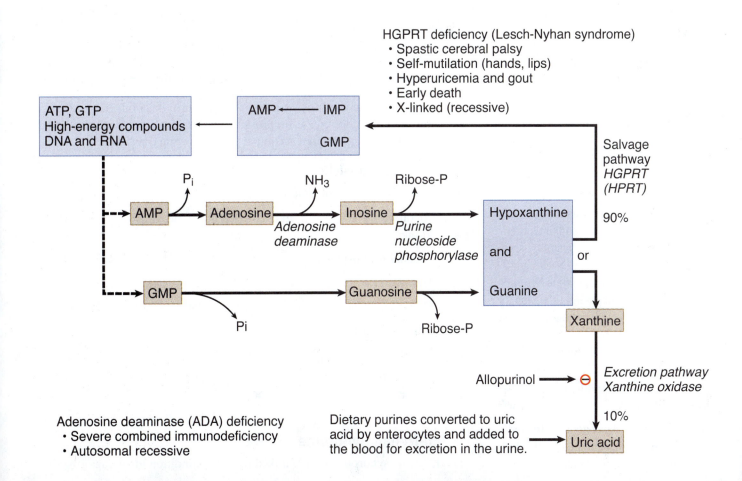

Figure I-18-5. Purine Excretion and Salvage Pathways

Section I • Biochemistry

Bridge to Pharmacology
Thiazide diuretics (hydrochlorothiazide and chlorthalidone) may cause hyperuricemia.

Bridge to Pathology
Treatment of large tumors with chemotherapeutic regimens or radiation may cause "tumor lysis syndrome" and excessive excretion of uric acid, resulting in gout. The cause of the excessive uric acid is the destruction of the cancer cell's nucleic acid into purines undergoing turnover.

Clinical Correlate
Gout

Acute gouty arthritis, seen most commonly in males, results from precipitation of monosodium urate crystals in joints. The crystals, identified as negatively birefringent and needle-shaped, initiate neutrophil-mediated and acute inflammation, often first affecting the big toe. Chronic gout may manifest over time as tophi (deposits of monosodium urate) develop in soft tissue around joints, leading to chronic inflammation involving granulomas.

- Acute attacks of gout are treated with colchicine or indomethacin to reduce the inflammation.
- Chronic hyperuricemia, because of underexcretion, is treated with a uricosuric drug (probenecid).
- Overproduction of uric acid and chronic gout are treated with allopurinol.

Adenosine Deaminase Deficiency

Adenosine deaminase (ADA) deficiency, an autosomal recessive disorder, causes a type of severe combined immunodeficiency (SCID). Lacking both B-cell and T-cell function, children are multiply infected with many organisms (*Pneumocystis carinii, Candida*) and do not survive without treatment. Enzyme replacement therapy and bone marrow transplantation may be used. Experimental gene therapy trials have not yet yielded completely successful cures.

High levels of dATP accumulate in red cells of ADA patients and inhibit ribonucleotide reductase, thereby inhibiting the production of other essential deoxynucleotide precursors for DNA synthesis (see Figure I-18-3). Although it is believed that the impaired DNA synthesis contributes to dysfunction of T cells and B cells, it is not known why the main effects are limited to these cell types.

Hyperuricemia and Gout

Hyperuricemia may be produced by overproduction of uric acid or underexcretion of uric acid by the kidneys. Hyperuricemia may progress to acute and chronic gouty arthritis if uric acid (monosodium urate) is deposited in joints and surrounding soft tissue, where it causes inflammation. Uric acid is produced from excess endogenous purines as shown in Figure I-18-5, and is also produced from dietary purines (digestion of nucleic acid in the intestine) by intestinal epithelia. Both sources of uric acid are transported in the blood to the kidneys for excretion in urine.

Allopurinol inhibits xanthine oxidase and also can reduce purine synthesis by inhibiting PRPP amidotransferase, provided HGPRT is active (see Figure I-18-4). Hyperuricemia and gout often accompany the following conditions:

- Lesch-Nyhan syndrome (no purine salvage)
- Partial deficiency of HGPRT
- Alcoholism (lactate and urate compete for same transport system in the kidney)
- Glucose 6-phosphatase deficiency
- Hereditary fructose intolerance (aldolase B deficiency)
- Galactose 1-phosphate uridyl transferase deficiency (galactosemia)
- Mutations in PRPP synthetase that lower *Km*

In the last two diseases, phosphorylated sugars accumulate, decreasing the available P_i and increasing AMP (which cannot be phosphorylated to ADP and ATP). The excess AMP is converted to uric acid.

Lesch-Nyhan Syndrome

Lesch-Nyhan syndrome is an X-linked recessive condition involving:

- Near-complete deficiency of HGPRT activity
- Mental retardation
- Spastic cerebral palsy with compulsive biting of hands and lips
- Hyperuricemia
- Death often in first decade

Over 100 distinct mutations of the HGPRT gene located on the X chromosome have been reported to give rise to Lesch-Nyhan syndrome. These mutations include complete deletions of the gene, point mutations that result in an increased K_m for hypoxanthine and guanine for the enzyme, and mutations that cause the encoded enzyme to have a short half-life.

Lesch-Nyhan syndrome

The parents of a 9-month-old male infant were concerned that their son appeared generally weak, had difficulty moving his arms and legs, repeatedly bit his lips, and frequently seemed to be in pain. The infant was brought to the pediatrician. The parents mentioned that since the baby was born, they often noticed tiny, orange-colored particles when they changed the infant's diapers. Laboratory analysis of uric acid in urine was normalized to the urinary creatinine in the infant, and it was found that the amount was 3 times greater than the normal range.

One of the earliest signs of Lesch-Nyhan syndrome is the appearance of orange crystals in diapers. They are needle-shaped sodium urate crystals. Without the salvaging of hypoxanthine and guanine by HGPRT, the purines are shunted toward the excretion pathway. This is compounded by the lack of regulatory control of the PRPP amidotransferase in the purine synthesis pathway, resulting in the synthesis of even more purines in the body. The large amounts of urate will cause crippling, gouty arthritis and urate nephropathy. Renal failure is usually the cause of death. Treatment with allopurinol will ease the amount of urate deposits formed.

Bridge to Pharmacology
Febuxostat is a nonpurine inhibitor of xanthine oxidase.

Bridge to Medical Genetics
There are a large number of known mutations in the HGPRT gene. These have varying effects on the K_m for the enzyme product, generating varying degrees of severity. This concept is known as allelic heterogeneity.

Chapter Summary

Nucleotide Synthesis
- **Ribose 5-P from HMP shunt**

    PRPP synthetase activates

- **Salvage pathway**

    Utilizes pre-formed purine or pyrimidine

- **De novo synthesis pathway**

    Includes synthesis of purine or pyrimidine

Pyrimidine De Novo Synthesis
- UMP, CMP, dTMP

Important Vitamin
- Folate for dTMP synthesis

Amino Acids Used
- Aspartate and glutamine

(Continued)

Section I • Biochemistry

Chapter Summary (continued)

Important Enzymes

- Ribonucleotide reductase
  - Inhibited by hydroxyurea
- Thymidylate synthase
  - Inhibited by 5-fluorouracil
- Dihydrofolate reductase
  - Inhibited by methotrexate (euk), trimethoprim (prok), pyrimethamine (protozoal)

Genetic Disease

- Orotic aciduria with megaloblastic anemia
  - Enzyme deficiency: UMP synthase

Purine De Novo Synthesis

- GMP, AMP (IMP)

Important Vitamin

- Folate

Amino Acids Used

- Aspartate, glutamine, glycine

Rate-Limiting Enzyme

- PRPP amidotransferase
  - Inhibited by GMP, AMP, and IMP
  - Inhibited by allopurinol (nucleotide) and 6-mercaptopurine (nucleotide)

Purine Salvage Pathway Enzyme

- HGPRT (HPRT)

Genetic Deficiency

- Lesch-Nyhan

Purine Catabolism

End Product

- Uric acid

(Continued)

Chapter Summary (continued)

Causes of Hyperuricemia

- Excessive cell death
- Excessive alcohol consumption
- Excessive dietary nucleic acid
- Secondary to genetic disease:
  - Lesch-Nyhan
  - Glucose-6-phosphatase deficiency
  - Galactose uridyltransferase deficiency
  - Fructose 1-P aldolase (aldolase B) deficiency
- Underexcretion by kidney

Review Questions

Select the ONE best answer.

1. A 6-month-old boy becomes progressively lethargic and pale and shows delayed motor development. Laboratory evaluation reveals normal blood urea nitrogen (BUN), low serum iron, hemoglobin 4.6 g/dL, and leukopenia. His bone marrow shows marked megaloblastosis, which did not respond to treatment with iron, folic acid, vitamin B_{12}, or pyridoxine. His urine developed abundant white precipitate identified as orotic acid. The underlying defect causing the megaloblastic anemia in this child is most likely in which of the following pathways?

   A. Homocysteine metabolism
   B. Pyrimidine synthesis
   C. Urea synthesis
   D. Uric acid synthesis
   E. Heme synthesis

2. Patients with Lesch-Nyhan syndrome have hyperuricemia, indicating an increased biosynthesis of purine nucleotides, and markedly decreased levels of hypoxanthine phosphoribosyl transferase (HPRT). The hyperuricemia can be explained on the basis of a decrease in which regulator of purine biosynthesis?

   A. ATP
   B. GDP
   C. Glutamine
   D. IMP
   E. PRPP

Section I • Biochemistry

3. A 12-week-old infant with a history of persistent diarrhea and candidiasis is seen for a respiratory tract infection with *Pneumocystis jiroveci*. A chest x-ray confirms pneumonia and reveals absence of a thymic shadow. Trace IgG is present in his serum, but IgA and IgM are absent. His red blood cells completely lack an essential enzyme in purine degradation. The product normally formed by this enzyme is

   A. guanine monophosphate
   B. hypoxanthine
   C. inosine
   D. xanthine
   E. xanthine monophosphate

Items 4 and 5

The anticancer drug 6-mercaptopurine is deactivated by the enzyme xanthine oxidase. A cancer patient being treated with 6-mercaptopurine develops hyperuricemia, and the physician decides to give the patient allopurinol.

4. What effect will allopurinol have on the activity of 6-mercaptopurine?

   A. Enhanced deactivation of 6-mercaptopurine
   B. Enhanced elimination of 6-mercaptopurine as uric acid
   C. Enhanced retention and potentiation of activity
   D. Decreased inhibition of PRPP glutamylamidotransferase

5. Resistance of neoplastic cells to the chemotherapeutic effect of 6-mercaptopurine would most likely involve loss or inactivation of a gene encoding

   A. thymidylate synthase
   B. hypoxanthine phosphoribosyltransferase
   C. purine nucleoside pyrophosphorylase
   D. orotic acid phosphoribosyltransferase
   E. adenosine deaminase

Answers

1. **Answer: B.** Accumulation of orotic acid indicates megaloblastic anemia arises because pyrimidines are required for DNA synthesis.

2. **Answer: D.** IMP is a feedback inhibitor of PRPP amidophosphoribosyl transferase, the first reaction in the biosynthesis of purines. IMP is formed by the HPRT reaction in the salvage of hypoxanthine.

3. **Answer: C.** The child most likely has severe combined immunodeficiency caused by adenosine deaminase deficiency. This enzyme deaminates adenosine (a nucleoside) to form inosine (another nucleoside). Hypoxanthine and xanthine are both purine bases, and the monophosphates are nucleotides.

4. **Answer: C.** Because allopurinol inhibits xanthine oxidase, the 6-mercaptopurine will not be deactivated as rapidly.

5. **Answer: B.** HPRT is required for activation of 6-mercaptopurine to its ribonucleotide and inhibition of purine synthesis. The other enzymes listed are not targets for this drug.

SECTION II

Medical Genetics

Single-Gene Disorders 1

Learning Objectives

❏ Interpret scenarios about basic definitions
❏ Use knowledge of major modes of inheritance
❏ Use knowledge of important principles that can characterize single-gene diseases

BASIC DEFINITIONS

Chromosomes

Humans are composed of two groups of cells:

- **Gametes.** Ova and sperm cells, which are haploid, have one copy of each type of chromosome (1–22, X or Y). This DNA is transmitted to offspring.
- **Somatic cells** (cells other than gametes). Nearly all somatic cells are diploid, having two copies of each type of autosome (1–22) and either XX or XY.

Diploid cells

- **Homologous chromosomes.** The two chromosomes in each diploid pair are said to be homologs, or homologous chromosomes. They contain the same genes, but because one is of paternal origin and one is of maternal origin, they may have different alleles at some loci.
- **X and Y chromosomes,** or the sex chromosomes, have some homologous regions but the majority of genes are different. The regions that are homologous are sometimes referred to as pseudoautosomal regions. During meiosis-1 of male spermatogenesis, the X and Y chromosomes pair in the pseudoautosomal regions, allowing the chromosomes to segregate into different cells.

Genes

- **Gene.** Physically a gene consists of a sequence of DNA that encodes a specific protein (or a nontranslated RNA; for example: tRNA, rRNA, or snRNA).
- **Locus.** The physical location of a gene on a chromosome is termed a locus.
- **Alleles.** Variation (mutation) in the DNA sequence of a gene produces a new allele at that locus. Many genes have multiple alleles. Although this term has been used most frequently with genes, noncoding DNA can also have alleles of specific sequences.
- **Polymorphism.** When a specific site on a chromosome has multiple alleles in the population, it is said to be polymorphic (many forms).

Note

- **Gene**—basic unit of inheritance
- **Locus**—location of a gene on a chromosome
- **Allele**—different forms of a gene
- **Genotype**—alleles found at a locus
- **Phenotype**—physically observable features
- **Homozygote**—alleles at a locus are the same
- **Heterozygote**—alleles at a locus are different
- **Dominant**—requires only one copy of the mutation to produce disease
- **Recessive**—requires two copies of the mutation to produce disease

Section II • Medical Genetics

For example, the β-globin gene encodes a protein (β-globin). It has been mapped to chromosome 11p15.5 indicating its locus, a specific location on chromosome 11. Throughout human history there have been many mutations in the β-globin gene, and each mutation has created a new allele in the population. The β-globin locus is therefore polymorphic. Some alleles cause no clinical disease, but others, like the sickle cell allele, are associated with significant disease. Included among the disease-causing alleles are those associated with sickle cell anemia and several associated with β-thalassemia.

Genotype

The specific DNA sequence at a locus is termed a genotype. In diploid somatic cells a genotype may be:

- **Homozygous** if the individual has the same allele on both homologs (homologous chromosomes) at that locus.
- **Heterozygous** if the individual has different alleles on the two homologs (homologous chromosomes) at that locus.

Phenotype

The phenotype is generally understood as the expression of the genotype in terms of observable characteristics.

Mutations

> **Note**
> Major types of single-gene mutations are:
> - Missense
> - Nonsense
> - Deletion
> - Insertion
> - Frameshift

A *mutation* is an alteration in DNA sequence (thus, mutations produce new alleles). When mutations occur in cells giving rise to gametes, the mutations can be transmitted to future generations. *Missense* mutations result in the substitution of a single amino acid in the polypeptide chain (e.g., sickle cell disease is caused by a missense mutation that produces a substitution of valine for glutamic acid in the β-globin polypeptide). *Nonsense* mutations produce a stop codon, resulting in premature termination of translation and a truncated protein. Nucleotide bases may be inserted or deleted. When the number of inserted or deleted bases is a multiple of three, the mutation is said to be *in-frame*. If not a multiple of three, the mutation is a *frameshift,* which alters all codons downstream of the mutation, typically producing a truncated or severely altered protein product. Mutations can occur in promoter and other regulatory regions or in genes for transcription factors that bind to these regions. This can decrease or increase the amount of gene product produced in the cell. (For a complete description of these and other mutations, see Section I, Chapter 4: Translation; Mutations.)

Mutations can also be classified according to their phenotypic effects. Mutations that cause a missing protein product or cause decreased activity of the protein are termed *loss-of-function*. Those that produce a protein product with a new function or increased activity are termed *gain-of-function*.

Recurrence risk

The *recurrence risk* is the probability that the offspring of a couple will express a genetic disease. For example, in the mating of a normal homozygote with a heterozygote who has a dominant disease-causing allele, the recurrence risk for each offspring is 1/2, or 50%. It is important to remember that each reproductive event is statistically independent of all previous events. Therefore, the recurrence risk remains the same regardless of the number of previously affected or unaffected offspring. Determining the mode of inheritance of a disease (e.g., autosomal dominant versus autosomal recessive) enables one to assign an appropriate recurrence risk for a family.

Pedigrees

A patient's family history is diagrammed in a pedigree (see symbols in Figure II-1-1). The first affected individual to be identified in the family is termed the **proband**.

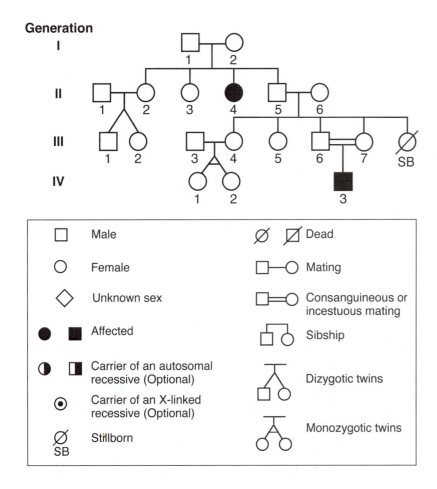

Figure II-1-1. Pedigree Nomenclature

MAJOR MODES OF INHERITANCE

Autosomal Dominant Inheritance

A number of features in a pedigree help identify autosomal dominant inheritance:

- Because affected individuals must receive a disease-causing gene from an affected parent, the disease is typically observed in multiple generations of a pedigree (see Figure II-1-2).

- Skipped generations are not typically seen because two unaffected parents cannot transmit a disease-causing allele to their offspring (an exception occurs when there is reduced penetrance, discussed below).

- Because these genes are located on autosomes, males and females are affected in roughly equal frequencies.

Autosomal dominant alleles are relatively rare in populations, so the typical mating pattern is a heterozygous affected individual (Aa genotype) mating with a homozygous normal individual (aa genotype), as shown in Figure II-1-3. Note that, by convention, the dominant allele is shown in uppercase (A) and the recessive allele is shown in lowercase (a). The recurrence risk is thus 50%, and half the children, on average, will be affected with the disease. If both parents are heterozygous, the recurrence risk is 75%.

Note
Autosomal Dominant Diseases

- Familial hypercholesterolemia (LDL receptor deficiency)
- Huntington disease
- Neurofibromatosis type 1
- Marfan syndrome
- Acute intermittent porphyria

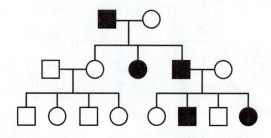

Figure II-1-2. Autosomal Dominant Inheritance

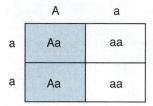

A Punnett square: Affected offspring (Aa) are shaded.

Figure II-1-3. Recurrence Risk for the Mating of Affected Individual (Aa) with a Homozygous Unaffected Individual (aa) using a Punnett Square

Autosomal Recessive Inheritance

Important features that distinguish autosomal recessive inheritance:

- Because autosomal recessive alleles are clinically expressed only in the homozygous state, the offspring must inherit one copy of the disease-causing allele from each parent.

- In contrast to autosomal dominant diseases, autosomal recessive diseases are typically seen in only one generation of a pedigree (see Figure II-1-4).

- Because these genes are located on autosomes, males and females are affected in roughly equal frequencies.

Most commonly, a homozygote is produced by the union of two heterozygous (*carrier*) parents. The recurrence risk for offspring of such matings is 25% (see Figure II-1-5).

Consanguinity (the mating of related individuals) is sometimes seen in recessive pedigrees because individuals who share common ancestors are more likely to carry the same recessive disease-causing alleles.

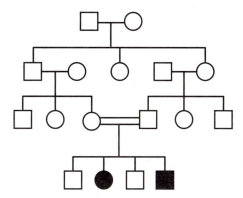

A consanguineous mating has produced two affected offspring.

Figure II-1-4. Pedigree for an Autosomal Recessive Disease

Note
Autosomal Recessive Diseases

Examples include:

- Sickle cell anemia
- Cystic fibrosis
- Phenylketonuria (PKU)
- Tay-Sachs disease (hexosaminidase A deficiency)

	A	a
A	AA	Aa
a	Aa	aa

The affected genotype (aa) is shaded.

Figure II-1-5. Recurrence Risk for the Mating of Two Heterozygous Carriers (Aa) of a Recessive Mutation

Determining the Recurrence Risk for an Individual Whose Phenotype Is Known. In Figure II-1-4, Individual IV-1 may wish to know his risk of being a carrier. Because his phenotype is known, there are only three possible genotypes he can have, assuming complete penetrance of the disease-producing allele. He cannot be homozygous for the recessive allele (aa). Two of the remaining three possibilities are carriers (Aa and aA), and one is homozygous normal (AA). Thus, his risk of being a carrier is 2/3, or 0.67 (67%).

Section II • Medical Genetics

X-Linked Recessive Inheritance

Properties of X-linked recessive inheritance

Because males have only one copy of the X chromosome, they are said to be **hemizygous** (*hemi* = "half") for the X chromosome. If a recessive disease-causing mutation occurs on the X chromosome, a male will be affected with the disease.

- Because males require only one copy of the mutation to express the disease and females require two copies, X-linked recessive diseases are seen much more commonly in males than in females (see Figure II-1-6).

- Skipped generations are commonly seen because an affected male can transmit the disease-causing mutation to a heterozygous daughter, who is unaffected but who can transmit the disease-causing allele to her sons.

- Male-to-male transmission is not seen in X-linked inheritance; this helps distinguish it from autosomal inheritance.

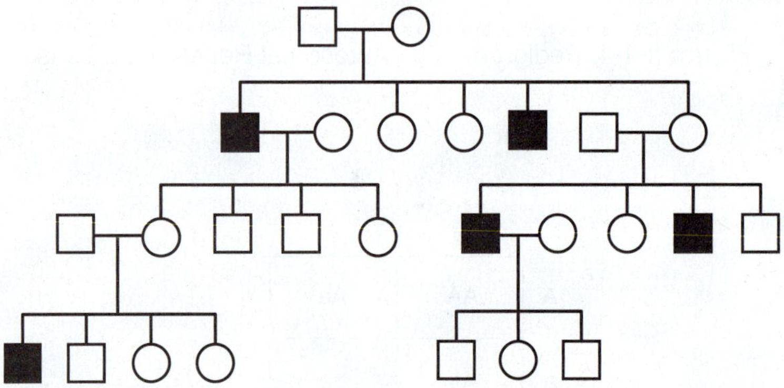

Note
X-Linked Recessive Diseases

- Duchenne muscular dystrophy
- Lesch-Nyhan syndrome (hypoxanthine-guanine phosphoribosyltransferase [HGPRT] deficiency)
- Glucose-6-phosphate dehydrogenase deficiency
- Hemophilia A and B
- Red-green color blindness
- Menke's disease
- Ornithine transcarbamoylase (OTC) deficiency
- SCID (IL-receptor γ-chain deficiency)

Figure II-1-6. X-Linked Recessive Inheritance

Recurrence Risks. Figure II-1-7 shows the recurrence risks for X-linked recessive diseases.

- Affected male–homozygous normal female: All of the daughters will be heterozygous carriers; all of the sons will be homozygous normal.

- Normal male–carrier female: On average, half of the sons will be affected and half of the daughters will be carriers. Note that in this case, the recurrence rate is different depending on the sex of the child. If the fetal sex is known, the recurrence rate for a daughter is 0, and that for a son is 50%. **If the sex of the fetus is not known, then the recurrence rate is multiplied by 1/2, the probability that the fetus is a male versus a female. Therefore if the sex is unknown, the recurrence risk is 25%.**

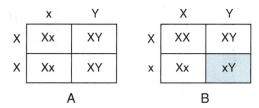

A. Affected male–homozygous normal female
   (X chromosome with mutation is in lower case)
B. Normal male–carrier female

Figure II-1-7. Recurrence Risks for X-Linked Recessive Diseases

X inactivation

Normal males inherit an X chromosome from their mother and a Y chromosome from their father, whereas normal females inherit an X chromosome from each parent. Because the Y chromosome carries only about 50 protein-coding genes and the X chromosome carries hundreds of protein-coding genes, a mechanism must exist to equalize the amount of protein encoded by X chromosomes in males and females. This mechanism, termed X inactivation, occurs in the blastocyst (~100 cells) during the development of female embryos (Figure II-1-8). When an X chromosome is inactivated, its DNA is not transcribed into mRNA, and the chromosome is visualized under the microscope as a highly condensed *Barr body* in the nuclei of interphase cells. X inactivation has several important characteristics:

- It is *random*—in some cells of the female embryo, the X chromosome inherited from the father is inactivated, and in others the X chromosome inherited from the mother is inactivated. Like coin tossing, this is a random process. As shown in Figure II-1-6, most women have their paternal X chromosome active in approximately 50% of their cells and the maternal X chromosome active in approximately 50% of their cells. Thus, females are said to be *mosaics* with respect to the active X chromosome.
- It is *fixed*—once inactivation of an X chromosome occurs in a cell, the same X chromosome is inactivated in all descendants of the cell.
- It is *incomplete*—there are regions throughout the X chromosome, including the tips of both the long and short arms, that are not inactivated.
- X-chromosome inactivation is permanent in somatic cells and reversible in developing germ line cells. Both X chromosomes are active during oogenesis.
- All X chromosomes in a cell are inactivated except one. For example, females with three X chromosomes in each cell (see Chapter 3) have two X chromosomes inactivated in each cell (thus, two Barr bodies can be visualized in an interphase cell).

X-chromosome inactivation is thought to be mediated by >1 mechanism.

- A gene called *XIST* has been identified as the primary gene that causes X inactivation. *XIST* produces an RNA product that coats the chromosome, helping produce its inactivation.
- Condensation into heterochromatin
- Methylation of gene regions on the X chromosome

Note

X inactivation occurs early in the female embryo and is random, fixed, and incomplete. In a cell, all X chromosomes but one are inactivated.

Note

Genetic Mosaicism

Genetic mosaicism is the presence of 2 or more cell lines with different karyotypes in an individual. It arises from mitotic nondisjunction. The number of cell lines that develop and their relative proportions are influenced by the *timing* of nondisjunction during embryogenesis and the *viability* of the aneuploid cells produced.

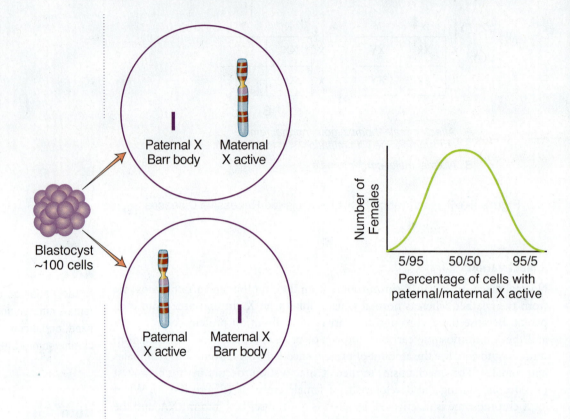

Figure II-1-8. Inactivation of the X Chromosome during Embryogenesis Is a Random Process

Manifesting (female) heterozygotes

Normal females have two copies of the X chromosome, so they usually require two copies of the mutation to express the disease. However, because X inactivation is a random process, a heterozygous female will occasionally express an X-linked recessive mutation because, by random chance, most of the X chromosomes carrying the normal allele have been inactivated. Such females are termed *manifesting heterozygotes*. Because they usually have at least a small population of active X chromosomes carrying the normal allele, their disease expression is typically milder than that of hemizygous males.

Y Chromosome Highlights

- The *SRY* (sex determining region) gene is a transcription factor that initiates male development.
- The q arm of Y chromosomes contains a large block of heterochromatin.
- Microdeletions of Yq in males result in nonobstructive azoospermia.

X-Linked Dominant Inheritance

There are relatively few diseases whose inheritance is classified as X-linked dominant. Fragile X syndrome is an important example. In this condition, females are differently affected than males, and whereas penetrance in males is 100%, that in females is approximately 60% (see margin note). The typical fragile X patient described is male.

As in X-linked recessive inheritance, male–male transmission of the disease-causing mutation is not seen (see Figure II-1-9).

- Heterozygous females are affected. Because females have two X chromosomes (and thus two chances to inherit an X-linked disease-causing mutation) and males have only one, X-linked dominant diseases are seen about twice as often in females as in males.

- As in autosomal dominant inheritance, the disease phenotype is seen in multiple generations of a pedigree; skipped generations are relatively unusual.

- Examine the children of an affected male (II-1 in Figure II-I-9). None of his sons will be affected, but all of his daughters have the disease (assuming complete penetrance).

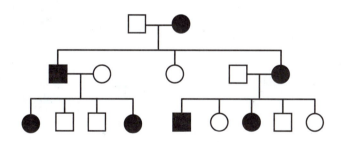

Figure II-1-9. X-Linked Dominant Inheritance

Recurrence Risks

Figure II-1-10 shows the recurrence risks for X-linked dominant inheritance.

- Affected male–homozygous normal female: None of the sons are affected; all of the daughters are affected. Note that in this case, the recurrence rate is different depending on the sex of the child. If the fetal sex is known, the recurrence rate for a daughter is 100%, and that for a son is 0%. **If the sex of the fetus is not known, then the recurrence rate is multiplied by 1/2, the probability that the fetus is a male versus a female. Therefore if the sex is unknown, the recurrence risk is 50%.**

- Normal male–heterozygous affected female: On average, 50% of sons are affected and 50% of daughters are affected.

Clinical Correlate
Fragile X Syndrome

Males: 100% penetrance
- Mental retardation
- Large ears
- Prominent jaw
- Macro-orchidism (usually postpubertal)

Females: 60% penetrance
- Mental retardation

Note
Penetrance in Genetic Diseases

The penetrance of a disease-causing mutation is the percentage of individuals who are known to have the disease-causing genotype who display the disease phenotype (develop symptoms).

Section II • Medical Genetics

Note

X-Linked Dominant Diseases

- Hypophosphatemic rickets
- Fragile X syndrome

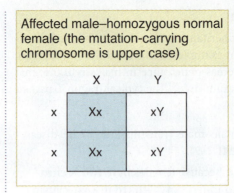
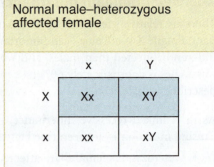

Figure II-1-10. Recurrence Risks for X-Linked Dominant Inheritance

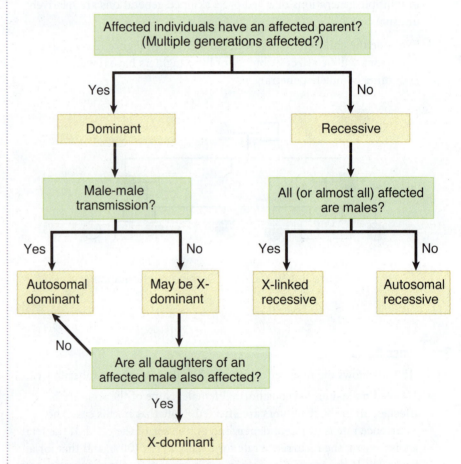

Note: If transmission occurs *only* through affected mothers and never through affected sons, the pedigree is likely to reflect mitochondrial inheritance.

Figure II-I-11. A Basic Decision Tree for Determining the Mode of Inheritance in a Pedigree

Mitochondrial Inheritance

Mitochondria, which are cytoplasmic organelles involved in cellular respiration, have their own chromosomes, each of which contains 16,569 DNA base pairs (bp) arranged in a circular molecule. This DNA encodes 13 proteins that are subunits of complexes in the electron transport and oxidative phosphorylation processes (see Section I, Chapter 13). In addition, mitochondrial DNA encodes 22 transfer RNAs and 2 ribosomal RNAs.

Because a sperm cell contributes no mitochondria to the egg cell during fertilization, mitochondrial DNA is inherited exclusively through females. Pedigrees for mitochondrial diseases thus display a distinct mode of inheritance: Diseases are transmitted only from affected females to their offspring (see Figure II-1-12).

- Both males and females are affected.
- Transmission of the disease is only from a female.
- All offspring of an affected female are affected.
- None of the offspring of an affected male is affected.
- Diseases are typically neuropathies and/or myopathies (see margin note).

Heteroplasmy

A typical cell contains hundreds of mitochondria in its cytoplasm, and each mitochondrion has its own copy of the mitochondrial genome. When a specific mutation occurs in some of the mitochondria, this mutation can be unevenly distributed into daughter cells during cell division: Some cells may inherit more mitochondria in which the normal DNA sequence predominates, while others inherit mostly mitochondria with the mutated, disease-causing gene. This condition is known as *heteroplasmy*. Variations in heteroplasmy account for substantial variation in the severity of expression of mitochondrial diseases.

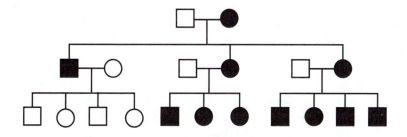

Figure II-1-12. Pedigree for a Mitochondrial Disease

Note
Mitochondrial Diseases

- Leber hereditary optic neuropathy
- MELAS: mitochondrial encephalomyopathy, lactic acidosis, and stroke-like episodes
- Myoclonic epilepsy with ragged red muscle fibers

IMPORTANT PRINCIPLES THAT CAN CHARACTERIZE SINGLE-GENE DISEASES

Variable Expression

> **Hemochromatosis**
>
> Mary B. is a 45-year-old white female with hip pain of 2 years' duration. She also experiences moderate chronic fatigue. Routine blood work shows that liver function tests (LFTs) are slightly elevated. She does not drink alcohol. She takes no prescription drugs although she does use aspirin for the hip pain. She takes no vitamin or mineral supplements.
>
> Mary B.'s 48-year-old brother has recently been diagnosed with hereditary hemochromatosis. Her brother's symptoms include arthritis for which he takes Tylenol (acetaminophen), significant hepatomegaly, diabetes, and "bronze" skin. His transferrin saturation is 75% and ferritin 1300 ng/mL. A liver biopsy revealed stainable iron in all hepatocytes and initial indications of hepatic cirrhosis. He was found to be homozygous for the most common mutation (C282Y) causing hemochromatosis. Subsequently Mary was tested and also proved to be homozygous for the C282Y mutation. Following diagnosis, both individuals were treated with periodic phlebotomy to satisfactorily reduce iron load.

Most genetic diseases vary in the degree of phenotypic expression: Some individuals may be severely affected, whereas others are more mildly affected. This can be the result of several factors:

Environmental Influences. In the case of hemochromatosis described above, Mary's less-severe phenotype may in part be attributable to loss of blood during regular menses throughout adulthood. Her brother's use of Tylenol may contribute to his liver problems.

The autosomal recessive disease xeroderma pigmentosum will be expressed more severely in individuals who are exposed more frequently to ultraviolet radiation.

Allelic Heterogeneity. Different mutations in the disease-causing locus may cause more- or less-severe expression. Most genetic diseases show some degree of allelic heterogeneity. For example, missense mutations in the factor VIII gene tend to produce less severe hemophilia than do nonsense mutations, which result in a truncated protein product and little, if any, expression of factor VIII.

Allelic heterogeneity usually results in phenotypic variation between families, not within a single family. Generally the same mutation is responsible for all cases of the disease within a family. In the example of hemochromatosis above, both Mary and her brother have inherited the same mutation; thus, allelic heterogeneity is not responsible for the variable expression in this case.

It is relatively uncommon to see a genetic disease in which there is no allelic heterogeneity.

Heteroplasmy in mitochondrial pedigrees.

Modifier Loci. Disease expression may be affected by the action of other loci, termed modifier loci. Often these may not be identified.

Incomplete Penetrance

A disease-causing mutation is said to have incomplete penetrance when some individuals who have the disease genotype (e.g., one copy of the mutation for an autosomal dominant disease or two copies for an autosomal recessive disease) do not display the disease phenotype (see Figure II-1-13). Incomplete penetrance is distinguished from variable expression in that the nonpenetrant gene has no phenotypic expression at all. In the pedigree shown in Figure II-1-13, Individual II-4 must have the disease-causing allele (he passed it from his father to his son) but shows no symptoms. He is an example of nonpenetrance.

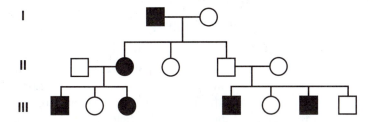

The unaffected male in generation II (II-4) has an affected father and two affected sons. He must have the disease-causing mutation, although it shows incomplete penetrance.

Figure II-1-13. Incomplete Penetrance for an Autosomal Dominant Disease

The penetrance of a disease-causing mutation is quantified by examining a large number of families and calculating the percentage of individuals who are known to have the disease-causing genotype who display the disease phenotype.

Suppose that we had data from several different family studies of the disease affecting the family in Figure II-1-13 and had identified 50 individuals with the disease-producing genotype. Of these individuals only 40 had any symptom(s). Penetrance would be calculated as:

$$40/50 = 0.80, \text{ or } 80\%$$

Penetrance must be taken into account when predicting recurrence risks. For instance, if II-1 and II-2 have another child, the recurrence risk is:

$$0.50 \times 0.80 = 0.40, \text{ or } 40\%$$

Both dominant diseases (as shown in Figure II-1-13) and recessive diseases can show incomplete (reduced) penetrance.

- Although 1 in 300 whites inherits the homozygous genotype for hemochromatosis, a much smaller percentage of individuals develop the disease (approximately 1 in 1,000–2,000). Penetrance for this autosomal recessive disease is only about 15%.

Notice that hereditary hemochromatosis is an example of incomplete penetrance and also an example of variable expression. Expression of the disease phenotype in individuals homozygous for the disease-causing mutation can run the gamut from severe symptoms to none at all. Among the 15% of individuals with at least some phenotypic expression, that expression can be more or less severe (variable expression). However, 85% of individuals homozygous for the disease-causing mutation never have any symptoms (nonpenetrance). The same factors that contribute to variable expression in hemochromatosis can also contribute to incomplete penetrance.

It is necessary to be able to:

- Define incomplete (reduced) penetrance.
- Identify an example of incomplete penetrance in an autosomal dominant pedigree as shown in Figure II-1-13.
- Include penetrance in a simple recurrence risk calculation.

Incomplete Penetrance in Familial Cancer. Retinoblastoma is an autosomal dominant condition caused by an inherited loss-of-function mutation in the *Rb* tumor suppressor gene. In 10% of individuals who inherit this mutation, there is no additional somatic mutation in the normal copy and retinoblastoma does not develop, although they can pass the mutation to their offspring. Penetrance of retinoblastoma is therefore 90%.

Pleiotropy

Pleiotropy exists when a single disease-causing mutation affects multiple organ systems. Pleiotropy is a common feature of genetic diseases.

Pleiotropy in Marfan Syndrome

Marfan syndrome is an autosomal dominant disease that affects approximately 1 in 10,000 individuals. It is characterized by skeletal abnormalities (thin, elongated limbs; pectus excavatum; pectus carinatum), hypermobile joints, ocular abnormalities (frequent myopia and detached lens), and most importantly, cardiovascular disease (mitral valve prolapse and aortic aneurysm). Dilatation of the ascending aorta is seen in 90% of patients and frequently leads to aortic rupture or congestive heart failure. Although the features of this disease seem rather disparate, they are all caused by a mutation in the gene that encodes fibrillin, a key component of connective tissue. Fibrillin is expressed in the periosteum and perichondrium, the suspensory ligament of the eye, and the aorta. Defective fibrillin causes the connective tissue to be "stretchy" and leads to all of the observed disease features. Marfan syndrome thus provides a good example of the principle of pleiotropy.

Locus Heterogeneity

Locus heterogeneity exists when the same disease phenotype can be caused by mutations in different loci. Locus heterogeneity becomes especially important when genetic testing is performed by testing for mutations at specific loci.

Locus Heterogeneity in Osteogenesis Imperfecta Type 2

Osteogenesis imperfecta (OI) is a disease of bone development that affects approximately 1 in 10,000 individuals. It results from a defect in the collagen protein, a major component of the bone matrix. Four major forms of OI have been identified. The severe perinatal form (type 2) is the result of a defect in type 1 collagen, a trimeric molecule that has a triple helix structure. Two members of the trimer are encoded by a gene on chromosome 17, and the third is encoded by a gene on chromosome 7. Mutations in either of these genes give rise to a faulty collagen molecule, causing type 2 OI. Often, patients with chromosome 17 mutations are clinically indistinguishable from those with chromosome 7 mutations. This exemplifies the principle of locus heterogeneity.

New Mutations

In many genetic diseases, particularly those in which the mortality rate is high or the fertility rate is low, a large proportion of cases are caused by a new mutation transmitted from an unaffected parent to an affected offspring. There is thus no family history of the disease (for example, 100% of individuals with osteogenesis imperfecta type 2, discussed above, are the result of a new mutation in the family). A pedigree in which there has been a new mutation is shown in Figure II-1-14. Because the mutation occurred in only one parental gamete, the recurrence risk for other offspring of the parents remains very low. However, the recurrence risk for future offspring of the affected individual would be the same as that of any individual who has inherited the disease-causing mutation.

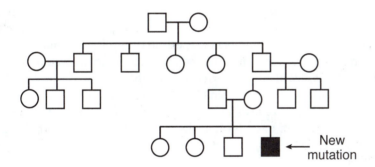

Figure II-1-14. Pedigree with a New Mutation

Delayed Age of Onset

Many individuals who carry a disease-causing mutation do not manifest the phenotype until later in life. This can complicate the interpretation of a pedigree because it may be difficult to distinguish genetically normal individuals from those who have inherited the mutation but have not yet displayed the phenotype.

Section II • Medical Genetics

Clinical Correlate

Diseases with Delayed Age of Onset

- Acute intermittent porphyria (peri- or postpubertal)
- Huntington disease
- Hemochromatosis
- Familial breast cancer

Delayed Age of Onset in Huntington Disease

Huntington disease, an autosomal dominant condition, affects approximately 1 in 20,000 individuals. Features of the disease include progressive dementia, loss of motor control, and affective disorder. This is a slowly progressing disease, with an average duration of approximately 15 years. Common causes of death include aspiration pneumonia, head trauma (resulting from loss of motor control), and suicide. Most patients first develop symptoms in their 30s or 40s, so this is a good example of a disease with delayed age of onset. The mutation produces a buildup of toxic protein aggregates in neurons, eventually resulting in neuronal death.

Examples of diseases with delayed age of onset are listed in the margin note.

Anticipation

Anticipation refers to a pattern of inheritance in which individuals in the most recent generations of a pedigree develop a disease at an earlier age or with greater severity than do those in earlier generations. For a number of genetic diseases, this phenomenon can be attributed to the gradual expansion of trinucleotide repeat polymorphisms within or near a coding gene. Huntington disease was cited above as an example of delayed age of onset. This disease is also a good example of anticipation.

The condition results from a gain-of-function mutation on chromosome 4 and is an example of a trinucleotide repeat expansion disorder. Normal *huntingin* genes have fewer than 27 CAG repeats in the 5′ coding region, and the number is stable from generation to generation. In families who eventually present with Huntington disease, premutations of 27–35 repeats are seen, although these individuals do not have Huntington disease. Some of these individuals (generally males) may then transmit an expanded number of repeats to their offspring. Individuals with more than 39 repeats are then seen, and these individuals develop symptoms. Within this group, age of onset is correlated with the number of repeats and ranges from a median age of 66 years old (39 repeats) to less than 20 years old (more than 70 repeats). Figure II-1-15 illustrates anticipation in a family with Huntington disease. The ages of onset for the affected individuals are shown along with the number of CAG repeats (in parentheses).

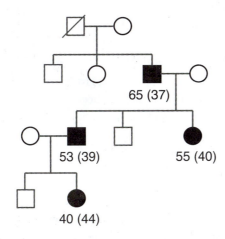

Numbers under pedigree symbols identify age of onset (CAG repeats).

Figure II-1-15. Anticipation for Huntington Disease, an Autosomal Dominant Disorder

Table II-1-1. Examples of Diseases Showing Anticipation Associated with Triplet Repeat Expansions

Disease	Symptoms	Repeat
Huntington disease (autosomal dominant)	Movement abnormality Emotional disturbance Cognitive impairment Death 10–15 years after onset	CAG 5′ coding
Fragile X syndrome (X dominant)	Mental retardation Large ears and jaw Post-pubertal macro-orchidism (males) Attention deficit disorder (in females)	CGG 5′ UTR
Myotonic dystrophy (autosomal dominant)	Muscle loss Cardiac arrhythmia Testicular atrophy Frontal baldness Cataracts	CTG 3′ UTR
Friedreich ataxia (autosomal recessive)	Early onset progressive gait and limb ataxia Areflexia in all 4 limbs Hypertrophic cardiomyopathy Axonal sensory neuropathy Kyphoscoliosis	GAA Intron 1

Clinical Correlate

Friedreich Ataxia

A 16-year-old female is seen by her neurologist for increasing weakness in her arms. She was apparently normal at birth, began walking at age 13 months, and had normal development until age 6. At that time her parents noted increasing clumsiness and stumbling. After undergoing neurologic testing, she was diagnosed with Friedreich ataxia.

She began using a wheelchair at 8 years old and currently cannot stand or walk unaided.

She has developed hypertrophic obstructive cardiomyopathy. She is breathless upon exertion but not at rest. She has kyphoscoliosis that has been progressive since 12 years old but does not impair her breathing.

Deep tendon reflexes are absent and there was an extensor plantar response bilaterally.

Friedreich ataxia is caused by expansion of a GAA repeat in the *frataxin* gene and is an autosomal recessive condition. Average life expectancy is approximately 40 years of age, but can vary significantly in different patients.

Imprinting

Imprinting refers to the fact that a small number of genes are transcriptionally active only when transmitted by one of the two sexes. The homologous locus in the other parent is rendered transcriptionally inactive. Thus, for imprinted loci, it is normal to have only the maternal (for some loci) active, or only the paternal (for other loci) active.

Imprinting:

- Occurs during gametogenesis.
- Is maintained in all somatic cells of the offspring.
- During gametogenesis in the offspring, is erased and re-established according to the sex of the individual.
- Involves methylation and possibly other mechanisms to imprint or inactivate the appropriate loci.
- Occurs in specific loci on several chromosomes.

Prader-Willi and Angelman Syndromes. On rare occasion, the transcriptionally active gene may be deleted from the chromosome (perhaps by unequal crossover) during gametogenesis. This leaves the offspring with no active gene at that locus. The gene from one parent is inactivated due to normal imprinting, and the gene from the other parent deleted by a mutation. This situation, as shown in Figure II-1-16, may result in a genetic disease.

Prader-Willi Syndrome

A 3-year-old boy is evaluated for obesity. At birth he fed poorly and was somewhat hypotonic and lethargic. At that time he was diagnosed with failure to thrive, cause unknown, and was given intragastric feedings until he regained his birth weight. He continued to gain weight slowly but remained in the lowest quartile for age-appropriate weight and height. Walking was delayed until he was 26 months old. Over the last year his appetite has increased dramatically. He has begun having temper tantrums of increasing frequency and violence, causing his withdrawal from preschool. His current evaluation reveals an obese boy with mental and developmental delay. The physician also notes underdeveloped genitalia, and she refers the boy to a genetics clinic for karyotype analysis. The result shows a deletion from one copy of chromosome 15q11-q13 consistent with Prader-Willi syndrome.

Prader-Willi syndrome is caused by loss from the paternal chromosome of an imprinted locus mapping to 15q11-13 that includes the gene *SNRPN*. This gene, normally active from the paternal copy of chromosome 15, encodes a component of mRNA splicing. Interestingly, a different genetic disease, Angelman syndrome, is produced if there is a deletion of 15q11-13 from the maternal chromosome. In this case the locus imprinted in the maternal chromosome includes a gene involved in the ubiquitin pathway known as *UBE3A*, for which the maternal gene is normally expressed while the paternal gene is silenced. This has led to the conclusion that there are at least two imprinted genes within this region, one active on the paternal chromosome 15 and the other normally active on the maternal chromosome 15. Loss, usually by deletion of paternal 15q11-13, causes Prader-Willi, whereas loss of the maternal 15q11-13 causes Angelman syndrome (see margin notes on next page).

Uniparental Disomy

Uniparental disomy is a rare condition in which both copies of a particular chromosome are contributed by one parent. This may cause problems if the chromosome contains an imprinted region or a mutation. For example, 25–30% of Prader-Willi cases are caused by maternal uniparental disomy of chromosome 15. A smaller percentage of Angelman syndrome is caused by paternal uniparental disomy of chromosome 15.

Section II • Medical Genetics

Clinical Correlate
Prader-Willi Syndrome

- Affects males and females
- Neonatal hypotonia
- Poor feeding in neonatal period
- Behavior problems
- Moderate mental and developmental retardation
- Hypogonadism, underdeveloped genitalia
- Hyperphagia (overeating) and obesity by ages 2–4 years
- Small hands and feet
- Deletion from paternal 15q
- Very low recurrence risk

Clinical Correlate
Angelman Syndrome

- Affects males and females
- Severe mental retardation
- Seizures
- Ataxia
- Puppet-like posture of limbs
- Happy disposition
- Deletion from maternal 15q
- Very low recurrence risk

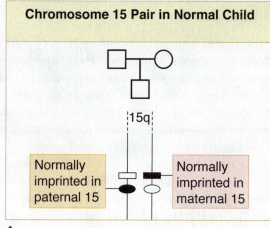

A.

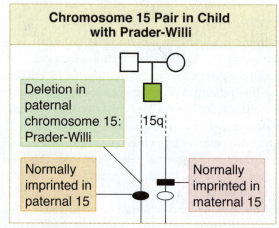

B.

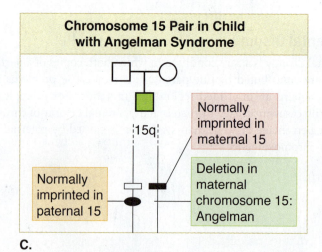

C.

A. Loci normally imprinted on chromosome 15
B. Deletion causing Prader-Willi syndrome
C. Deletion causing Angelman syndrome

Figure II-1-16. Prader-Willi and Angelman Syndromes: Diseases Involving Imprinted Loci

Chapter Summary

- Single-gene diseases have clear inheritance patterns.

  Modes of inheritance:
  - Autosomal dominant
  - Autosomal recessive
  - X-linked dominant
  - X-linked recessive
  - Mitochondrial (maternal)

- Recurrence risks can be predicted by drawing Punnett squares.

- Principles that can characterize single gene diseases:
  - Variable expression in severity of symptoms
  - Incomplete penetrance (individuals with the disease genotype don't have the disease phenotype)
  - Delayed age of onset for diseases that don't appear until later in life
  - Locus heterogeneity for diseases that can be caused by mutations in two or more different genes
  - New mutations (not inherited from a parent)
  - Anticipation caused by trinucleotide repeat expansion
  - Imprinting (symptoms depend on whether the mutant gene was inherited from the father or mother)

Review Questions

1. A 25-year-old woman has mild expression of hemophilia A. A genetic diagnosis reveals that she is a heterozygous carrier of a mutation in the X-linked factor VIII gene. What is the most likely explanation for mild expression of the disease in this individual?

   A. A high proportion of the X chromosomes carrying the mutation are active in this woman
   B. Her father is affected, and her mother is a heterozygous carrier
   C. Nonsense mutation causing truncated protein
   D. One of her X chromosomes carries the SRY gene
   E. X inactivation does not affect the entire chromosome

Section II • Medical Genetics

2. A 20-year-old man has had no retinoblastomas but has produced two offspring with multiple retinoblastomas. In addition, his father had two retinoblastomas as a young child, and one of his siblings has had three retinoblastomas. What is the most likely explanation for the absence of retinoblastomas in this individual?

   A. A new mutation in the unaffected individual, which has corrected the disease-causing mutation
   B. Highly variable expression of the disorder
   C. Incomplete penetrance
   D. Multiple new mutations in other family members
   E. Pleiotropy

3. A 30-year-old man is phenotypically normal, but two of his siblings died from infantile Tay-Sachs disease, an autosomal recessive condition that is lethal by the age of five. What is the risk that this man is a heterozygous carrier of the disease-causing mutation?

   A. 1/4
   B. 1/2
   C. 2/3
   D. 3/4
   E. Not elevated above that of the general population

4. A large, three-generation family in whom multiple members are affected with a rare, undiagnosed disease is being studied. Affected males never produce affected children, but affected females do produce affected children of both sexes when they mate with unaffected males. What is the most likely mode of inheritance?

   A. Autosomal dominant, with expression limited to females
   B. Y-linked
   C. Mitochondrial
   D. X-linked dominant
   E. X-linked recessive

5. A man who is affected with hemophilia A (X-linked recessive) mates with a woman who is a heterozygous carrier of this disorder. What proportion of this couple's daughters will be affected, and what proportion of the daughters will be heterozygous carriers?

   A. 0%; 50%
   B. 100%; 0%
   C. 0%; 100%
   D. 50%; 50%
   E. 2/3; 1/3

6. The clinical progression of Becker muscular dystrophy is typically much slower than that of Duchenne muscular dystrophy. This is usually the result of
   A. gain-of-function mutations in the Duchenne form; loss-of-function mutations in the Becker form
   B. in-frame deletions or insertions in the Becker form; frameshift deletions or insertions in the Duchenne form
   C. mis-sense mutations in the Becker form; nonsense mutations in the Duchenne form
   D. mutations at two distinct loci for these two forms of muscular dystrophy
   E. nonsense mutations in the Becker form; missense mutations in the Duchenne form

7. A 10-year-old girl is diagnosed with Marfan syndrome, an autosomal dominant condition. An extensive review of her pedigree indicates no previous family history of this disorder. The most likely explanation for this pattern is
   A. highly variable expression of the disease phenotype
   B. incomplete penetrance
   C. mitochondrial compensation in the mother
   D. new mutation transmitted by one of the parents to the affected girl
   E. pleiotropy

8. In assessing a patient with osteogenesis imperfecta, a history of bone fractures, as well as blue sclerae, are noted. These findings are an example of
   A. allelic heterogeneity
   B. gain-of-function mutation
   C. locus heterogeneity
   D. multiple mutations
   E. pleiotropy

9. In studying a large number of families with a small deletion in a specific chromosome region, it is noted that the disease phenotype is distinctly different when the deletion is inherited from the mother as opposed to the father. What is the most likely explanation?
   A. Imprinting
   B. Mitochondrial inheritance
   C. Sex-dependent penetrance
   D. X-linked dominant inheritance
   E. X-linked recessive inheritance

Section II • Medical Genetics

10. A man and woman are both affected by an autosomal dominant disorder that has 80% penetrance. They are both heterozygotes for the disease-causing mutation. What is the probability that they will produce phenotypically normal offspring?

    A. 20%
    B. 25%
    C. 40%
    D. 60%
    E. 80%

11. The severe form of alpha-1 antitrypsin deficiency is the result of a single nucleotide substitution that produces a single amino acid substitution. This is best described as a

    A. Frameshift mutation
    B. In-frame mutation
    C. Missense mutation
    D. Nonsense mutation
    E. Splice-site mutation

12. Waardenburg syndrome is an autosomal dominant disorder in which patients may exhibit a variety of clinical features, including patches of prematurely grey hair, white eyelashes, a broad nasal root, and moderate to severe hearing impairment. Occasionally, affected individuals display two eyes of different colors and a cleft lip and/or palate. Patients who possess a mutation in the *PAX3* gene on chromosome 2 can present with all of these disparate signs and symptoms. Which of the following characteristics of genetic traits is illustrated by this example?

    A. Anticipation
    B. Imprinting
    C. Incomplete penetrance
    D. Locus heterogeneity
    E. Pleiotropy

13. Hunter disease is an X-linked recessive condition in which a failure of mucopolysaccharide breakdown results in progressive mental retardation, deafness, skeletal abnormalities, and hepatosplenomegaly. In the family pedigree shown, all affected individuals were diagnosed biochemically by assaying activity of iduronate 2-sulfatase, the enzyme encoded by the gene involved in Hunter syndrome. Activity of the enzyme relative to the normal range is displayed below the symbol for selected individuals in the pedigree. What is the most likely explanation for the presence of the syndrome in individual III-2?

    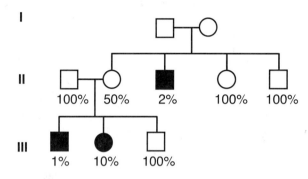

    A. She is a manifesting heterozygote.
    B. She is homozygous for the disease-producing allele.
    C. She is not the daughter of II-1.
    D. The trait has incomplete penetrance.
    E. The trait has variable expression.

14. A 9-year-old boy is referred to a pediatric clinic by his school psychologist because of poor academic performance, cognitive delay, and hyperkinetic behavior. Family history is significant for early dementia and ataxia in the maternal father. Physical examination reveals that the boy has a long thin face with prominent ears, some facial asymmetry, and a prominent forehead and jaw. His vital signs are normal, his lungs are clear to auscultation, and heart sounds are normal. His abdomen is soft, nontender, and nondistended. Examination of the extremities showed hyperextensible finger joints. The examining physician suspects a possible genetic disorder. What would be the best test to diagnose this disease?

    A. Brain MRI
    B. Cytogenetic testing for fragile X
    C. Developmental evaluation by a speech/language therapist
    D. EEG
    E. Measurement of testicular volume
    F. Southern blot analysis

Answers

1. **Answer: A.** The most likely explanation for mild expression in a heterozygous carrier is that when X inactivation occurred in the affected individual, the random process happened to inactivate most of the X chromosomes that carried the normal version of the factor VIII gene. Thus, most of the active X chromosomes in this individual would carry the mutation and would not produce factor VIII, leading to a clinically expressed deficiency.

   If the woman's father is affected and her mother is a carrier (**choice B**), she has a 50% chance of being an affected homozygote, but her expression is more likely to be severe.

   A nonsense mutation (**choice C**) is likely to produce severe expression if it is inherited from both the mother and the father.

   The SRY gene (**choice D**) is involved in sex determination and would not affect factor VIII expression.

   Although it is true that X inactivation does not affect the entire X chromosome (**choice E**), it consistently affects the factor VIII gene and thus could not explain the status of this woman.

2. **Answer: C.** Because multiple family members are affected and because mutations at the retinoblastoma gene are known to be sometimes nonpenetrant, the man in question is most likely an obligate carrier of the mutation who did not experience a second mutation in this gene during his fetal development.

   A new mutation correcting the defect could occur (**choice A**), but then the man's two sons would both have experienced new mutations. The combination of three mutations affecting three different individuals in the family is highly unlikely.

   Variable expression (**choice B**) refers to differences in the severity of a disorder but does not refer to the complete absence of the disorder, which is incomplete penetrance.

   The number of affected individuals in this family (four) makes multiple new mutations in so many individuals extremely unlikely (**choice D**). Remember that inherited mutations are rare events.

   Pleiotropy is observed in retinoblastoma (**choice E**), in that mutation carriers can develop other cancers, such as osteosarcoma. This, however, does not explain the lack of a tumor in the 20-year-old man.

3. **Answer: C.** Because two of the man's siblings had Tay-Sachs disease, his parents must both be carriers. This clearly elevates his risk above the general population and excludes **choice E**. He is not affected, so this excludes **choice A**, which is the probability of inheriting two copies of the disease allele. His risk of inheriting one copy of the disease gene at conception is 1/2 (**choice B**). However, the fact that he is phenotypically normal at age 30 means that he cannot have inherited copies of the disease gene from both parents. Only three possibilities remain: Either he inherited no copies of the mutation, he inherited a copy from his father, or he inherited a copy from his mother. Each of these three possibilities is equally likely, and two of them lead to heterozygosity. Thus, the risk that he is a carrier is 2/3.

4. **Answer: C.** This is a pattern expected of mitochondrial inheritance because only females transmit mitochondrial DNA to their offspring. Thus, an affected female can transmit the mutation to her offspring of both sexes, but an affected male cannot transmit it.

   Choice A is excluded because, although the disease is not transmitted by males, it is seen in them.

   Under Y-linked inheritance (**choice B**), affected males would transmit the mutation and would transmit it only to their sons.

   X-linked dominant inheritance (**choice D**) is excluded because affected males can transmit X-linked dominant mutations to their daughters.

   X-linked recessive inheritance (**choice E**) could explain this pattern because affected males typically produce only heterozygous carrier daughters and unaffected sons (unless they mate with a carrier female). However, affected homozygous females, who will produce affected sons, would produce an affected daughter only if they mated with an affected male.

5. **Answer: D.** Because the man transmits his X chromosome to all of his daughters, all of the daughters must carry at least one copy of the mutation. The mother will transmit a mutation-carrying X chromosome half the time and a normal X chromosome half the time. Thus, half of the daughters will be heterozygous carriers, and half will be affected homozygotes, having received a mutation from both parents.

6. **Answer: B.** In-frame deletions or insertions typically produce an altered protein product (dystrophin), but the alteration is mild enough so that Becker muscular dystrophy results. Frame-shifts usually produce a truncated protein because a stop codon is eventually encountered. The truncated protein is degraded, resulting in an absence of dystrophin and a more severe disease phenotype.

   Both types of muscular dystrophy are X-linked recessive mutations, making a gain-of-function highly unlikely for either type (**choice A**).

   Because approximately 2/3 of all mutations leading to these diseases are insertions or deletions, differences in single-base mutations (i.e., missense or nonsense mutations) would not be the most likely explanation, excluding **choice C** and **choice E**.

   These two forms of muscular dystrophy are known to be encoded by the same locus, so locus heterogeneity (**choice D**) is excluded.

7. **Answer: D.** For an autosomal dominant condition, the first occurrence in a family is usually the result of a new mutation that occurred in one of the gametes transmitted by a parent of the affected individual.

   Although variable expression (**choice A**) is a characteristic of this disease, other family members (including a parent) would be likely to manifest at least mild expression of the disorder.

   The penetrance of Marfan mutations is high, so it is highly unlikely that all other gene carriers in the family would be nonpenetrant carriers (**choice B**).

   Mitochondrial genes are not known to affect the expression of Marfan syndrome (**choice C**).

Section II • Medical Genetics

Marfan syndrome is an excellent example of pleiotropy (**choice E**), but this principle refers to the fact that a single mutation can affect multiple aspects of the phenotype, so it would not explain the pattern observed in this pedigree.

8. **Answer: E.** Pleiotropy refers to the multiple effects exerted by a single mutation and thus describes the two features observed in this patient.

    Allelic heterogeneity is observed in osteogenesis imperfecta (**choice A**), but allelic heterogeneity causes variable expression in patients and is not the principle described here.

    Osteogenesis imperfecta is a good example of a disease in which locus heterogeneity (**choice C**) is observed, but this principle refers to the fact that a mutation in either the type 1 procollagen gene on chromosome 7 or the type 1 procollagen gene on chromosome 17 can result in imperfect formation of the trimeric protein. This principle does not explain the co-occurrence of fractures and blue sclerae.

    A single mutation at either the chromosome 7 or chromosome 17 locus is sufficient to cause the disease, so multiple mutations (**choice D**) do not explain the pattern.

9. **Answer: A.** Imprinting refers to the differential transcriptional activity of genes inherited from the father versus the mother.

    Under mitochondrial inheritance (**choice B**), only an affected mother can transmit the disease phenotype; the offspring of affected males are always unaffected.

    The other modes of inheritance can influence the relative proportions of affected individuals who belong to one gender or the other (e.g., more affected males under X-linked recessive inheritance, more affected females under X-linked dominant inheritance), but they do not involve any differences in expression depending on the transmitting parent.

10. **Answer: C.** If both parents are heterozygotes, there is a 75% chance that their offspring will receive one or two copies of the disease-causing gene (i.e., a 50% chance that the offspring will receive one copy and a 25% chance that the offspring will receive two copies). With 80% penetrance, the probability that the offspring will be affected is 0.75×0.8, or 0.6 (60%). The probability that the offspring will be phenotypically normal is $1 - 0.60$, or 0.40 (40%).

11. **Answer: C.** A missense mutation results in the change of only a single amino acid.

    Frameshift mutations (**choice A**) are the result of the deletion or insertion of a series of nucleotides that are not a multiple of three (thus altering the reading frame). Although the insertion or deletion of a single nucleotide would produce a frameshift, it is highly unlikely that it would alter only a single amino acid. The shift in the reading frame typically alters a number of amino acids subsequent to the insertion or deletion site.

    An in-frame mutation (**choice B**) is the insertion or deletion of a multiple of three nucleotides, so this single-nucleotide substitution cannot be an in-frame mutation.

A nonsense mutation (**choice D**) is a single nucleotide substitution that produces a stop codon and thus truncation of the polypeptide. Therefore, it typically alters more than a single amino acid.

Splice-site mutations (**choice E**) occur at intron-exon boundaries and typically result in the loss of an exon or the inclusion of part of an intron in the coding sequence. Thus, more than a single amino acid would be altered in a typical splice-site mutation.

12. **Answer: E.** Pleiotropy refers to the appearance of apparently unrelated characteristics resulting from a single genetic defect. It is often the result of the presence of a single altered molecule in multiple locations in the body, so that the single mutation has effects in multiple organ systems. In Marfan syndrome, for example, a defect in the fibrillin gene causes manifestations of the disease in the eye, aorta, and joints.

    Anticipation (**choice A**) describes the finding that in some pedigrees, a disease trait occurs in earlier and earlier age groups as the generations progress. It is often a finding in pedigrees in which trinucleotide repeat expansions are linked to disease expression.

    Imprinting (**choice B**) refers to the selective inactivation of a gene in one of the parental sexes during gametogenesis. Males and females inactivate different regions on several autosomal chromosomes, so that the maternal or paternal source of such a chromosome may have different results in the progeny.

    Incomplete penetrance (**choice C**) indicates that a certain fraction of individuals with a disease-producing genotype develop no symptoms. An example is hemochromatosis in which 1/300 people in the United States have the disease-producing genotype, but only about 1/2,000 ever show symptoms of the disease.

    Locus heterogeneity (**choice D**) refers to the case in which a mutation in any one of several distinct genetic loci can result in a single disease phenotype. It is common in cases where a single molecule is composed of multiple subunits. The alteration of any one of the subunits results in the formation of a molecule with altered function; thus, several different mutations can yield the same phenotypic result.

13. **Answer: A.** X-linked recessive diseases should be expressed much more commonly in males than in females because males are hemizygous for the X chromosome (they have only one copy). In the pedigree shown, Individuals I-2 and II-2 are obligate carriers of the trait and have a 1 in 2 chance of transmitting the disease gene to their offspring. Male offspring who receive the X chromosome with the disease-causing allele will develop the disease (Individuals II-3 and III-1), and female offspring who receive the X chromosome with the disease-causing allele will be carriers of the trait. In most cases, the presence of a second, normal X chromosome in these female heterozygotes will prevent the expression of the disease. In some cases, however, inactivation of the normal X-chromosome may occur in an unusually high percentage of her cells. If this happens, most cells will have the X-chromosome with the mutation, and even though she is heterozygous she may manifest symptoms (manifesting heterozygote). That this is the case with III-2 is confirmed by finding lower than expected activity of the enzyme. One would expect a heterozygote to have approximately 50% normal enzyme activity. This woman has only 10%.

Section II • Medical Genetics

She is not homozygous for the disease-producing allele (**choice B**). Her father is unaffected by this X-linked recessive trait and therefore necessarily has the normal allele. The woman has inherited the disease-causing allele from her mother but as a carrier should have 50% normal enzyme activity and should not show symptoms.

She is not the daughter of II-1 (**choice C**) is not the best answer because this X-linked recessive trait is clearly segregating normally in this family. In most genetic diseases, which are relatively rare, it would be uncommon for a person entering the family through marriage (a different, biologic father to replace Individual II-1) to have the same rare genetic trait that is being expressed in the family studied.

That the trait has incomplete penetrance (**choice D**) is not a valid answer because incomplete penetrance results in diminished numbers of affected individuals, not increased numbers as shown here. You are asked in this question to explain why the female in Generation III expresses the disease trait when she would not be expected to do so, not to explain why someone who does not have the disease trait lacks it.

Variable expression (**choice E**) refers to the situation in which individuals with the disease-producing genotype have varying degrees of phenotypic expression. Individual III-2 does not have the disease-producing genotype.

14. **Answer: F.** This patient has fragile X syndrome, which is the most common cause of inherited mental retardation and, after trisomy 21, is the second most common cause of genetically associated mental deficiencies. The genetic basis of this disease is a triplet (CGG) repeat expansion in the 5′ untranslated region of a gene (FMR-1) on the X chromosome. The standard diagnostic testing for fragile X syndrome uses molecular genetic techniques. The exact number of CGG triplet repeats can be determined by Southern blotting or by amplification of the repeat with a polymerase chain reaction and gel electrophoresis. Southern blot analysis provides a more accurate estimation of the number of CGG triplet repeats if a full mutation is present (with a large CGG expansion).

Males with a permutation (moderate expansion but not sufficient to cause classic symptoms of fragile X) may have a fragile X tremor/ataxia syndrome (FXTAS) that presents later in life, usually after 50 years of age. Fragile X is also seen in females where learning disabilities and mild mental retardation characterize the syndrome.

Brain MRI (**choice A**) and EEG (**choice D**) are not useful in diagnosis of fragile X syndrome, but may be indicated when patient presents with seizures.

Fragile X chromosomes may show breakage when cultured in a medium containing folate; however, this cytogenetic testing for fragile X (**choice B**) is not as sensitive as molecular testing and cannot be considered as the best test with a false-negative result rate of approximately 20%.

Developmental evaluation by a speech/language therapist (**choice C**) will allow one to detect mental retardation; however, it does not help to establish the diagnosis of fragile X syndrome.

Measurement of testicular volume (**choice E**) may be helpful in postpubertal males when fragile X syndrome is suspected. In normal males, average testicular volume is 17 mL; in patients with fragile X syndrome, testicular volume is more than 25 mL and can be as high as 120 mL. However, measurement of testicular volume cannot be considered as a best diagnostic test, and this patient is only 9 years old.

Population Genetics   2

Learning Objectives

❏ Solve problems concerning definition
❏ Solve problems concerning genotype and allele frequencies
❏ Explain information related to Hardy-Weinberg equilibrium
❏ Interpret scenarios about factors responsible for genetic variation in/among populations

DEFINITION

Population genetics is the study of genetic variation in populations. Basic concepts of population genetics allow us to understand how and why the prevalence of various genetic diseases differs among populations.

GENOTYPE AND ALLELE FREQUENCIES

An essential step in understanding genetic variation is to measure it in populations. This is done by estimating genotype and allele frequencies.

Genotype Frequencies

For a given locus, the genotype frequency measures the proportion of each genotype in a population. For example, suppose that a population of 100 individuals has been assayed for an autosomal restriction fragment length polymorphism (RFLP; *see* Chapter 7 in Section I). If the RFLP has two possible alleles, labeled 1 and 2, there are three possible genotypes: 1-1, 1-2, and 2-2. Visualization of a Southern blot allows us to determine the genotype of each individual in our population, and we find that the genotypes are distributed as follows:

Table II-2-1. Genotype Frequency

Genotype	Count	Genotype Frequency
1-1	49	0.49
1-2	42	0.42
2-2	9	0.09
Total	100	1.00

Section II • Medical Genetics

The genotype frequency is then obtained by dividing the count for each genotype by the total number of individuals. Thus, the frequency of genotype 1-1 is 49/100 = 0.49, and the frequencies of genotypes 1-2 and 2-2 are 0.42 and 0.09, respectively.

Allele Frequencies

The allele frequency measures the proportion of chromosomes that contain a specific allele. To continue the RFLP example given above, we wish to estimate the frequencies of alleles 1 and 2 in our population. Each individual with the 1-1 genotype has two copies of allele 1, and each heterozygote (1-2 genotype) has one copy of allele 1. Because each diploid somatic cell contains two copies of each autosome, our denominator is 200. Thus, the frequency of allele 1 in the population is:

$$\frac{(2 \times 49) + 42}{200} = 0.7$$

The same approach can be used to estimate the frequency of allele 2, which is 0.3. A convenient shortcut is to remember that the allele frequencies for all of the alleles of a given locus must add up to 1. Therefore, we can obtain the frequency of allele 2 simply by subtracting the frequency of allele 1 (0.7) from 1.

HARDY-WEINBERG EQUILIBRIUM

If a population is large and if individuals mate at random with respect to their genotypes at a locus, the population should be in Hardy-Weinberg equilibrium. This means that there is a constant and predictable relationship between genotype frequencies and allele frequencies. This relationship, expressed in the Hardy-Weinberg equation, allows one to estimate genotype frequencies if one knows allele frequencies, and vice versa.

The Hardy-Weinberg Equation

$$p^2 + 2pq + q^2 = 1$$

In this equation:

p = frequency of allele 1 (conventionally the most common, normal allele)

q = frequency of allele 2 (conventionally a minor, disease-producing allele)

p^2 = frequency of genotype 1-1 (conventionally homozygous normal)

$2pq$ = frequency of genotype 1-2 (conventionally heterozygous)

q^2 = frequency of genotype 2-2 (conventionally homozygous affected)

In most cases where this equation is used, a simplification is possible. Generally p, the normal allele frequency in the population, is very close to 1 (e.g., most of the alleles of this gene are normal). In this case, we may assume that $p \sim 1$, and the equation simplifies to:

$$1 + 2q + q^2 \sim 1$$

> **Note**
>
> Genotype frequencies measure the proportion of each genotype in a population. Allele frequencies measure the proportion of chromosomes that contain a specific allele (of a gene).

The frequency of the disease-producing allele, q, in question is a very small fraction. This simplification would not necessarily be used in actual medical genetics practice, but for answering test questions, it works quite well. However, if the disease prevalence is greater than $1/100$, e.g., q is greater than $1/10$, the complete Hardy-Weinberg equation should be used to obtain an accurate answer. In this case, $p = 1 - q$. Although the Hardy-Weinberg equation applies equally well to autosomal dominant and recessive alleles, genotypes, and diseases, the equation is most frequently used with autosomal recessive conditions. In these instances, a large percentage of the disease-producing allele is "hidden" in heterozygous carriers who cannot be distinguished phenotypically (clinically) from homozygous normal individuals.

A Practical Application of the Hardy-Weinberg Principle

A simple example is illustrated by the following case.

> A 20-year-old female college student is taking a course in human genetics. She is aware that she has an autosomal recessive genetic disease that has required her lifelong adherence to a diet low in natural protein with supplements of tyrosine and restricted amounts of phenylalanine. She also must avoid foods artificially sweetened with aspartame (Nutrasweet™). She asks her genetics professor about the chances that she would marry a man with the disease-producing allele.

The geneticist tells her that the known prevalence of PKU in the population is 1/10,000 live births, but the frequency of carriers is much higher, approximately 1/50. Her greatest risk comes from marrying a carrier for two reasons. First, the frequency of carriers for this condition is much higher than the frequency of affected homozygotes, and second, an affected person would be identifiable clinically. The geneticist used the Hardy-Weinberg equation to estimate the carrier frequency from the known prevalence of the disease in the following way:

> Disease prevalence = q^2 = 1/10,000 live births
>
> Carrier frequency = $2q$ (to be calculated)
>
> q = square root of 1/10,000, which is 1/100
>
> $2q$ = 2/100, or **1/50, the carrier frequency**

> The woman now asks a second question: "Knowing that I have a 1/50 chance of marrying a carrier of this allele, what is the probability that I will have a child with PKU?"

The geneticist answers, "The chance of you having a child with PKU is 1/100." This answer is based on the joint occurrence of two nonindependent events:
- The probability that she will marry a heterozygous carrier (1/50), and
- If he is a carrier, the probability that he will pass his PKU allele versus the normal allele to the child (1/2).

These probabilities would be multiplied to give:
- 1/50 × 1/2 = **1/100, the probability that she will have a child with PKU**.

Note
Hardy-Weinberg Equilibrium in Phenylketonuria (PKU)

- Prevalence of PKU is 1/10,000 live births
- Allele frequency = $\sqrt{1/10,000}$ = 1/100 = 0.01
- Carrier frequency = 2(1/100) = 1/50

Bridge to Statistics
If events are nonindependent, multiply the probability of one event by the probability of the second event, assuming that the first has occurred. For example, what is the probability that the student's husband will pass the disease-producing allele to the child? It is the probability that he will be a carrier (1/50, event 1) multiplied by the probability that he will pass the disease-causing gene along (1/2, event 2), assuming that he is a carrier.

Section II • Medical Genetics

Note

Assuming random mating, the Hardy-Weinberg principle specifies a predictable relationship between allele frequencies and genotype frequencies in populations. This principle can be applied to estimate the frequency of heterozygous carriers of an autosomal recessive mutation.

In summary, there are three major terms one usually works with in the Hardy-Weinberg equation applied to autosomal recessive conditions:

- q^2, the disease prevalence
- $2q$, the carrier frequency
- q, the frequency of the disease-causing allele

When answering questions involving Hardy-Weinberg calculations, it is important to identify which of these terms has been given in the stem of the question and which term you are asked to calculate.

This exercise demonstrates two important points:

- The Hardy-Weinberg principle can be applied to estimate the prevalence of heterozygous carriers in populations when we know only the prevalence of the recessive disease.
- For autosomal recessive diseases, such as PKU, the prevalence of heterozygous carriers is much higher than the prevalence of affected homozygotes. In effect, the vast majority of recessive genes are hidden in the heterozygotes.

Hardy-Weinberg Equilibrium for Dominant Diseases

The calculations for dominant diseases must acknowledge that most of the affected individuals will be heterozygous. In this case, the prevalence is $2q$. (One can again use the assumption that $p \sim 1$.) The term q^2 represents the prevalence of homozygous affected individuals who, although much less commonly seen, may have more severe symptoms. For example,

- 1/500 people in the United States have a form of LDL-receptor deficiency and are at increased risk for cardiovascular disease and myocardial infarction.
- Taking $2q = 1/500$, one can calculate that $q^2 = 1/10^6$, or one in a million live births are homozygous for the condition. These individuals have greatly elevated LDL-cholesterol levels, a much-higher risk for cardiovascular disease than heterozygotes, and are more likely to present with characteristic xanthomas, xanthelasmas, and corneal arcus.

In contrast, in Huntington disease (autosomal dominant), the number of triplet repeats correlates much more strongly with disease severity than does heterozygous or homozygous status.

Sex Chromosomes and Allele Frequencies

When considering X-linked recessive conditions, one must acknowledge that most cases occur in hemizygous males (xY). Therefore, q = disease-producing allele frequency but, paradoxically, it also equals the prevalence of affected males. Thus, the statement "1/10,000 males has hemophilia A" also gives the allele frequency for the disease-producing allele: 1/10,000.

- q^2 = prevalence of disease in females (1/10^8, or 1/100,000,000)
- $2q$ = prevalence of female carriers (1/5,000)

This exercise demonstrates that:

- As with autosomal recessive traits, the majority of X-linked recessive genes are hidden in female heterozygous carriers (although a considerable number of these genes are seen in affected males).
- X-linked recessive traits are seen much more commonly in males than in females.

FACTORS RESPONSIBLE FOR GENETIC VARIATION IN/AMONG POPULATIONS

Although human populations are typically in Hardy-Weinberg equilibrium for most loci, deviations from equilibrium can be produced by new mutations, the introduction of a new mutation into a population from outside (founder effect), nonrandom mating (for example, consanguinity), the action of natural selection, genetic drift, and gene flow. Although these factors are discussed independently, often more than one effect contributes to allele frequencies in a population.

Mutation

Mutation, discussed previously, is ultimately the source of all new genetic variation in populations. In general, mutation rates do not differ very much from population to population.

Founder Effect. In some cases, a new mutation can be introduced into a population when someone carrying the mutation is one of the early founders of the community. This is referred to as a founder effect. As the community rapidly expands through generations, the frequency of the mutation can be affected by natural selection, by genetic drift (*see* below), and by consanguinity.

Note

The four evolutionary factors responsible for genetic variation in populations are:

- Mutation
- Natural selection
- Genetic drift
- Gene flow

> **Branched Chain Ketoacid Dehydrogenase Deficiency**
>
> Branched chain ketoacid dehydrogenase deficiency (maple syrup urine disease) occurs in 1/176 live births in the Mennonite community of Lancastershire, Pennsylvania. In the U.S. population at large, the disease occurs in only 1/180,000 live births. The predominance of a single mutation (allele) in the branched chain dehydrogenase gene in this group suggests a common origin of the mutation. This may be due to a founder effect.

Natural Selection

Natural selection acts upon genetic variation, increasing the frequencies of alleles that promote survival or fertility (referred to as fitness) and decreasing the frequencies of alleles that reduce fitness. The reduced fitness of most disease-producing alleles helps explain why most genetic diseases are relatively rare. Dominant diseases, in which the disease-causing allele is more readily exposed to the effects of natural selection, tend to have lower allele frequencies than do recessive diseases, where the allele is typically hidden in heterozygotes.

Section II • Medical Genetics

> ### Sickle Cell Disease and Malaria
>
> Sickle cell disease affects 1/600 African Americans and up to 1/50 individuals in some parts of Africa. How could this highly deleterious disease-causing mutation become so frequent, especially in Africa? The answer lies in the fact that the falciparum malaria parasite, which has been common in much of Africa, does not survive well in the erythrocytes of sickle cell heterozygotes. These individuals, who have no clinical signs of sickle cell disease, are thus protected against the lethal effects of malaria. Consequently, there is a heterozygote advantage for the sickle cell mutation, and it maintains a relatively high frequency in some African populations.

There is now evidence for heterozygote advantages for several other recessive diseases that are relatively common in some populations. Examples include:

- Cystic fibrosis (heterozygote resistance to typhoid fever)
- Hemochromatosis (heterozygote advantage in iron-poor environments)
- Glucose-6-phosphate dehydrogenase deficiency, hemolytic anemia (heterozygote resistance to malaria)

Genetic Drift

Mutation rates do not vary significantly from population to population, although they can result in significant differences in allele frequencies when they occur in small populations or are introduced by a founder effect. Mutation rates and founder effects act along with genetic drift to make certain genetic diseases more common (or rarer) in small, isolated populations than in the world at large. Consider the pedigrees (very small populations) shown in Figure II-2-1.

Chapter 2 • Population Genetics

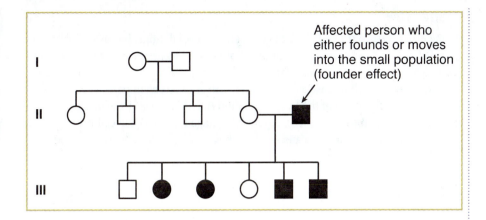

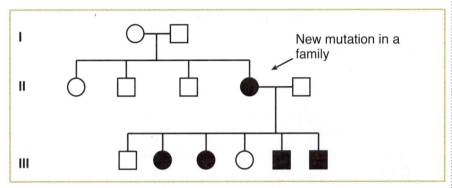

Genetic drift begins. In both examples the frequency of affected persons in generation III is 2/3, higher than the 1/2 predicted by statistics.

Figure II-2-1. Genetic Drift in Two Small Populations
(Illustrated with a Dominant Disease)

If the woman and the affected man (II-5) in the top panel had 1,000 children rather than 6, the prevalence of the disease in their offspring (Generation III) would be closer to 1/2, the statistical mean. Although genetic drift affects populations larger than a single family, this example illustrates two points:

- When a new mutation or a founder effect occurs in a small population, genetic drift can make the allele more or less prevalent than statistics alone would predict.

- A relatively large population in Hardy-Weinberg equilibrium for an allele or many alleles can be affected by population "bottlenecks" in which natural disaster or large-scale genocide dramatically reduces the size of the population. Genetic drift may then change allele frequencies and a new Hardy-Weinberg equilibrium is reached.

Gene Flow

Gene flow refers to the exchange of genes among populations. Because of gene flow, populations located close to one another often tend to have similar gene frequencies. Gene flow can also cause gene frequencies to change through time: The frequency of sickle cell disease is lower in African Americans in part because of gene flow from other sectors of the U.S. population that do not carry the disease-causing mutation; in addition, the heterozygote advantage for the sickle cell mutation (*see* text box) has disappeared because malaria has become rare in North America.

Consanguinity and Its Health Consequences

Consanguinity refers to the mating of individuals who are related to one another (typically, a union is considered to be consanguineous if it occurs between individuals related at the second-cousin level or closer). Figure II-2-2 illustrates a pedigree for a consanguineous union. Because of their mutual descent from common ancestors, relatives are more likely to share the same disease-causing genes. Statistically,

- Siblings (II-2 and II-3 or II-4) share 1/2 of their genes.
- First cousins (III-3 and III-4) share 1/8 of their genes (1/2 × 1/2 × 1/2).
- Second cousins (IV-1 and IV-2) share 1/32 of their genes (1/8 × 1/2 × 1/2).

These numbers are referred to as the coefficients of relationship. Thus, if individual III-1 carries a disease-causing allele, there is a 1/2 chance that individual III-3 (his brother) has it and a 1/8 chance that individual III-4 (his first cousin) has it.

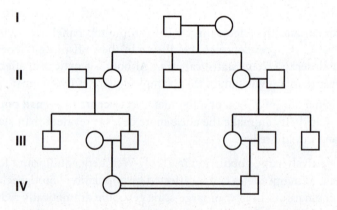

Figure II-2-2. A Pedigree Illustrating Consanguinity

Consequently, there is an increased risk of genetic disease in the offspring of consanguineous matings. Dozens of empirical studies have examined the health consequences of consanguinity, particularly first-cousin matings. These studies show that the offspring of first-cousin matings are approximately twice as likely to present with a genetic disease as are the offspring of unrelated matings. The frequency of genetic disease increases further in the offspring of closer unions (e.g., uncle/niece or brother/sister matings).

> **Note**
>
> Consanguineous matings are more likely to produce offspring affected with recessive diseases because individuals who share common ancestors are more liable to share disease-causing mutations.

Chapter Summary

- Population genetics allows predictions about the prevalence of diseases in populations.
- Genotype frequency measures the proportion of each genotype in a population.
- Gene (allele) frequency measures the proportion of each allele at a particular locus.
- Hardy-Weinberg equilibrium:
  - $p^2 + 2pq + q^2 = 1$
  - p and q are the allele frequencies at a locus
  - allows calculations of carrier frequency and prevalence of genetic diseases
  - p^2 = homozygous normal; $2pq$ = heterozygous carrier; q^2 = homozygous affected (for autosomal recessive diseases)
- Factors responsible for genetic variation:
  - Mutation is the source of new genetic variations
  - Natural selection increases or decreases allele frequencies, depending on their survival value (e.g., heterozygote advantage for the sickle cell mutation)
  - Genetic drift can change allele frequencies in small populations by chance
  - Gene flow occurs when populations exchange genes with each other
- Consanguinity (mating of related individuals) increases the likelihood of genetic disease in the offspring.

Section II • Medical Genetics

Review Questions

1. A population has been assayed for a four-allele polymorphism, and the following genotype counts have been obtained:

Genotype	Count
1,1	4
1,3	8
1,4	3
2,3	5
2,4	9
3,3	4
3,4	6
4,4	11

   On the basis of these genotype counts, what are the gene frequencies of alleles 1 and 2?

   A. 0.38, 0.28
   B. 0.19, 0.14
   C. 0.095, 0.07
   D. 0.25, 0.25
   E. 0.38, 0.20

2. Which of the following best characterizes Hardy-Weinberg equilibrium?

   A. Consanguinity has no effect on Hardy-Weinberg equilibrium.
   B. Genotype frequencies can be estimated from allele frequencies, but the reverse is not true.
   C. Natural selection has no effect on Hardy-Weinberg equilibrium.
   D. Once a population deviates from Hardy-Weinberg equilibrium, it takes many generations to return to equilibrium.
   E. The frequency of heterozygous carriers of an autosomal recessive mutation can be estimated if one knows the incidence of affected homozygotes in the population.

3. In a genetic counseling session, a healthy couple has revealed that they are first cousins and that they are concerned about health risks for their offspring. Which of the following best characterizes these risks?

   A. Because the couple shares approximately half of their genes, most of the offspring are likely to be affected with some type of genetic disorder.
   B. The couple has an increased risk of producing a child with an autosomal dominant disease.
   C. The couple has an increased risk of producing a child with an autosomal recessive disease.
   D. The couple has an increased risk of producing a child with Down syndrome.
   E. There is no known increase in risk for the offspring.

4. An African American couple has produced two children with sickle cell disease. They have asked why this disease seems to be more common in the African American population than in other U.S. populations. Which of the following factors provides the best explanation?

   A. Consanguinity
   B. Genetic drift
   C. Increased gene flow in this population
   D. Increased mutation rate in this population
   E. Natural selection

5. If the incidence of cystic fibrosis is 1/2,500 among a population of Europeans, what is the predicted incidence of heterozygous carriers of a cystic fibrosis mutation in this population?

   A. 1/25
   B. 1/50
   C. 2/2,500
   D. 1/2,500
   E. $(1/2,500)^2$

6. A man is a known heterozygous carrier of a mutation causing hyperprolinemia, an autosomal recessive condition. Phenotypic expression is variable and ranges from high urinary excretion of proline to neurologic manifestations including seizures. Suppose that 0.0025% (1/40,000) of the population is homozygous for the mutation causing this condition. If the man mates with somebody from the general population, what is the probability that he and his mate will produce a child who is homozygous for the mutation involved?

   A. 1% (1/100)
   B. 0.5% (1/200)
   C. 0.25% (1/400)
   D. 0.1% (1/1,000)
   E. 0.05% (1/2,000)

Section II • Medical Genetics

7. The incidence of Duchenne muscular dystrophy in North America is about 1/3,000 males. On the basis for this figure, what is the gene frequency of this X-linked recessive mutation?

   A. 1/3,000
   B. 2/3,000
   C. $(1/3,000)^2$
   D. 1/6,000
   E. 1/9,000

Answers

1. **Answer: B.** The denominator of the gene frequency is 100, which is obtained by adding the number of genotyped individuals (50) and multiplying by 2 (because each individual has two alleles at the locus). The numerator is obtained by counting the number of alleles of each type: the 4 homozygotes with the 1,1 genotype contribute 8 copies of allele 1; the 1,3 heterozygotes contribute another 8 alleles; and the 1,4 heterozygotes contribute 3 alleles. Adding these together, we obtain 19 copies of allele 1. Dividing by 100, this yields a gene frequency of 0.19 for allele 1. For allele 2, there are two classes of heterozygotes that have a copy of the allele: those with the 2,3 and 2,4 genotypes. These 2 genotypes yield 5 and 9 copies of allele 2, respectively, for a frequency of 14/100 = 0.14.

2. **Answer: E.** The incidence of affected homozygotes permits the estimation of the frequency of the recessive mutation in the population. Using the Hardy-Weinberg equilibrium relationship between gene frequency and genotype frequency, the gene frequency can then be used to estimate the frequency of the heterozygous genotype in the population.

    Consanguinity (**choice A**) affects Hardy-Weinberg equilibrium by increasing the number of homozygotes in the population above the equilibrium expectation (i.e., consanguinity results in a violation of the assumption of random mating).

    Genotype frequencies can be estimated from gene frequencies (**choice B**), but gene frequencies can also be estimated from genotype frequencies (as in **choice A**).

    By eliminating a specific genotype from the population (e.g., affected homozygotes), natural selection can cause deviations from equilibrium (**choice C**).

    Only one generation of random mating is required to return a population to equilibrium (**choice D**).

3. **Answer: C.** Because the couple shares common ancestors (i.e., one set of grandparents), they are more likely to be heterozygous carriers of the same autosomal recessive disease-causing mutations. Thus, their risk of producing a child with an autosomal recessive disease is elevated above that of the general population.

    First cousins share approximately 1/8 of their genes, not 1/2 (**choice A**).

    Because both members of the couple are healthy, neither one is likely to harbor a dominant disease-causing mutation (**choice B**). In addition, consanguinity itself does not elevate the probability of producing a child with a dominant disease because only one copy of the disease-causing allele is needed to cause the disease.

    Down syndrome (**choice D**) typically is the result of a new mutation. When it is transmitted by an affected female, it acts like a dominant mutation and thus would not be affected by consanguinity.

    Empirical studies indicate that the risk of genetic disease in the offspring of first cousin couples is approximately double that of the general population (**choice E**).

Section II • Medical Genetics

4. **Answer: E.** The frequency of sickle cell disease is elevated in many African populations because heterozygous carriers of the sickle cell mutation are resistant to malarial infection but do not develop sickle cell disease, which is autosomal recessive. Thus, there is a selective advantage for the mutation in heterozygous carriers, elevating its frequency in the population.

    Consanguinity (**choice A**) could elevate the incidence of this autosomal recessive disease in a specific family, but it does not account for the elevated incidence of this specific disease in the African American population in general.

    The African American population is large and consequently would not be expected to have experienced elevated levels of genetic drift (**choice B**).

    Although there has been gene flow (**choice C**) from other populations into the African American population, this would be expected to decrease, rather than increase, the frequency of sickle cell disease because the frequency of this disease is highest in some African populations.

    There is no evidence that the mutation rate (**choice D**) is elevated in this population. In contrast, the evidence for natural selection is very strong.

5. **Answer: A.** This answer is obtained by taking the square root of the incidence (i.e., the frequency of affected homozygotes) to get a gene frequency for the disease-causing mutation (q) of 1/50 (0.02). The carrier frequency is given by 2pq, or approximately 2q, or 1/25.

6. **Answer: C.** One must first determine the probability that the man's mate will also be a heterozygous carrier. If the frequency of affected homozygotes (q^2) is 1/40,000, then the allele frequency, q, is 1/200. The carrier frequency in the population (approximately 2q) is 1/100. Three independent events must happen for their child to be homozygous for the mutation. The mate must be a carrier (probability 1/100), the mate must pass along the mutant allele (probability 1/2), and the man must also pass along the mutant allele (probability 1/2). Multiplying the 3 probabilities to determine the probability of their joint occurrence gives $1/100 \times 1/2 \times 1/2 = 1/400$.

7. **Answer: A.** Because males have only a single X chromosome, each affected male has one copy of the disease-causing recessive mutation. Thus, the incidence of an X-linked recessive disease in the male portion of a population is a direct estimate of the gene frequency in the population.

Cytogenetics 3

Learning Objectives

❏ Interpret scenarios about basic definitions and terminology
❏ Solve problems concerning numerical chromosome abnormalities
❏ Demonstrate understanding of structural chromosome abnormalities
❏ Demonstrate understanding of other chromosome abnormalities
❏ Solve problems concerning advances in molecular cytogenetics

OVERVIEW

This chapter reviews diseases that are caused by microscopically observable alterations in chromosomes. These alterations may involve the presence of extra chromosomes or the loss of chromosomes. They may also consist of structural alterations of chromosomes. Chromosome abnormalities are seen in approximately 1 in 150 live births and are the leading known cause of mental retardation. The vast majority of fetuses with chromosome abnormalities are lost prenatally: Chromosome abnormalities are seen in 50% of spontaneous fetal losses during the first trimester of pregnancy, and they are seen in 20% of fetuses lost during the second trimester. Thus, chromosome abnormalities are the leading known cause of pregnancy loss.

Note
X chromosome contains ~1,200 genes

Y chromosome contains ~50 genes

BASIC DEFINITIONS AND TERMINOLOGY

Karyotype

Chromosomes are most easily visualized during the metaphase stage of mitosis, when they are maximally condensed. They are photographed under the microscope to create a karyotype, an ordered display of the 23 pairs of human chromosomes in a typical somatic cell (Figure II-3-1). In Figure II-3-1A, a karyogram represents a drawing of each type of chromosome; the presentation is haploid (only one copy of each chromosome is shown). Figure II-3-1B is a karyotype of an individual male. It is diploid, showing both copies of each autosome, the X and the Y chromosome. Chromosomes are ordered according to size, with the sex chromosomes (X and Y) placed in the lower right portion of the karyotype.

Metaphase chromosomes can be grouped according to size and to the position of the centromere, but accurate identification requires staining with one of a variety of dyes to reveal characteristic banding patterns.

Section II • Medical Genetics

Chromosome banding

To visualize chromosomes in a karyotype unambiguously, various stains are applied so that banding is evident.

- **G-banding.** Mitotic chromosomes are partially digested with trypsin (to digest some associated protein) and then stained with Giemsa, a dye that binds DNA.

G-banding reveals a pattern of light and dark (G-bands) regions that allow chromosomes to be accurately identified in a karyotype. There are several other stains that can be used in a similar manner. The chromosomes depicted in Figure II-3-1 have been stained with Giemsa.

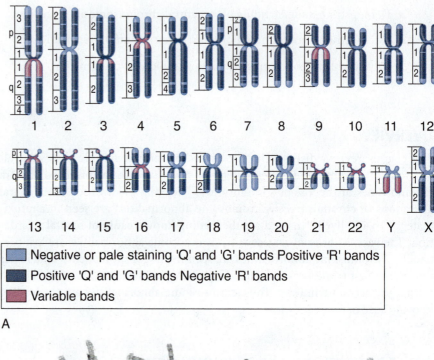

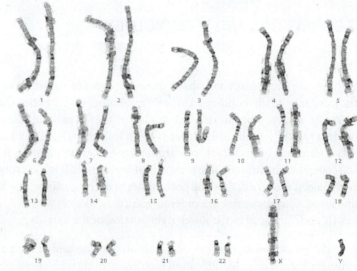

Figure II-3-1. Human Metaphase Chromosomes. (*A*) Idealized Drawing (Karyogram) and (*B*) Photograph of Metaphase Chromosomes (Karyotype)

Chromosome abnormalities in some cases can be identified visually by looking at the banding pattern, but this technique reveals differences (for instance, larger deletions) only to a resolution of about 4 Mb. Smaller abnormalities (microdeletions) must be identified in other ways (FISH), discussed at the end of the chapter.

Chromosome nomenclature

Each mitotic chromosome contains a centromere and two sister chromatids because the cell has gone through interphase and has entered mitosis when the karyotype analysis is performed (metaphase). The long arm of the chromosome is labeled q, and the short arm is labeled p. One of the characteristics described is the relative position of the centromere.

- **Metacentric** chromosomes (for instance, chromosome 1) have the centromere near the middle. The p and q arms are of roughly equal length.
- **Submetacentric** chromosomes have the centromere displaced toward one end (for example, chromosome 4). The p and q arms are evident.
- **Acrocentric** chromosomes have the centromere far toward one end. In these chromosomes, the p arm contains little genetic information, most of it residing on the q arm. Chromosomes 13, 14, 15, 21, and 22 are the acrocentric chromosomes. Only the acrocentric chromosomes are involved in **Robertsonian translocations**, which will be discussed in this chapter.

The tips of the chromosomes are termed telomeres.

Table II-3-1 contains some standard nomenclature applied to chromosomes.

Table II-3-1. Common Symbols Used in Karyotype Nomenclature

1-22	Autosome number
X, Y	Sex chromosomes
(+) or (−)	When placed before an autosomal number, indicates that chromosome is extra or missing
p	Short arm of the chromosome
q	Long arm of the chromosome
t	Translocation
del	Deletion

NUMERICAL CHROMOSOME ABNORMALITIES

Euploidy

When a cell has a multiple of 23 chromosomes, it is said to be **euploid**. Gametes (sperm and egg cells) are euploid cells that have 23 chromosomes (one member of each pair); they are said to be **haploid**. Most somatic cells are **diploid**, containing both members of each pair, or 46 chromosomes. Two types of euploid cells with abnormal numbers of chromosomes are seen in humans: triploidy and tetraploidy.

Note

Euploid Cells (multiple of 23 chromosomes)

- Haploid (23 chromosomes): gametes
- Diploid (46 chromosomes): most somatic cells
- Triploid (69 chromosomes): rare lethal condition
- Tetraploid (92 chromosomes): very rare lethal condition

Triploidy. Triploidy refers to cells that contain three copies of each chromosome (69 total). Triploidy, which usually occurs as a result of the fertilization of an ovum by two sperm cells, is common at conception, but the vast majority of these conceptions are lost prenatally. However, about 1 in 10,000 live births is a triploid. These babies have multiple defects of the heart and central nervous system, and they do not survive.

Tetraploidy. Tetraploidy refers to cells that contain four copies of each chromosome (92 total). This lethal condition is much rarer than triploidy among live births: Only a few cases have been described.

Aneuploidy

Aneuploidy, a deviation from the euploid number, represents the gain (+) or loss (−) of a specific chromosome. Two major forms of aneuploidy are observed:

- Monosomy (loss of a chromosome)
- Trisomy (gain of a chromosome)

Autosomal aneuploidy

Two generalizations are helpful:

- All autosomal monosomies are inconsistent with a live birth.
- Only three autosomal trisomies (trisomy 13, 18, and 21) are consistent with a live birth.

Trisomy 21 (47,XY,+21 or 47,XX,+21); Down Syndrome

- Most common autosomal trisomy
- Mental retardation
- Short stature
- Hypotonia
- Depressed nasal bridge, upslanting palpebral fissures, epicanthal fold
- Congenital heart defects in approximately 40% of cases
- Increased risk of acute lymphoblastic leukemia
- Alzheimer disease by fifth or sixth decade (*amyloid precursor protein, APP* gene on chromosome 21)
- Reduced fertility
- Risk increases with increased maternal age

Trisomy 18 (47,XY,+18 or 47,XX,+18); Edward Syndrome

- Clenched fist with overlapping fingers
- Inward turning, "rocker-bottom" feet
- Congenital heart defects
- Low-set ears, micrognathia (small lower jaw)
- Mental retardation
- Very poor prognosis

Trisomy 13 (47,XY,+13 or 47,XX,+13); Patau Syndrome

- Polydactyly (extra fingers and toes)
- Cleft lip, palate
- Microphthalmia (small eyes)
- Microcephaly, mental retardation
- Cardiac and renal defects
- Very poor prognosis

Sex chromosome aneuploidy

Aneuploidy involving the sex chromosomes is relatively common and tends to have less severe consequences than does autosomal aneuploidy. Some generalizations are helpful:

- At least one X chromosome is required for survival.
- If a Y chromosome is present, the phenotype is male (with minor exceptions).
- If more than one X chromosome is present, all but one will become a Barr body in each cell.

The two important sex chromosome aneuploidies are Turner syndrome and Klinefelter syndrome.

Klinefelter Syndrome (47,XXY)

- Testicular atrophy
- Infertility
- Gynecomastia
- Female distribution of hair
- Low testosterone
- Elevated FSH and LH
- High-pitched voice

Turner Syndrome (45,X or 45,XO)

- Only monosomy consistent with life
- 50% are 45,X
- Majority of others are mosaics for 45,X and one other cell lineage (46,XX, 47,XXX, 46,XY)
- Females with 45,X;46,XY are at increased risk for gonadal blastoma.
- Short stature
- Edema of wrists and ankles in newborn
- Cystic hygroma *in utero* resulting in excess nuchal skin and "webbed" neck
- Primary amenorrhea
- Coarctation of the aorta or other congenital heart defect in some cases
- Infertility
- Gonadal dysgenesis

Note

Trisomy is the most common genetic cause of spontaneous loss of pregnancy.

Note

Genetic Mosaicism in Turner Syndrome

Genetic mosaicism is defined as a condition in which there are cells of different genotypes or chromosome constitutions within a single individual. Some women with Turner syndrome have somatic cells that are 45,X and others that are 46,XX or 47,XXX. Mosaicism in Turner syndrome is thought to arise in early embryogenesis by mechanisms that are not completely understood.

Section II • Medical Genetics

Nondisjunction is the usual cause of aneuploidies

Germ cells undergo meiosis to produce the haploid egg or sperm. Normal meiosis is illustrated in Figure II-3-2A. The original cell is diploid for all chromosomes, although only one homologous pair is shown in the figure for simplicity. The same events would occur for each pair of homologs within the cell.

Figure II-3-2B shows the result of nondisjunction of one homologous pair (for example, chromosome 21) during meiosis 1. All other homologs segregate (disjoin) normally in the cell. Two of the gametes are diploid for chromosome 21. When fertilization occurs, the conception will be a trisomy 21 with Down syndrome. The other gametes with no copy of chromosome 21 will result in conceptions that are monosomy 21, a condition incompatible with a live birth.

Figure II-3-2C shows the result of nondisjunction during meiosis 2. In this case, the sister chromatids of a chromosome (for example, chromosome 21) fail to segregate (disjoin). The sister chromatids of all other chromosomes segregate normally. One of the gametes is diploid for chromosome 21. When fertilization occurs, the conception will be a trisomy 21 with Down syndrome. One gamete has no copy of chromosome 21 and will result in a conception that is a monosomy 21. The remaining two gametes are normal haploid ones.

Some important points to remember:

- Nondisjunction is the usual cause of aneuploidies including Down, Edward, and Patau syndromes, as well as Turner and Klinefelter syndromes.
- Nondisjunction is more likely to occur during oogenesis than during spermatogenesis.
- Nondisjunction is more likely with increasing maternal age. No environmental agents (e.g., radiation, alcohol) have been shown to have measurable influence.
- Nondisjunction is more likely in meiosis I than meiosis II.

> ### Clinical Correlate: Maternal Age, Risk of Down Syndrome, and Prenatal Diagnosis
>
> Surveys of babies with trisomy 21 show that approximately 90–95% of the time, the extra copy of the chromosome is contributed by the mother (similar figures are obtained for trisomies of the 18th and 13th chromosomes). The increased risk of Down syndrome with maternal age is well documented. The risk of bearing a child with Down is less than 1/1,000 for women age <30. The risk increases to about 1/400 at age 35, 1/100 at age 40, and 3–4% or age >45. This increase reflects an elevated rate of nondisjunction in older ova (recall that all of a woman's egg cells are formed during her fetal development, and they remain suspended in prophase I until ovulation). There is no corresponding increase in risk with advanced paternal age; sperm cells are generated continuously throughout the life of the male.
>
> The increased risk of trisomy with advanced maternal age motivates more than half of pregnant women in North America to undergo prenatal diagnosis (most commonly, amniocentesis or chorionic villus sampling, discussed in Chapter 6). Down syndrome can also be screened by assaying maternal serum levels of α-fetoprotein, chorionic gonadotropin, and unconjugated estriol. This so-called *triple screen* can detect approximately 70% of fetuses with Down.

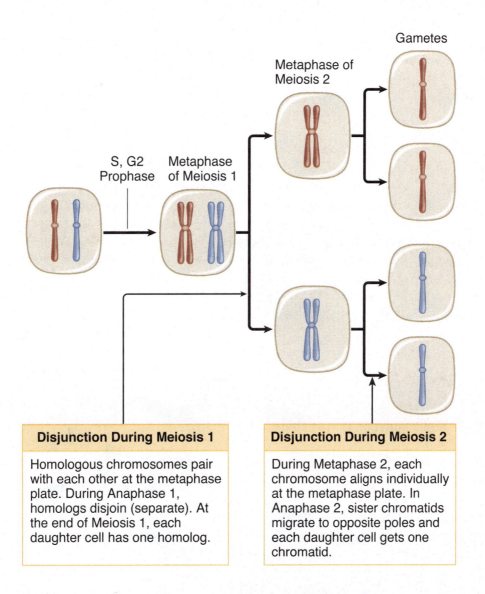

Figure II-3-2A. Disjunction During Normal Meiosis

Section II • Medical Genetics

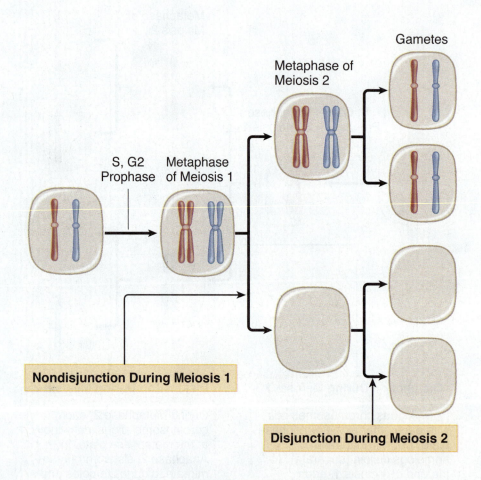

Figure II-3-2B. Nondisjunction During Meiosis 1

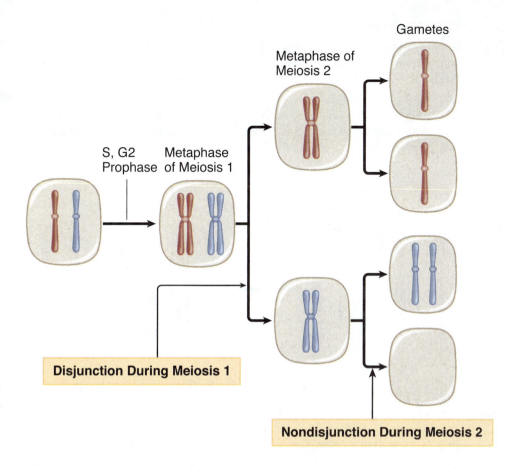

Figure II-3-2C. Nondisjunction During Meiosis 2

STRUCTURAL CHROMOSOME ABNORMALITIES

Structural alterations of chromosomes occur when chromosomes are broken by agents termed **clastogens** (e.g., radiation, some viruses, and some chemicals). Some alterations may result in a loss or gain of genetic material and are called **unbalanced** alterations; **balanced** alterations do not result in a gain or loss of genetic material and usually have fewer clinical consequences. As with other types of mutations, structural alterations can occur either in the germ line or in somatic cells. The former can be transmitted to offspring. The latter, although not transmitted to offspring, can alter genetic material such that the cell can give rise to cancer.

Translocations

Translocations occur when chromosomes are broken and the broken elements reattach to other chromosomes. Translocations can be classified into two major types: reciprocal and Robertsonian.

Reciprocal translocation

Reciprocal translocations occur when genetic material is exchanged between non-homologous chromosomes; for example, chromosomes 2 and 8 (Figure II-3-3). If this happens during gametogenesis, the offspring will carry the reciprocal translocation in all his or her cells and will be called a **translocation carrier**. The karyotype would be 46,XY,t(2p;8p) or 46,XX,t(2p;8p). Because this individual has all of the genetic material (balanced, albeit some of it misplaced because of the translocation), there are often no clinical consequences other than during reproduction.

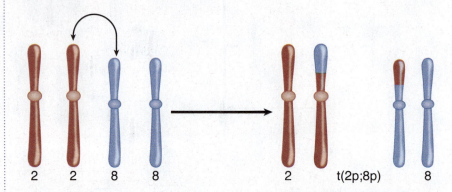

Figure II-3-3. A Reciprocal Translocation

In a translocation carrier, during gametogenesis and meiosis, unbalanced genetic material can be transmitted to the offspring, causing partial trisomies and partial monosomies typically resulting in pregnancy loss. During meiosis 1, the translocated chromosomes may segregate as chromosome 8 or as chromosome 2, producing a variety of possible gametes with respect to these chromosomes. For example, see Figure II-3-4, which depicts a man who is a translocation carrier mating with a normal woman. The diagram in the upper right is used to depict the possible sperm the father can produce. It acknowledges that the translocated chromosomes can potentially pair with either of the two homologs (2 or 8) during meiosis.

Sperm that contain balanced chromosomal material (labeled alternate segregation in the diagram) produce either a normal diploid conception or another translocation carrier. Both are likely to be live births.

Sperm that contain unbalanced chromosomal material (labeled adjacent segregation in the diagram) produce conceptions that have partial monosomies and partial trisomies. These conceptions are likely to result in pregnancy loss.

Note
Alternate Versus Adjacent Segregation

Alternate and adjacent segregation refer to diagrams (Figure II-3-4, upper right) used to predict the possible gametes produced by a translocation carrier.

- Adjacent segregation—chromosomes from adjacent quadrants (next to each other) enter a gamete.
- Alternate segregation—chromosomes from alternate (diagonally opposed) quadrants enter a gamete.

Chapter 3 • Cytogenetics

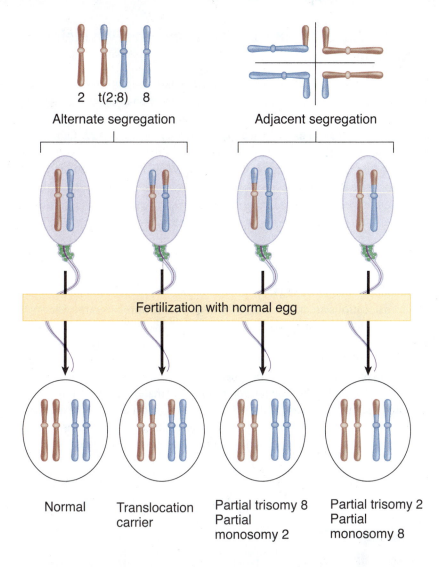

Figure II-3-4. Consequences of a Reciprocal Translocation (Illustrated with Male)

Note
Reciprocal Translocations and Pregnancy Loss

When one parent is a reciprocal translocation carrier:

- Adjacent segregation produces unbalanced genetic material and most likely loss of pregnancy.

- Alternate segregation produces a normal haploid gamete (and diploid conception) or a liveborn who is a phenotypically normal translocation carrier.

Reciprocal Translocations After Birth. Reciprocal translocations may occur by chance at the somatic cell level throughout life. Because these translocations involve only a single cell and the genetic material is balanced, there is often no consequence. Rarely, however, a reciprocal translocation may alter the expression or structure of an oncogene or a tumor suppressor gene, conferring an abnormal growth advantage to the cell.

Section II • Medical Genetics

Bridge to Pathology
Translocations Involving Oncogenes

Translocations are seen in a variety of cancers. Important examples presented in pathology include:

- t(9;22) chronic myelogenous leukemia (*c-abl*)
- t(15;17) acute myelogenous leukemia (*retinoid receptor-α*)
- t(14;18) follicular lymphomas (*bcl-2* that inhibits apoptosis)
- t(8;14) Burkitt lymphoma (*c-myc*)
- t(11;14) mantle cell lymphoma (*cyclin D*)

Chronic Myelogenous Leukemia and the Philadelphia Chromosome

Although most of our discussion deals with inherited chromosome alterations, rearrangements in somatic cells can lead to the formation of cancers by altering the genetic control of cellular proliferation. A classic example is a reciprocal translocation of the long arms of chromosomes 9 and 22, termed the *Philadelphia chromosome*. This translocation alters the activity of the *abl* proto-oncogene (proto-oncogenes can lead to cancer). When this alteration occurs in hematopoietic cells, it can result in chronic myelogenous leukemia. More than 100 different chromosome rearrangements involving nearly every chromosome have been observed in more than 40 types of cancer.

Robertsonian translocations

These translocations are much more common than reciprocal translocations and are estimated to occur in approximately 1 in 1,000 live births. They occur only in the acrocentric chromosomes (13, 14, 15, 21, and 22) and involve the loss of the short arms of two of the chromosomes and subsequent fusion of the long arms. An example of a Robertsonian translocation involving chromosomes 14 and 21 is shown in Figure II-3-5. The karyotype of this (male) translocation carrier is designated 45,XY,−14,−21,+t(14q;21q). Because the short arms of the acrocentric chromosomes contain no essential genetic material, their loss produces no clinical consequences, and the translocation carrier is not clinically affected.

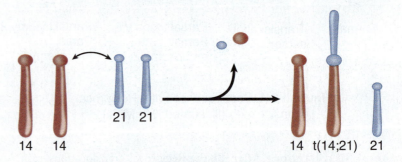

Figure II-3-5. A Robertsonian Translocation

When the carrier's germ cells are formed through meiosis, the translocated chromosome must pair with its homologs. If **alternate segregation** occurs, the offspring will inherit either a normal chromosome complement or will be a normal carrier like the parent (Figure II-3-6). If **adjacent segregation** occurs, the offspring will have an unbalanced chromosome complement (an extra or missing copy of the long arm of chromosome 21 or 14). Because only the long arms of these chromosomes contain genetically important material, the effect is equivalent to a trisomy or monosomy.

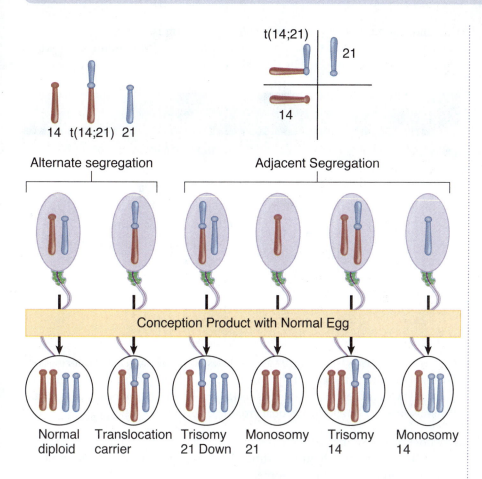

Figure II-3-6. Consequences of a Robertsonian Translocaton in One Parent (Illustrated with Male)

Robertsonian Translocation and Down Syndrome. Approximately 5% of Down syndrome cases are the result of a Robertsonian translocation affecting chromosome 14 and chromosome 21. When a translocation carrier produces gametes, the translocation chromosome can segregate with the normal 14 or with the normal 21. A diagram can be drawn to represent the six possible gametes that could be produced. Figure II-3-6 shows the diagram, the six sperm (in this example, the translocation carrier is a male), and the outcome of conception with a genetically normal woman.

Although adjacent segregation usually results in pregnancy loss, one important exception is that which produces trisomy 21. This may be a live birth, resulting in an infant with Down syndrome.

One can determine the mechanism leading to Down syndrome by examining the karyotype. Trisomy 21 due to nondisjunction during meiosis (95% of Down syndrome cases) has the karyotype 47,XX,+21 or 47,XY,+21. In the 5% of cases where Down syndrome is due to a Robertsonian translocation in a parent, the karyotype will be 46,XX,–14,+t(14q;21q) or 46,XY,–14,+t(14q;21q). The key difference is 47 versus 46 chromosomes in the individual with Down syndrome.

Although the recurrence risk for trisomy 21 due to nondisjunction during meiosis is very low, the recurrence risk for offspring of the Robertsonian translocation carrier parent is significantly higher. The recurrence risk (determined empirically) for female translocation carriers is 10–15%, and that for male translocation carriers is 1–2%. The reason for the difference between males and females is not

Note

Robertsonian Translocations

When one parent is a Robertsonian translocation carrier:

- Adjacent segregation produces unbalanced genetic material and most likely loss of pregnancy. Important exception: Down syndrome: 46,XX or 46XY,–14 +t(14q;21q)

- Alternate segregation produces a normal haploid gamete (and diploid conception) or a liveborn who is a phenotypically normal translocation carrier.

well understood. The elevated recurrence risk for translocation carriers versus noncarriers underscores the importance of ordering a chromosome study when Down syndrome is suspected in a newborn.

Down syndrome (nondisjunction during meiosis)	Down syndrome (parent carries a Robertsonian translocation)
• 47,XX,+21 or 47,XY,+21 • No association with prior pregnancy loss • Older mother • Very low recurrence rate	• 46,XX,–14,+t(14;21), or 46,XY,–14,+t(14;21) • *May* be associated with prior pregancy loss • *May* be a younger mother • Recurrence rate 10–15% if mom is translocation carrier; 1–2% if dad is translocation carrier

Deletions

A deletion occurs when a chromosome loses some of its genetic information. Terminal deletions (the end of the chromosome is lost) and interstitial deletions (material within the chromosome is lost) may be caused by agents that cause chromosome breaks and by unequal crossover during meiosis.

Deletions can be large and microscopically visible in a stained preparation. Figure II-3-7 shows both an interstitial deletion and a terminal deletion of 5p. Both result in Cri-du-chat syndrome.

- 46,XX or 46,XY, del(5p)
- High-pitched, cat-like cry
- Mental retardation, microcephaly
- Congenital heart disease

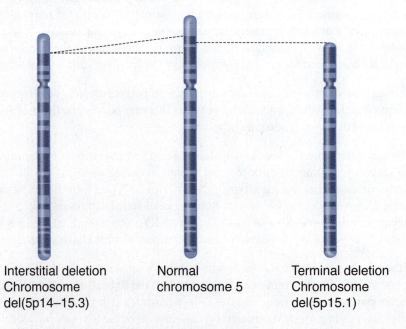

Figure II-3-7. Terminal and Interstitial Deletions of Chromosome 5p

Microdeletions

Some deletions may be so small that they are not readily apparent microscopically without special fluorescent probes (FISH). Examples include:

- Prader-Willi syndrome
- Angelman syndrome

If a microdeletion includes several contiguous genes, a variety of phenotypic outcomes may be part of the genetic syndrome. Examples are

- DiGeorge syndrome: congenital absence of the thymus and parathyroids, hypocalcemic tetany, T-cell immunodeficiency, characteristic facies with cleft palate, heart defects
- Wilms tumor: aniridia, genital abnormalities, mental retardation (WAGR)
- Williams syndrome: hypercalcemia, supravalvular aortic stenosis, mental retardation, characteristic facies

OTHER CHROMOSOME ABNORMALITIES

Several other types of structural abnormalities are seen in human karyotypes. In general, their frequency and clinical consequences tend to be less severe than those of translocations and deletions.

Inversions

Inversions occur when the chromosome segment between two breaks is reinserted in the same location but in reverse order. Inversions that include the centromere are termed **pericentric**, whereas those that do not include the centromere are termed **paracentric**. The karyotype of the inversion shown in Figure II-3-8, extending from 3p21 to 3q13 is 46,XY,inv(3)(p21;q13). Inversion carriers still retain all of their genetic material, so they are usually unaffected (although an inversion may interrupt or otherwise affect a specific gene and thus cause disease). Because homologous chromosomes must line up during meiosis, inverted chromosomes will form loops that, through recombination, may result in a gamete that contains a deletion or a duplication, which may then be transmitted to the offspring.

Note
Structural Abnormalities

- Translocations (Robertsonian and reciprocal)
- Deletions and duplications
- Inversions (pericentric and paracentric)
- Ring chromosomes
- Isochromosomes

Pericentric Inversion of Chromosome 16

A male infant, the product of a full-term pregnancy, was born with hypospadias and ambiguous genitalia. He had a poor sucking reflex, fed poorly, and had slow weight gain. He had wide-set eyes, a depressed nasal bridge, and microcephaly. The father stated that several members of his family, including his brother, had an abnormal chromosome 16. His brother had two children, both healthy, and the father assumed that he would also have normal children. Karyotype analysis confirmed that the father had a pericentric inversion of chromosome 16 and that his infant son had a duplication of material on 16q, causing a small partial trisomy.

Section II • Medical Genetics

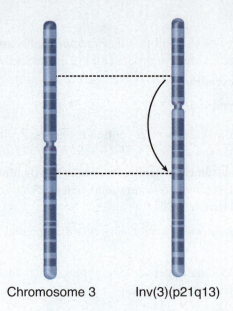

Figure II-3-8. A Pericentric Inversion of Chromosome 3

Ring Chromosome

A ring chromosome can form when a deletion occurs on both tips of a chromosome and the remaining chromosome ends fuse together. The karyotype for a female with a ring chromosome X would be 46,X,r(X). An example of this chromosome is shown in Figure II-3-9. Ring chromosomes are often lost, resulting in a monosomy (e.g., loss of a ring X chromosome would produce Turner syndrome). These chromosomes have been observed at least once for each human chromosome.

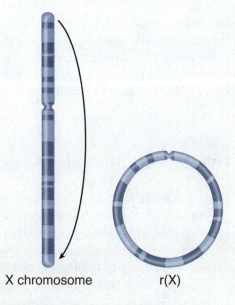

Figure II-3-9. Ring X-Chromosome

Isochromosome

When a chromosome divides along the axis perpendicular to its normal axis of division, an **isochromosome** is created (i.e., two copies of one arm but no copy of the other). Because of the lethality of autosomal isochromosomes, most isochromosomes that have been observed in live births involve the X chromosome, as shown in Figure II-3-10. The karyotype of an isochromosome for the long arm of the X chromosome would be 46,X,i(Xq); this karyotype results in an individual with Turner syndrome, indicating that most of the critical genes responsible for the Turner phenotype are on Xp.

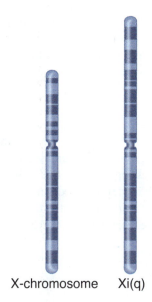

Figure II-3-10. Isochromosome Xq

ADVANCES IN MOLECULAR CYTOGENETICS

Although chromosome abnormalities are still commonly visualized by examining metaphase chromosomes under a microscope, several powerful new techniques combine cytogenetics with modern molecular methods. Two of the most important techniques are described here.

Note
FISH analysis detects:

- Aneuploidies
- Translocations
- Deletions, including microdeletions

Fluorescence *in situ* Hybridization (FISH)

In fluorescence *in situ* hybridization (FISH), a chromosome-specific DNA segment is labeled with a fluorescent tag to create a **probe**. This probe is then hybridized with the patient's chromosomes, which are visualized under a fluorescence microscope. Because the probe will hybridize only with a complementary DNA sequence, the probe will mark the presence of the chromosome segment being tested. For example, a probe that is specific for chromosome 21 will hybridize in three places in the cells of a trisomy 21 patient, providing a diagnosis of Down syndrome. FISH is also commonly used to detect deletions: An analysis using a probe that hybridizes to the region of 15q corresponding to Prader-Willi syndrome (*see* Chapter 1) will show only a single signal in a patient, confirming the diagnosis of this deletion syndrome. An advantage of FISH is that chromosomes do not have to be in the metaphase stage for accurate diagnosis: Even though interphase and prophase chromosomes cannot be clearly visualized themselves, the number of hybridization signals can still be counted accurately.

Spectral Karyotyping

Spectral karyotyping involves the use of five different fluorescent probes that hybridize differentially to different sets of chromosomes. In combination with special cameras and image-processing software, this technique produces a karyotype in which every chromosome is "painted" a different color. This allows the ready visualization of chromosome rearrangements, such as small translocations, e.g., the Philadelphia chromosome rearrangement t(9;22) involved in chronic myelogenous leukemia.

Chapter Summary

- Cytogenetics is the study of microscopically observable chromosomal abnormalities.
- Diseases can be caused by abnormalities in chromosome number or structure.
- Numerical chromosome abnormalities
- Euploidy (multiple of 23 chromosomes):
  - Haploid (23, normal gametes)
  - Diploid (46, normal somatic cells)
  - Triploid (69, lethal)
  - Tetraploid (92, lethal)
- Aneuploidy (loss or gain of specific chromosomes, usually caused by nondisjunction during meiosis):
  - Trisomy 21 (Down syndrome)
  - Trisomy 18 (Edwards syndrome)
  - Trisomy 13 (Patau syndrome)
  - 47,XXY (Klinefelter syndrome, male)
  - 45,X (Turner syndrome, female)
- Structural chromosome abnormalities
- Translocations:
  - Reciprocal (chronic myelogenous leukemia)
  - Robertsonian (5% of Down syndrome cases)
- Deletions (cri-du-chat syndrome)
- Inversions
- Ring chromosomes
- Isochromosomes
- New methods for studying chromosomes:
  - FISH
  - Spectral karyotyping

Section II • Medical Genetics

Review Questions

1. A 26-year-old woman has produced two children with Down syndrome, and she has also had two miscarriages. Which of the following would be the best explanation?

    (A) Her first cousin has Down syndrome.

    (B) Her husband is 62 years old.

    (C) She carries a reciprocal translocation involving chromosomes 14 and 18.

    (D) She carries a Robertsonian translocation involving chromosomes 14 and 21.

    (E) She was exposed to multiple x-rays as a child.

2. A 6-year-old boy has a family history of mental retardation and has developmental delay and some unusual facial features. He is being evaluated for possible fragile X syndrome. Which of the following would be most useful in helping establish the diagnosis?

    (A) Genetic test for a trinucleotide repeat expansion in the fragile X gene

    (B) IQ test

    (C) Karyotype of the child's chromosomes

    (D) Karyotype of the father's chromosomes

    (E) Measurement of testicular volume

3. A couple has one son, who is age 7. Multiple attempts to have a second child have ended in miscarriages and spontaneous abortions. Karyotypes of the mother, the father, and the most recently aborted fetus are represented schematically below. What is the most likely explanation for the most recent pregnancy loss?

    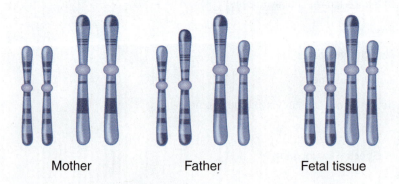

    Mother   Father   Fetal tissue

    (A) Aneuploidy in the fetus

    (B) Fetus identified as a reciprocal translocation carrier

    (C) Nondisjunction during oogenesis in the mother

    (D) Partial monosomy and trisomy in the fetus

    (E) Unbalanced chromosomal material in the father

4. A woman brings her 16-year-old daughter to a physician because she has not yet begun menstruating. Although her parents are both 1.75 meters, the patient is 1.5 meters and has always been below the 50th percentile in height. Physical examination reveals no breast development. She has no problems in school and is of normal intelligence. What is the most likely underlying basis for her condition?

    (A) A 45,X karyotype
    (B) A balanced reciprocal translocation
    (C) A balanced Robertsonian translocation
    (D) Two Barr bodies
    (E) Deletion of an imprinted locus

5. A 38-year-old woman in her 15th week of pregnancy undergoes ultrasonography that reveals an increased area of nuchal transparency. Amniocentesis is recommended and performed at 16 weeks' gestation. The amniotic karyotype is 46,XYadd(18)(p.11.2), indicating additional chromosomal material on the short arm of one chromosome 18 at band 11.2. All other chromosomes are normal. What is the most likely cause of this fetal karyotype?

    (A) A balanced reciprocal translocation in one of the parents
    (B) A balanced Robertsonian translocation in one of the parents
    (C) An isochromosome 18i(p) in one of the parents
    (D) Nondisjunction during meiosis 1 in one of the parents
    (E) Nondisjunction during meiosis 2 in one of the parents

6. A 37-year-old woman is brought to emergency department because of crampy abdominal pain and vaginal bleeding for 3 hours. She is 11 weeks pregnant. This is her first pregnancy. Her pregnancy has been unremarkable until this episode. Her temperature is 36.8 C (98.2 F), pulse is 106/min, blood pressure is 125/70 mm Hg, and respiration rate is 22/min. Speculum examination shows the presence of blood in the vagina and cervical dilatation. Inevitable spontaneous abortion is suspected. After discussing the condition with the patient, she gave her consent for dilatation and curettage. What is the most common cause of spontaneous abortions?

    (A) Chromosomal abnormality, polyploidy
    (B) Chromosomal abnormality, monosomy X
    (C) Chromosomal abnormality, trisomy
    (D) Effects of environmental chemicals
    (E) Immunologic rejection
    (F) Infection
    (G) Maternal endocrinopathies
    (H) Physical stresses
    (I) Teratogenic drugs

Section II • Medical Genetics

Answers

1. **Answer: D.** As a translocation carrier, it is possible that she can transmit the translocated chromosome, containing the long arms of both 14 and 21, to each of her offspring. If she also transmits her normal copy of chromosome 21, then she will effectively transmit two copies of chromosome 21. When this egg cell is fertilized by a sperm cell carrying another copy of chromosome 21, the zygote will receive three copies of the long arm of chromosome 21. The miscarriages may represent fetuses that inherited three copies of the long arm and were spontaneously aborted during pregnancy.

    Although the risk for Down syndrome increases if a woman has had a previous child, there is no evidence that the risk increases if a more distant relative, such as a first cousin, is affected (**choice A**).

    Although there is no conclusive evidence for an increased risk of Down syndrome with advanced maternal age, there is little or no evidence for a paternal age effect on Down syndrome risk (**choice B**).

    An extra copy of material from chromosome 14 or 18 (**choice C**) could result in a miscarriage, but neither would produce children with Down syndrome, which is caused by an extra copy of the long arm of chromosome 21.

    Heavy irradiation has been shown to induce nondisjunction in some experimental animals, but there is no good evidence for a detectable effect on human trisomy (**choice E**).

2. **Answer: A.** The presence of an expanded trinucleotide repeat in the 5′ untranslated region of the gene is an accurate test for fragile X syndrome.

    An IQ test (**choice B**) would be useful because the IQ is typically much lower than average in fragile X syndrome patients. However, many other syndromes also include mental retardation as a feature, so this would not be a specific test.

    A karyotype of the child's chromosomes (**choice C**) might reveal X chromosomes with the decondensed long arm characteristic of this syndrome, but not all chromosomes have this appearance in affected individuals. Thus, the karyotype may yield a false-negative diagnosis.

    The father's chromosomes (**choice D**) will not be relevant because this is an X-linked disorder.

    Testicular volume (**choice E**) is increased in males with fragile X syndrome, but this is observed in postpubertal males.

3. **Answer: D.** The fetal karyotype shows a partial trisomy and a partial monosomy.

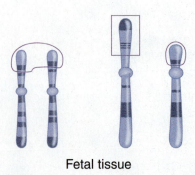

Fetal tissue

The fetus has 46 chromosomes, indicating euploidy (a multiple of 23), not aneuploidy (**choice A**). The father is the reciprocal translocation carrier, not the fetus (**choice B**). Nondisjunction during meiosis (**choice C**) produces full trisomies and chromosomes have normal structure. Although the father is a translocation carrier, his genetic material is balanced, not unbalanced (**choice E**). He is diploid for all loci.

4. **Answer: A.** The daughter most likely has Turner syndrome, monosomy X, or 45,X. It should be high on the differential diagnosis list for a female adolescent of short stature who presents with primary amenorrhea. Women with Turner syndrome have streak gonads, and the absence of ovarian function is responsible for failure to develop many secondary sex characteristics.

   Balanced translocations (**choices B and C**) have few, if any, consequences on the phenotype, although they may result in pregnancy loss of conceptions with unbalanced chromosome material.

   Women with Turner syndrome have no Barr body. Two Barr bodies (**choice D**) would be consistent with a 47,XXX karyotype or a 48,XXXY karyotype, neither of which produces the phenotype described.

   Deletion of a locus subject to imprinting (**choice E**) is consistent with Prader-Will syndrome or Angelman syndrome but is not associated with the phenotype described.

5. **Answer: A.** The fetus has unbalanced chromosomal material (additional chromosomal material on one copy of chromosome 18). One of the parents is likely to be a carrier of a reciprocal translocation involving chromosome 18 and one other chromosome (unspecified in stem).

   A Robertsonian translocation (**choice B**) would result in fusion of q arms from two acrocentric chromosomes. This is not what is described in the fetal karyotype.

   Isochromosome 18(p) indicates a chromosome 18 with two p arms and no q arms (**choice C**). This is not the abnormality described in the fetal karyotype.

   Nondisjunction during either meiosis 1 or meiosis 2 (**choices D and E**) would produce a full trisomy.

6. **Answer: C.** Chromosomal abnormalities are responsible for about 50% of first trimester spontaneous abortions, and of these the most common cause is trisomy (52%). The most common trisomy in spontaneous abortion is trisomy 16. Polyploidy (**choice A**) is seen in 22% and monosomy (**choice B**) in 19%.

   All other listed causes can also cause miscarriage; however, these problems are less common than chromosomal anomalies.

Genetics of Common Diseases 4

Learning Objectives

❏ Interpret scenarios about multifactorial inheritance

OVERVIEW

Previous discussion has dealt with diseases caused by an alteration in a single gene or in a specific chromosome. Most common diseases (heart disease, cancer, diabetes, etc.) have substantial genetic components, but their causation is complex. These diseases tend to cluster in families (familial), but they do not conform to mendelian pedigree patterns. This chapter reviews some basic principles of the genetics of common, complex diseases.

MULTIFACTORIAL INHERITANCE

The term *multifactorial inheritance* refers to the fact that most common diseases are caused by multiple genes (i.e., a polygenic component) and expression is often influenced by environmental factors. The genetic and environmental factors involved are referred to as **risk factors,** and the summation of these in an individual represents that person's **liability** for the disease. Because several genes and influential environmental factors contribute to the liability, its distribution in the population can be represented as a Gaussian ("bell-shaped") curve. Figure II-4-1A shows an example of a distribution curve for body mass index (BMI), a multifactorial trait, in the U.S. adult population. The mean BMI is 26 ± 6 kg/m^2. Because obesity is defined in terms of BMI (BMI ≥ 30 kg/m^2), this graph can also represent a liability curve for obesity.

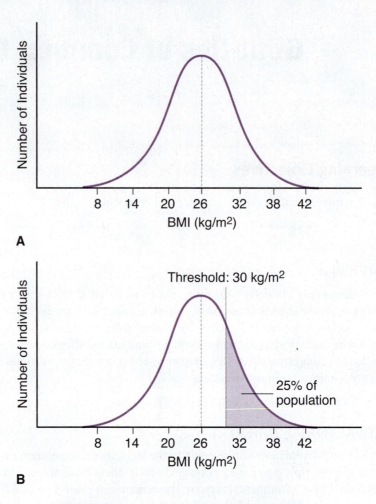

Figure II-4-1. Obesity in the U.S. Population.
(A) Distribution of BMI in the U.S. Population
(B) Threshold for and Prevalence of Obesity

Multifactorial Threshold Model

Unlike liability for a disease, the multifactorial diseases themselves are not continuous traits. Either a person has the disease or does not; i.e., it is a discontinuous characteristic. Expression of the disease phenotype occurs only when a certain threshold of liability is reached. The threshold for a complex disease is set by the diagnostic criteria. As a simple example, obesity is a complex, multifactorial condition in which excess body fat may put a person at risk for a variety of other conditions, including type 2 diabetes and cardiovascular disease (see below). The clinical definition of obesity is a BMI ≥ 30 kg/m^2. If one plots BMI for the population of the United States and sets the "obesity threshold" at 30 kg/m^2, nearly 25% of adults over 20 years of age will be above this threshold. Thus, the prevalence of obesity in this population is 25% (0.25; 1 in 4).

For some common diseases, the male and female thresholds are different (Figure II-4-2.) For example, risk factors for atherosclerosis and myocardial infarction include:

- LDL-receptor deficiency
- Hyperlipidemia
- Smoking
- Diabetes
- Obesity
- Lack of exercise
- Elevated homocysteine
- Male sex

Some of these risk factors are more completely genetic (LDL-receptor deficiency), some are more completely environmental (lack of exercise and smoking), and some have substantial genetic and environmental contributions (obesity). The contributing factors and an individual's liability are usually determined empirically, as are the recurrence risks.

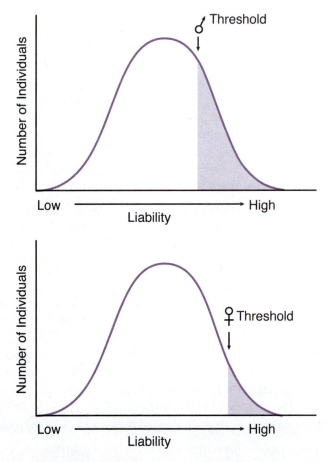

The male threshold is lower than the female threshold, so the prevalence of the disease is higher in males than in females.

Figure II-4-2. Multifactorial Diseases May Have Different Male and Female Thresholds

Section II • Medical Genetics

Assessing Recurrence Risks for Multifactorial Diseases

The inheritance patterns of multifactorial diseases differ from those of single-gene disorders in several important ways. Recurrence risks:

- **Are estimated empirically.** For single-gene disorders, the mechanism of gene action is understood (e.g., cystic fibrosis is caused by an autosomal recessive mutation, neurofibromatosis is produced by an autosomal dominant mutation, etc.), and recurrence risks can be derived based on known principles of inheritance. In contrast, the genes and environmental factors underlying multifactorial traits have not been identified specifically. Consequently, empirical recurrence risks (i.e., based on direct observation of data) must be derived. For example, if we wish to know the recurrence risk for siblings of individuals with cleft lip and/or palate, we ascertain a large cohort of individuals with cleft lip and/or palate and then measure the proportion of their siblings who are also affected with cleft lip and/or palate (in this case, the sibling recurrence risk is approximately 3%, which is considerably higher than the general population prevalence of 0.1%).

- **Increase as the number of affected relatives increases.** Recurrence risks for single-gene traits remain the same regardless of the number of affected individuals in the family (e.g., the recurrence risk for cystic fibrosis is 25% in a carrier-by-carrier mating, even if several previous siblings have all been affected). Multifactorial recurrence risks increase as the number of affected relatives (e.g., siblings) increases. This does not mean that the true risk has changed; rather, it reflects the fact that additional affected individuals provide more information about the true risk. The presence of multiple affected individuals indicates that the family is located higher on the liability distribution (i.e., they likely have more genetic and environmental risk factors). For example, one study showed that sibling recurrence risk for a neural tube defect (spina bifida or anencephaly; *see* Clinical Correlate) was 3% if one sibling was affected, 12% if two were affected, and 25% if three were affected.

- **Increase as the severity of the disease expression increases.** Again, this reflects the fact that the individual and his or her relatives are located higher on the liability distribution.

- **Increase if the affected individual (i.e., the proband) is a member of the less commonly affected sex.** This principle follows from the fact that an affected individual of the less commonly affected sex will be, on average, higher on the liability distribution (Figure II-4-2). For example, the prevalence of pyloric stenosis (congenital constriction of the pylorus) is approximately 1/1,000 for females and 1/200 for males. Thus, the average affected female is likely to be located higher on the liability distribution than is an affected male (i.e., the female has more genetic and environmental risk factors). The presence of more risk factors implies that the affected female's relatives are more likely to be affected than are the affected male's relatives.

- **Decrease rapidly for more remotely related relatives.** For example, one study of autism reported a sibling risk of 4.5%, an uncle–niece risk of 0.1%, and a first-cousin risk of 0.05%. In contrast, the risk of carrying a single-gene mutation decreases by only 1/2 with each successive degree of relationship (i.e., 50% chance for siblings, 25% for uncle–niece relationships, and 12.5% for first cousins).

Note

Recurrence Risks for Multifactorial Diseases

- Are estimated empirically
- Increase as the number of affected relatives increases
- Increase as the severity of the disease expression increases
- Increase if the affected individual is a member of the less commonly affected sex
- Decrease very rapidly for more remotely related relatives
- Increase as the prevalence of the disease increases in a population

- **Increase as the prevalence of the disease increases in a population.** Although the recurrence risk for a single-gene disorder remains the same regardless of the prevalence of the disease in a population, the empirical risk for multifactorial diseases increases as the population prevalence increases. This is because populations with higher prevalence rates have a higher preponderance of genetic and environmental risk factors. This in turn raises the risk for relatives of affected individuals.

Clinical Correlate: Neural Tube Defects

Neural tube defects (NTDs: anencephaly, spina bifida, and encephalocele) are one of the most common congenital malformations and are seen in approximately 1 in 1,000 births in the United States. Anencephaly (partial or complete absence of the brain) usually leads to a stillbirth, and anencephalics that survive to term do not live for more than a few days. Spina bifida, a protrusion of spinal tissue through the vertebral column, produces secondary hydrocephalus in 75% of cases and often produces some degree of paralysis. Improved intervention strategies have increased survival rates substantially for this condition, with more than two thirds of patients now surviving beyond 10 years of age. The sibling recurrence risk for NTDs is estimated to be 2–5%, which is much higher than the population prevalence. Thus, the disorder clusters in families. Recent epidemiologic studies show that 50–70% of NTDs can be prevented by periconceptional dietary folic acid supplementation. Folic acid deficiency is likely to be present in successive pregnancies, providing a nongenetic explanation for some of the familial clustering of this disease. However, there is also evidence for genetic variation in the ability to metabolize folic acid. Thus, NTDs provide an example in which familial clustering is likely related to both genetic and nongenetic factors.

Genetics of Common Diseases: Summary of Principles

Several key principles should emerge from this review of the genetics of common diseases:

- Common diseases generally have both genetic and environmental liability factors.
- Liability for common diseases in a population can be represented by a normal (Gaussian) distribution.
- The disease threshold is set by diagnostic criteria and may be different for males and females. The fraction (or percent) of the population above the threshold defines the prevalence of the disease in that population.
- Recurrence risks within a family are determined empirically. Recurrence risks increase with the number of affected relatives, the severity of disease expression in the family, the probands of the less commonly affected sex, and the prevalence of disease in the population. Recurrence risks decrease rapidly for remotely related relatives.
- Heritability represents the contribution of genes to the liability curve. Heritability can be estimated by twin studies and adoption studies.

Section II • Medical Genetics

- For many common diseases, subsets of cases exist in which genetic factors play an especially important role. These subsets tend to develop disease early in life (e.g., *BRCA1* and *BRCA2* mutations in breast cancer), and they often tend to have a more severe expression of the disease.

- In some cases, genes involved in the less common, strongly inherited subsets of common diseases (in cancer, specific oncogenes and tumor suppressor genes) are also involved in the common noninherited cases (but in different ways, such as a somatic mutation instead of a germ-line mutation).

> **Chapter Summary**
>
> - Many common diseases exhibit multifactorial inheritance.
>
> - Recurrence risks for multifactorial diseases are estimated empirically.
>
> - Twin and adoption studies are performed to determine the relative effects of genetics and environment on diseases.
>
> - Coronary heart disease can be caused by mutations in the LDL receptor (familial hypercholesterolemia).

Review Questions

1. Pyloric stenosis is five times more common in males than in females in certain Japanese populations. The liability curve for the development of this condition in that population is shown below:

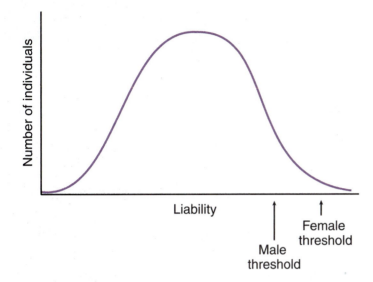

Within this population, which of the following is most at risk for the development of disease?

A. The daughters of affected fathers
B. The daughters of affected mothers
C. The sons of affected fathers
D. The sons of affected mothers

Answers

1. **Answer: D.** Because the trait in this case is five times more common in males in females, it means that males are found lower on the liability curve. Fewer factors are needed to cause the disease phenotype in the male. Therefore, a female with the disease is higher on the liability curve and has a larger number of factors promoting disease. The highest risk population in this model of multifactorial inheritance would be the sons (the higher risk group) of affected mothers (the lower risk group). The affected mother had an accumulation of more disease-promoting liabilities, so she is likely to transmit these to her sons, who need fewer liabilities to develop the syndrome.

Recombination Frequency 5

Learning Objectives

❏ Solve problems concerning polymorphic markers and linkage analysis
❏ Solve problems concerning gene mapping: linkage analysis
❏ Demonstrate understanding of determining recombination frequency accurately
❏ Explain information related to LOD scores

OVERVIEW

An important step in understanding the basis of an inherited disease is to locate the gene(s) responsible for the disease. This chapter provides an overview of the techniques that have been used to map and clone thousands of human genes.

POLYMORPHIC MARKERS AND LINKAGE ANALYSIS

A prerequisite for successful linkage analysis is the availability of a large number of highly polymorphic markers dispersed throughout the genome. There are several classes of these polymorphic markers (Figure II-5-1). Over 20,000 individual examples of these polymorphic markers at known locations have now been identified and are available for linkage studies. These markers collectively provide a marker map of each chromosome, so when one wishes to map the position of a gene—often one involved in a disease process—the gene's position can be located relative to one or more markers by recombination mapping. These high-density marker maps allow genome-wide screening for mapping genes. Chromosome gene and marker maps are available online at www.pubmed.gov.

Section II • Medical Genetics

In an RFLP, the presence or absence of a restriction site (▲) produces DNA fragments of varying lengths, reflecting sequence variation.

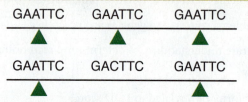

In a VNTR, variation in fragment lengths is produced by differences in the number of tandem repeats located between two restriction sites (▲).

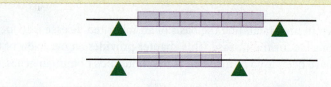

In an STRP, variation in fragment lengths is produced by differences in the number of microsatellite repeats found between two PCR primer sites (■).

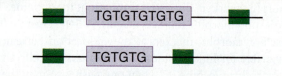

SNPs are single differences in a nucleotide sequence.

```
A C C G T C C G
A C C C T C C G
      ↑
```

Figure II-5-1. Different Types of DNA Polymorphisms

RFLPs (restriction fragment length polymorphisms)

Restriction endonuclease (RE) sites—palindromes recognized by specific restriction endonucleases—can serve as two-allele markers. A specific site may be present in some individuals (allele 1) and absent in others (allele 2), producing different-sized restriction fragments that can be visualized on a Southern blot. Alternatively, the area containing the restriction site can be amplified by using a PCR (polymerase chain reaction) and treating the PCR product with the restriction enzyme to determine whether one (RE site absent) or two (RE site present) fragments are produced. The PCR product(s) can be separated by agarose gel electrophoresis and visualized directly without using a blot (*see* RFLP Analysis of PCR Products in Medical Genetics Chapter 6 for an example).

VNTRs (variable number of tandem repeats)

These polymorphisms are the result of varying numbers of minisatellite repeats in a specific region of a chromosome. The minisatellite repeat units typically range in size from 20 to 70 bases each. The repeat is flanked on both sides by a restriction site, and variation in the number of repeats produces restriction fragments of varying size. VNTRs are used infrequently in current genetic mapping, as they tend to cluster near the ends of chromosomes.

STRPs (short tandem repeat polymorphisms, or microsatellites)

Short tandem repeat polymorphisms are repetitive sequences in which the repeated unit is generally two to six bases long. An example of a dinucleotide repeat (CA/TG) is shown in Figure II-5-1. These markers have many alleles in the population, with each different repeat length at a locus representing a different allele. STRPs can be amplified with a PCR by using primers designed to flank the repeat block. Variation in the number of repeats produces PCR products of varying length, which can then be visualized on agarose gel electrophoresis. STRPs are distributed throughout the chromosomes, making them very useful in mapping genes. As illustrated in Chapter 7 of Biochemistry, STRPs are used in paternity testing and in forensic cases, but these sequences can also be used in gene mapping.

SNPs (single nucleotide polymorphisms)

SNPs represent nucleotide positions in the human genome where only two nucleotides—for example, C or G—are found. These occur on average about once in every 1,000 base pairs (bp) and, like STRPs, are very useful in mapping genes. Unlike STRPs, which have multiple alleles at each locus, SNPs are usually two-allele markers (either G or C in the above example). These can be typed either by PCR amplification and identification by sequencing or through the use of probes on DNA chips, a process that can be automated.

GENE MAPPING: LINKAGE ANALYSIS

Crossing Over, Recombination, and Linkage

The first step in gene mapping is to establish linkage with a known polymorphic marker (one with at least two alleles in the population). This can be done by recombination mapping to determine whether the gene is near a particular marker. Multiple markers on different chromosomes are used to establish linkage (or the lack of it).

Recombination mapping is based on crossing over during meiosis, the type of cell division that produces haploid ova and sperm. During prophase I of meiosis, homologous chromosomes line up and occasionally exchange portions of their DNA. This process (shown in Figure II-5-2) is termed **crossover**.

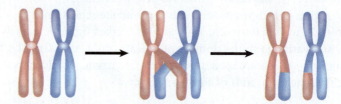

Figure II-5-2. The Process of Crossing Over Between Homologous Chromosomes

When a crossover event occurs between two loci, G and M, the resulting chromosomes **may** contain a new combination of alleles at loci G and M. When a new combination occurs, the crossover has produced a **recombination**. Because crossover events occur more or less randomly across chromosomes, loci that are located farther apart are more likely to experience an intervening crossover and thus a recombination of alleles. Recombination frequency provides a means of assessing the distance between loci on chromosomes, a key goal of gene mapping.

This process is illustrated in Figure II-5-3.

- If the gene of interest (with alleles G_1 and G_2) and the marker (with alleles M_1 and M_2) are on different chromosomes, the alleles will remain together in an egg or a sperm only about 50% of the time. They are **unlinked**.

- If the gene and the marker are on the same chromosome but are far apart, the alleles will remain together about 50% of the time. The larger distance between the gene and the marker allows multiple crossovers to occur between the alleles during prophase I of meiosis. An odd number of crossovers separates G_1 from M_1 (recombination), whereas an even number of crossovers places the alleles together on the same chromosome (no recombination). The gene and marker are again defined as **unlinked**.

- If the gene and the marker are close together on the same chromosome, a crossover between the two alleles is much less likely to occur. Therefore, G_1 and M_1 are likely to remain on the same chromosome more than 50% of the time. In other words, they show **less than 50% recombination**. The gene and the marker are now defined as **linked**.

Gene and marker on different chromosomes. If a cell gets G1, then 50% of the time it will get M$_1$ and 50% of the time it will get M2. Gene and marker are **unlinked**.

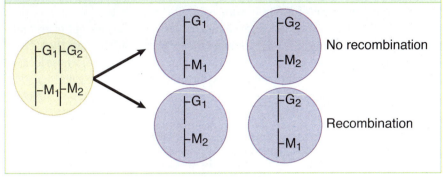

A

Gene and marker are far apart on same chromosome. If cell gets G1, then 50% of the time it will get M$_1$ (even number of crossovers) and 50% of the time it will get M2 (odd number of crossovers). Gene and marker are **unlinked**.

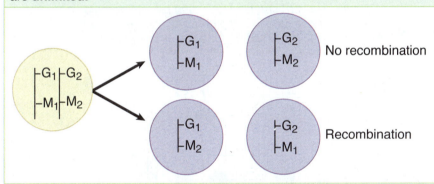

B

Note
- G1 and G2 are alleles of a gene to be mapped.
- M1 and M2 are alleles of a marker whose locus is known.

Gene and marker are close together on the same chromosome. If a cell gets G1 it is more likely to get M$_1$ also. Gene and marker are **linked**.

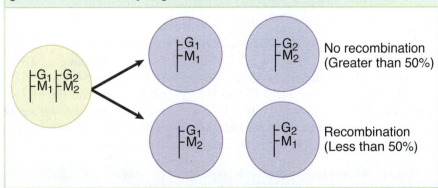

C

Figure II-5-3. Gene Mapping by Recombination Frequency with a Marker Whose Locus Is Known

Section II • Medical Genetics

Recombination Frequencies and Gene Mapping

The closer together two linked loci are—for instance, a gene and a marker—the lower the recombination frequency will be between them. Therefore, recombination frequency can be used to estimate proximity between a gene and a linked marker.

The following example of a family with neurofibromatosis type 1, an autosomal dominant disorder with complete penetrance, illustrates the concept of recombination frequency (Figure II-5-4). Some members of the family have the disease-producing allele of the gene (indicated by phenotype in the pedigree) whose location is to be determined. Other individuals have the normal allele of the gene.

Each individual has also been typed for his or her allele(s) of a two-allele marker (1 or 2). Three steps are involved in determining whether linkage exists and, if so, estimating the distance between the gene and the known marker.

1. Establish linkage phase between the disease-producing allele of the gene and an allele of the marker in the family.
2. Determine if linkage exists between the two alleles.
3. If linkage exists, estimate the recombination frequency.

A family in which a mutation causing neurofibromatosis type 1 is transmitted in three generations. The genotype of a marker locus is shown for each pedigree member.

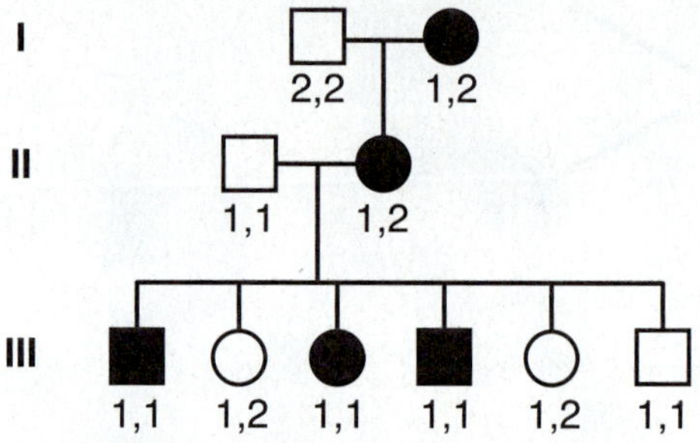

Figure II-5-4. Pedigree for Neurofibromatosis Type 1

Note

A **haplotype** is the combination of alleles on a single chromosome. With respect to the gene and the marker in Figure II-5-3, individual II-2 has two haplotypes, AM_1 and aM_2, depicted below, where A and a are alleles of the gene causing the disease. The marker has alleles 1 and 2.

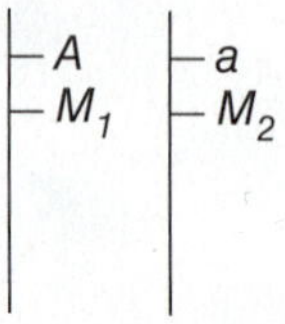

Linkage Phase. The pedigree indicates that the grandmother (I-2) had the disease-producing allele (A) of the gene, which she passed to her daughter (II-2). Is it also possible to determine which allele of the marker was passed from the grandmother to her daughter? Yes, allele 1. If linkage is present, the disease-producing allele (A) is linked to allele 1 of the marker. We can then designate the daughter's two haplotypes as AM_1/aM_2, indicating the chromosomes from her mother/father respectively.

Determine If Linkage Exists. Are the gene and the marker actually linked as we hypothesize? Looking at the children in generation III (each representing a meiotic event in their mother, II-2), we would expect a child who inherited marker allele 1 from the mother to have the disease. The children who inherited allele 2 from the mother should not have the disease. Examination of the six children's haplotypes shows that this assumption is true in all but one case (III-6). Because the AM_1 and aM_2 haplotypes remain together more than 50% of the time (or, conversely, are separated by recombination less than 50% of the time), our hypothesis of linkage is correct.

Estimate the Recombination Frequency. Out of six children, there is only one recombinant (III-6). The estimated recombination frequency in this family is 1/6, or 17%.

Recombination frequencies can be related to physical distance by the centimorgan (cM)

The recombination frequency provides a measure of genetic distance between any pair of linked loci. This distance is expressed in centimorgans. The centimorgan is equal to 1% recombination frequency. For example, if two loci show a recombination frequency of 2%, they are said to be 2 centimorgans apart. Physically, 1 cM is approximately equal to 1 million base pairs of DNA (1 Mb). This relationship is only approximate, however, because crossover frequencies are somewhat different throughout the genome, e.g., they are less common near centromeres and more common near telomeres.

Note
For Linked Loci:
- 1 centimorgan (cM) = 1% recombination frequency
- 1 cM ≈ 1 million base pairs

Determining Recombination Frequency Accurately: LOD Scores

In the previous example, a very small population (six children, or six meiotic events) was used to determine and calculate linkage, allowing only a very rough estimate of linkage distance. In fact, there is some small chance that the gene and the marker are not actually linked at all and the data were obtained by chance. We could be more confident that our conclusions were correct if we had used a much larger population. Because families don't have 100 or 200 children, the next best approach is to combine data from different families with this same disease to increase the number of meioses examined. These data can be combined by using LOD (log of the odds) calculations.

A LOD score, calculated by computer, compares the probability (P) that the data resulted from actual linkage with a recombination frequency of theta (θ) versus the probability that the gene and the marker are unlinked ($\theta = 50\%$) and that the data were obtained by chance alone. In the example calculation:

$$\text{Odds} = \frac{\text{Probability of observing pedigree data if } \theta = 0.17}{\text{Probability of observing pedigree data if } \theta = 0.5}$$

In practice, because 17% might not be the correct number, the computer calculates these probabilities assuming a variety of recombination frequencies from $\theta = 0$ (gene and marker are in the same location) to $\theta = 0.5$ (gene and marker are unlinked). The "odds of linkage" is simply the probability that each recombination frequency (θ) is consistent with the family data. If data from multiple families are combined, the numbers can be added by using the $\log_{10}$ of these odds.

$$\text{Log of the Odds (LOD)} = \log_{10} \frac{P \text{ (linkage at recombination frequency, } \theta)}{P \text{ (unlinked, recombination frequency, 50\%)}}$$

This equation need not be memorized. These calculations are done by computer and are displayed as a LOD table that gives the LOD score for each recombination frequency, θ (Table II-5-1).

Section II • Medical Genetics

Note

- A LOD score > 3 indicates linkage; a LOD score < –2 indicates no linkage.
- The value of υ at which the highest LOD score is seen is the most likely estimate of the recombination frequency.
- For any pair of loci, LOD scores obtained from different families can be added together.

Table II-5-1. LOD Scores for a Gene and a Marker

Recombination frequency (θ)	0.01	0.05	0.10	0.20	0.30	0.40
LOD score	0.58	1.89	3.47	2.03	–0.44	–1.20

When interpreting LOD scores, the following rules apply:

- A LOD score greater than 3.00 shows statistical evidence of linkage. (It is 1,000 times more likely that the gene and the marker are linked at that distance than unlinked.)
- A LOD score less than –2.00 shows statistical evidence of nonlinkage. (It is 100 times more likely that the gene and the marker are unlinked than linked at that distance.)
- A LOD score between –2.00 and 3.00 is indeterminate.

An examination of Table II-5-1 shows that in only one case is there convincing evidence for linkage and that score has a recombination frequency of 0.10. Therefore, the most likely distance between the gene and the marker is a recombination frequency of 10%, or 10 cM.

If no LOD score on the table is greater than 3.00, the data may be suggestive of linkage, but results from additional families with the disease would need to be gathered.

Gene mapping by linkage analysis serves several important functions:

- It can define the approximate location of a disease-causing gene.
- Linked markers can be used along with family pedigree information for genetic testing (*see* Chapter 6). In practice, markers that are useful for genetic testing must show less than 1% recombination with the gene involved (be less than 1 cM distant from the gene).
- Linkage analysis can identify locus heterogeneity (*see* Question 1 at the end of this chapter).

Review Questions

1. A family with an autosomal dominant disorder is typed for a 2 allele marker, which is closely linked to the disease locus. Based on the individuals in Generation III, what is the recombination rate between the disease locus and the marker locus?

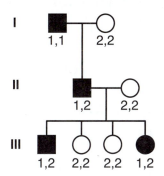

   (A) 0
   (B) 0.25
   (C) 0.50
   (D) 0.75
   (E) 1.0
   (F) The marker is uninformative

2. A man who has alkaptonuria marries a woman who has hereditary sucrose intolerance. Both are autosomal recessive diseases and both map to 3q with a distance of 10 cM separating the two loci. What is the chance they will have a child with alkaptonuria and sucrose intolerance?

   (A) 0%
   (B) 12.5%
   (C) 25%
   (D) 50%
   (E) 100%

Section II • Medical Genetics

3. In a family study following an autosomal dominant trait through three generations, two loci are compared for their potential linkage to the disease locus. In the following three-generation pedigree, shaded symbols indicate the presence of the disease phenotype, and the expression of ABO blood type and MN alleles are shown beneath each individual symbol.

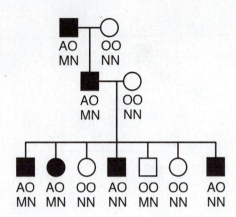

Which of the following conclusions can be made about the linkage of the disease allele, ABO blood group locus, and MN locus?

(A) The ABO and MN alleles are linked, but assort independently from the disease allele

(B) The ABO, MN, and disease alleles all assort independently

(C) The disease allele is linked to the ABO locus

(D) The disease allele is linked to the ABO and MN loci

(E) The disease allele is linked to the MN locus

Answers

1. **Answer: A.** In this pedigree, the disease allele is consistently transmitted with the 1 allele. There is no case in this small number of individuals where recombination between these two loci has occurred. Therefore, in Generation III, there is no recombination seen in any of the four individuals. Receiving the one allele always goes together with receiving the disease gene. Linked markers can be "uninformative" (**choice E**) in some pedigrees if, for example, the same alleles are expressed in all family members. In such a case, it would be impossible to determine any recombination frequency.

2. **Answer: A.** A child will inherit a gene for alkaptonuria from the father and the normal allele of this gene from the mother. Conversely, the child will inherit a gene for hereditary sucrose intolerance from the mother and a normal allele of this gene from the father. The child will therefore be a carrier for each disease but will not be affected with either one.

3. **Answer: C.** In this pedigree, the disease locus alleles are segregating with the ABO blood locus alleles. In each case, individuals who receive the A allele also receive the disease allele. The MN locus is not linked to the AO locus because individuals III-4, -5, and -7 are each recombinants between these loci. The MN locus is not linked to the disease allele because individuals III-4, -5, and -7 are each recombinants between these loci.

Genetic Diagnosis 6

Learning Objectives

❑ Demonstrate understanding of overview
❑ Explain information related to genetic diagnosis
❑ Explain information related to applications of genetic diagnosis

OVERVIEW

In this chapter, we review some of the practical clinical applications of genetic research. Once a gene is identified, the associated genetic disease in at-risk individuals can be diagnosed.

GENETIC DIAGNOSIS

The goal of genetic diagnosis is to determine whether an at-risk individual has inherited a disease-causing gene. Two major types of genetic diagnosis can be distinguished: direct diagnosis, in which the mutation itself is examined, and indirect diagnosis, in which linked markers are used to infer whether the individual has inherited the chromosome segment containing the disease-causing mutation.

Direct Genetic Diagnosis

PCR and allele-specific oligonucleotide (ASO) probes

ASO probes are short nucleotide sequences that bind specifically to a single allele of the gene. For example, the most common mutation causing hemochromatosis is the C282Y mutation that results from a G to A substitution in codon 282.

Codon:	280	281	282	283	284
Normal HFE allele:	TAT	ACG	T**G**C	CAG	GTG
			↑		
C282Y allele:	TAT	ACG	T**A**C	CAG	GTG
			↑		

The ASO for the normal allele would have the sequence

3′ ATA TGC A**C**G GTC CAC 5′

The ASO for the C282Y allele would have the sequence

$$3'\ \text{ATA}\ \text{TGC}\ \text{ATG}\ \text{GTC}\ \text{CAC}\ 5'$$

The two ASOs could be used to probe the PCR-amplified material on a dot blot (Figure II-6-1).

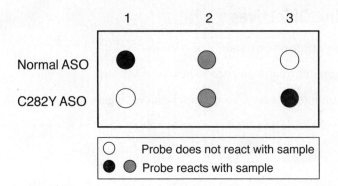

Figure II-6-1. Allele-Specific Oligonucleotide Probes in Hemochromatosis

The results show that individual 1 is homozygous for the normal HFE allele. Individual 2 is heterozygous for the normal and C282Y alleles. Individual 3 is homozygous for the C282Y allele. Only individual 3 would be expected to have symptoms. Note that this test merely determines genotype, and many considerations must be taken into account before predictions about phenotype could be made. Hemochromatosis has only about 15% penetrance, and in those who do have symptoms, variable expression is seen.

DNA chips

This approach involves embedding thousands of different oligonucleotides, representing various mutations and normal sequences, on a silicone chip. Patient DNA from specific regions is amplified by PCR, tagged with a fluorescent label, and exposed to the oligonucleotides on the chip. The sites of hybridization on the chip are recorded by a computer. This approach has the advantages of ready computerization and miniaturization (hundreds of thousands of oligonucleotides can be embedded on a single 2-cm^2 chip).

Restriction fragment length polymorphism (RFLP) analysis of PCR products (RFLP-PCR)

Occasionally a mutation that creates a disease-producing allele also destroys (or creates in some instances) a restriction enzyme site, as illustrated by the following case:

> A 14-year-old girl has been diagnosed with Gaucher disease (glucocerebrosidase A deficiency), an autosomal recessive disorder of sphingolipid catabolism. The mutation, T1448C, in this family also affects an HphI restriction site. PCR amplification of the area containing the mutation yields a 150-bp product. The PCR product from the normal allele of the gene is not cut by HphI. The PCR product of the mutant allele T1448C is cut by HphI to yield 114- and 36-bp fragments. The PCR product(s) is visualized directly by gel electrophoresis. Based on the results shown below in Figure II-6-3 using this assay on DNA samples from this family, what is the most likely conclusion about sibling 2?

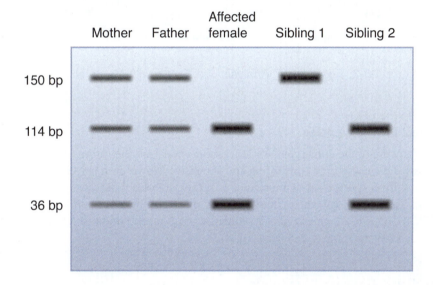

Figure II-6-2. PCR and RFLP for Gaucher Disease

(Ans.: Sibling 2 is also affected)

RFLP diagnosis of myotonic dystrophy

RFLP analysis is also useful in a few cases in which polymorphisms are too large to conveniently amplify with a PCR. One such case is myotonic dystrophy, in which the expanded sequence is within the gene region itself (a CTG in the 3′ untranslated region). This disease shows anticipation, and family members with a severe form of myotonic dystrophy may have several thousand copies of this repeat. As shown in Figure II-6-3, when *Eco*RI digests are analyzed by Southern blotting, a probe reveals 9- to 10-kb fragments in unaffected individuals. The size of the fragment can reach 20 kb in severely affected individuals.

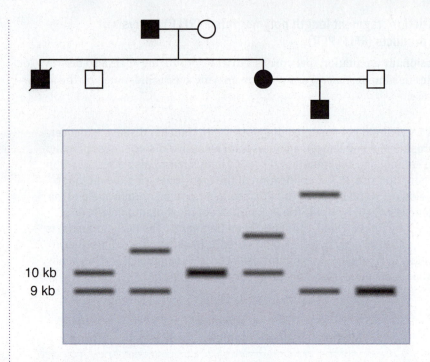

Figure II-6-3. *Eco*RI RFLP Analysis of a Family with Myotonic Dystrophy

Direct DNA sequencing

Sequencing of the entire gene (or at least the exons and the intron–exon boundaries) is relatively time consuming and expensive. However, it is sometimes necessary if no specific set of mutations is responsible for most cases of a disease (e.g., familial breast cancer caused by any of several hundred mutations of the *BRCA1* or *BRCA2* genes). DNA sequencing is typically done using automated sequencing machines (see Figure I-7-8).

Indirect Genetic Diagnosis

If the mutation causing a disease in a family is not known, indirect genetic analysis can often be used to infer whether a parent has transmitted the mutation to his or her offspring. Indirect genetic analysis uses genetic markers that are closely linked (showing less than 1% recombination) to the disease locus. The markers are the same ones used in genetic mapping studies: restriction fragment length polymorphisms (RFLPs), short tandem repeat polymorphisms (STRPs), and single nucleotide polymorphisms (SNPs). Because STRPs can have multiple alleles (with each allele representing a different number of repeats), they are often informative markers to use.

Indirect genetic diagnosis using STRPs

Figure II-6-4 portrays a three-generation pedigree in which Marfan syndrome is being transmitted. Each family member has been typed for a four-allele STRP that is closely linked to the disease locus. The affected father in Generation I transmitted the disease-causing mutation to his daughter, and he also transmitted allele 3 of the marker. This allows us to establish linkage phase in this family. Because of the close linkage between the marker and the disease locus, we can predict accurately that the offspring in Generation III who receive allele 3 from their mother will also receive the disease-causing mutation. Thus, the risk for each child, instead of being the standard 50% recurrence risk for an autosomal dominant disease, is much more definitive: nearly 100% or nearly 0%.

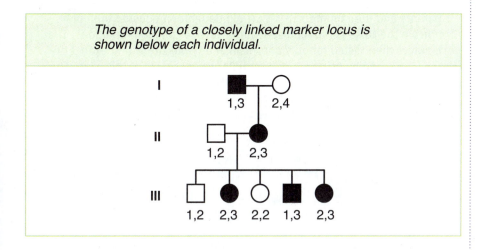

Figure II-6-4. A Three-Generation Family in Which Marfan Syndrome Is Being Transmitted

Recurrence risks may have to take into account the small chance of recombination between the marker allele and the disease-causing gene. If the STR and the disease-causing gene used in this case show 1% recombination, then the recurrence risk for a fetus in generation III whose marker genotype is 2,2 would be 1% rather than 0%. If a fetus in generation III had the marker genotype 2,3, the recurrence risk for that child would be 99%.

Indirect genetic testing using RFLPs

If an RFLP is used as a marker for a disease-causing gene, the data may be analyzed by using Southern blotting and a probe for the gene region.

A man and a woman seek genetic counseling because the woman is 8 weeks pregnant, and they had a previous child who died in the perinatal period. A retrospective diagnosis of long-chain acyl-CoA dehydrogenase (LCAD) deficiency was made based on the results of mass spectrometry performed on a blood sample. The couple also has an unaffected 4-year-old daughter with a normal level of LCAD activity consistent with homozygosity for the normal LCAD allele. The parents wish to know whether the current pregnancy will result in a child with the same rare condition as the previous child who died. DNA samples from both parents and their unaffected 4-year-old daughter are tested for mutations in the LCAD gene. All test negative for the common mutations. The family is then tested for polymorphism at a BamII site within exon 3 of the LCAD gene by using a probe for the relevant region of this exon. The RFLP marker proves informative. Fetal DNA obtained by amniocentesis is also tested in the same way. The results of the Southern blot are shown below in Figure II-6-6. What is the best conclusion about the fetus?

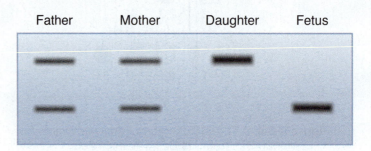

Figure II-6-5. RFLP Analysis for LCAD

(Ans: The fetus is homozygous for the LCAD mutation and should be clinically affected.)

Although RFLP analysis can be used as both an indirect test and a direct test, there is a significant difference between the two situations.

In the direct test, the mutation causing the disease is the same as the one that alters the restriction site. There is no distance separating the mutations and no chance for recombination to occur, which might lead to an incorrect conclusion.

In the indirect assay, the mutation in the restriction site (a marker) has occurred independently of the mutation causing the disease. Because the mutations are close together on the chromosome, the RFLP can be used as a surrogate marker for the disease-producing mutation. Linkage phase in each family must be established. Because the RFLP and the locus of the disease-producing mutation are some distance apart, there is a small chance for recombination and incorrect conclusions.

RFLP analysis for an X-linked disease

Individual II-2 in the family shown below has Lesch Nyhan disease. His sister, II-4, is pregnant and wants to know the likelihood that her child will be affected. The mutation in this family is uncharacterized, but is mapped to within 0.05 cM of an EcoR1 site that is informative in this family. DNA from all family members is obtained. Fetal DNA is obtained by chorionic villus sampling. What is the best conclusion about the fetus?

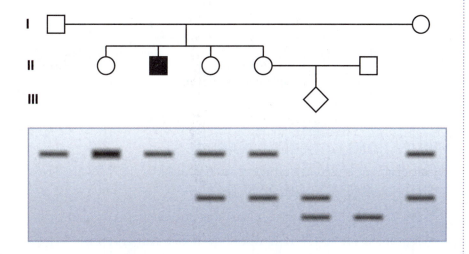

Figure II-6-6. RFLP Analysis of HGPRT Deficiency in a Family

(Ans: The fetus (a girl) will not be affected. She will not be a carrier either because her mother, II-4, is not a carrier)

Comparison of Direct and Indirect Genetic Diagnosis

Direct genetic diagnosis is used whenever possible. Its major limitation is that the disease-producing mutation(s) must be known if one is to test for them. If a family carries a mutation not currently documented, as in the family above with LCAD deficiency, it will not be detected by direct mutation testing. In these cases, indirect genetic testing can be used. A comparison of the key features of direct and indirect genetic diagnosis is summarized in Table II-6-1.

Table II-6-1. Key Features of Indirect and Direct Genetic Diagnosis

	Indirect Diagnosis	Direct Diagnosis
Family information needed	Yes	No
Errors possible because of recombination	Yes	No
Markers may be uninformative	Yes	No
Multiple mutations can be assayed with a single test	Yes	No
Disease-causing mutation itself must be known	No	Yes

APPLICATIONS OF GENETIC DIAGNOSIS

Genetic diagnosis is used in a variety of settings, including the ones listed below.

- Carrier diagnosis in recessive diseases
- Presymptomatic diagnosis for late-onset diseases
- Asymptomatic diagnosis for diseases with reduced penetrance
- Prenatal diagnosis
- Preimplantation testing

Prenatal Genetic Diagnosis

Prenatal diagnosis is one of the most common applications of genetic diagnosis. Diagnosis of a genetic disease in a fetus may aid in making an informed decision regarding pregnancy termination, and it often aids parents in preparing emotionally and medically for the birth of an affected child. There is a variety of types of prenatal diagnosis.

Amniocentesis

A small sample of amniotic fluid (10–20 mL) is collected at approximately 16 weeks' gestation. Fetal cells are present in the amniotic fluid and can be used to diagnose single-gene disorders, chromosome abnormalities, and some biochemical disorders. Elevated α-fetoprotein levels indicate a fetus with a neural tube defect. The risk of fetal demise due to amniocentesis is estimated to be approximately 1/200.

Chorionic villus sampling

This technique, typically performed at 10–12 weeks' gestation, involves the removal of a small sample of chorionic villus material (either a transcervical or a transabdominal approach may be used). The villi are of fetal origin and thus provide a large sample of actively dividing fetal cells for diagnosis. This technique has the advantage of providing a diagnosis earlier in the pregnancy. Disadvantages are a higher fetal mortality rate than with amniocentesis (about 1/100) and a small possibility of diagnostic error because of placental mosaicism (i.e., multiple cell types in the villi).

Preimplantation diagnosis

Embryos derived from *in vitro* fertilization can be diagnosed by removing a single cell, typically from the eight-cell stage (this does not harm the embryo). DNA is PCR amplified and is used to make a genetic diagnosis. The advantage of this technique is that pregnancy termination need not be considered: only embryos without the mutation are implanted. The primary disadvantage is potential diagnostic error as a result of PCR amplification from a single cell.

Review Questions

Select the ONE best answer.

1. The pedigree below shows a family in which hemophilia A, an X-linked disorder, is segregating. PCR products for each member of the family are also shown for a short tandem repeat polymorphism located within an intron of the factor VIII gene. What is the best explanation for the phenotype of individual II-1?

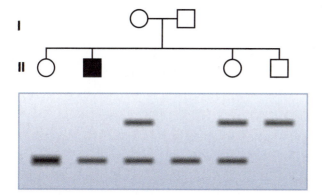

   (A) Heterozygous for the disease-producing allele
   (B) Homozygous for the disease-producing allele
   (C) Homozygous for the normal allele
   (D) Incomplete penetrance
   (E) Manifesting heterozygote

2. A 22-year-old woman with Marfan syndrome, a dominant genetic disorder, is referred to a prenatal genetics clinic during her tenth week of pregnancy. Her family pedigree is shown below (the arrow indicates the pregnant woman). PCR amplification of a short tandem repeat (STR) located in an intron of the fibrillin gene is carried out on DNA from each family member. What is the best conclusion about the fetus (III-1)?

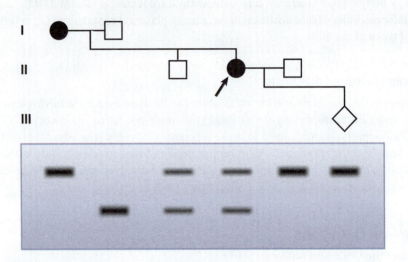

(A) Has a 25% change of having Marfan syndrome

(B) Has a 50% chance of having Marfan syndrome

(C) Will develop Marfan syndrome

(D) Will not develop Marfan syndrome

(E) Will not develop Marfan syndrome, but will be a carrier of the disease allele

3. The pedigree below represents a family in which phenylketonuria (PKU), an autosomal recessive disease, is segregating. Southern blots for each family member are also shown for an RFLP that maps 10 million bp upstream from the phenylalanine hydroxylase gene. What is the most likely explanation for the phenotype of II-3?

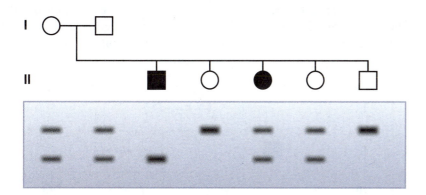

(A) A large percentage of her cells have the paternal X chromosome carrying the PKU allele active
(B) Heteroplasmy
(C) Male I-2 is not the biologic father
(D) PKU shows incomplete penetrance
(E) Recombination has occurred

Section II • Medical Genetics

4. A 14-year-old boy has Becker muscular dystrophy (BMD), an X-linked recessive disease. A maternal uncle is also affected. His sisters, aged 20 and 18, wish to know their genetic status with respect to the BMD. Neither the boy nor his affected uncle has any of the known mutations in the dystrophin gene associated with BMD. Family members are typed for a HindII restriction site polymorphism that maps to the 5′ end of intron 12 of the dystrophin gene. The region around the restriction site is amplified with a PCR. The amplified product is treated with the restriction enzyme HindII and the fragments separated by agarose gel electrophoresis. The results are shown below. What is the most likely status of individual III-2?

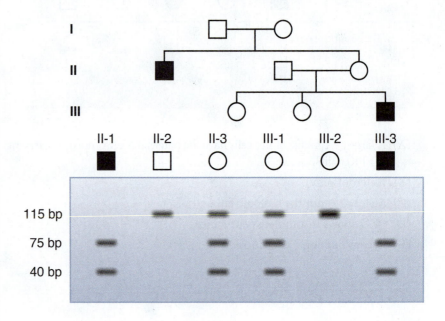

(A) Carrier of the disease-producing allele
(B) Hemizygous for the disease-producing allele
(C) Homozygous for the normal allele
(D) Homozygous for the disease-producing allele
(E) Manifesting heterozygote

5. Two phenotypically normal second cousins marry and would like to have a child. They are aware that one ancestor (great-grandfather) had PKU and are concerned about having an affected offspring. They request ASO testing and get the following results. What is the probability that their child will be affected?

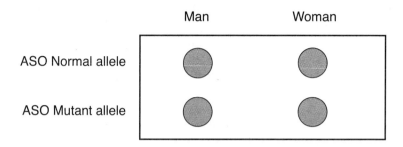

(A) 1.0
(B) 0.75
(C) 0.67
(D) 0.50
(E) 0.25

6. A 66-year-old man (I-2) has recently been diagnosed with Huntington disease, a late-onset, autosomal dominant condition. His granddaughter (III-1) wishes to know whether she has inherited the disease-producing allele, but her 48-year-old father (II-1) does not wish to be tested or to have his status known. The grandfather, his unaffected wife, the granddaughter, and her mother (II-2) are tested for alleles of a marker closely linked to the *huntingtin* gene on 4p16.3. The pedigree and the results of testing are shown below. What is the best information that can be given to the granddaughter (III-1) about her risk for developing Huntington disease?

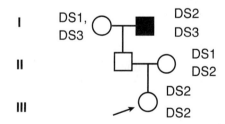

(A) 50%
(B) 25%
(C) Marker is not informative
(D) Nearly 100%
(E) Nearly 0%

Section II • Medical Genetics

Answers

1. **Answer: A.** The female II-1 in this family is heterozygous for the marker (from the gel) and also has an unaffected father. Her mother is a carrier and the bottom band in the mother's pattern is associated with the disease-producing allele of the factor VIII gene. All observations are consistent with II-1 being heterozygous (Xx) for the factor VIII gene. She has no symptoms, so she is not a manifesting heterozygote (**choice E**). She cannot be homozygous for the disease-producing allele (**choice B**) because her father is unaffected. Homozygosity for the normal allele (**choice C**) is inconsistent with the results shown on the gel. She has inherited the chromosome from her mother (bottom band) that carries the mutant factor VIII allele, but from her father she has received a chromosome carrying the normal allele. Note that her father is not affected, and the bottom band in his pattern is in linkage phase with the normal allele of the gene. This is a case where linkage phase is different in the mother and the father. Incomplete penetrance (**choice D**) is not a good choice because the female (II-1) does not have the disease-producing genotype. She is heterozygous for the recessive and (dominant) normal allele. One would expect from her genotype that she would be unaffected.

2. **Answer: C.** The blot shows the top band in the patterns of I-1 and II-2 (the proband) is associated with the disease-producing allele. Because the fetus has inherited this marker allele from the mother (II-2) and Marfan disease is dominant, the fetus will develop Marfan disease. **Choices A** and **B** are recurrence risks associated with the pedigree data. With no blot to examine, choice B, 50% risk would be correct. **Choice D** would be correct if the blot from the fetal DNA showed both the bottom band (must be from mother) and the top band (from the unaffected father). **Choice E** is incorrect because Marfan is a dominant disease with no "carrier" status.

3. **Answer: E.** Although II-3 has an RFLP pattern consistent with heterozygosity for the PKU allele, she has PKU. The best explanation offered is that recombination has occurred, and although she is heterozygous for the restriction site generating the RFLP pattern, she is homozygous for the mutation causing PKU. The restriction site is 10 million bp upstream from the phenylalanine hydroxylase gene so there is a minimum chance of recombination of 10%. Although this is small, it is the most likely of the options listed. The phenylalanine hydroxylase gene is not on the X chromosome (**choice A**). Heteroplasmy (**choice B**) is associated with mitochondrial pedigrees, and the phenylalanine hydroxylase gene is a nuclear one. The RFLP pattern is quite consistent with I-2 being the biologic father (**choice C**), and he is a known carrier of the PKU mutation because he has another affected child (II-1). If II-3's RFLP pattern showed homozygosity for the marker (identical to II-1), and she had no symptoms, incomplete penetrance (**choice D**) would be a good choice.

4. **Answer: C.** The disease-producing allele of the gene is associated with the presence of the *Hin*dII site. Notice that both affected males show two smaller bands (75 and 40 bp). II-3, a carrier female, also has these two smaller bands in her pattern, in addition to a larger PCR product (115 bp), representing the absence of the *Hin*dII site on her normal chromosome. III-2 has only the larger PCR product (notice the density because both chromosomes yielded this product). She is homozygous for the normal allele. **Choice A**, carrier, would be correct if her pattern had looked like

those of II-3 and III-1. All the males shown are hemizygous (**choice B**) for the dystrophin gene because they have only one copy. II-1 and III-3 are hemizygous for the disease-producing allele, and II-2 is hemizygous for the normal allele. No one in the family is homozygous for the disease-producing allele (**choice D**). In an X-linked pattern, this would be characteristic of a female with two copies of the disease-producing allele and is very rarely seen. III-2 is not a manifesting heterozygote (**choice E**) because she has no symptoms and is not a heterozygote.

5. **Answer: E.** The blot indicates that both parents are heterozygous for the mutant allele. Because both are phenotypically normal, the disease must be autosomal recessive. If it had been X-linked recessive, the man would be hemizygous. Thus, the chance they will have an affected child is 25% (0.25).

6. **Answer: A.** The affected grandfather has marker alleles DS2 and DS3. There is no information about which one is in linkage phase with his disease-producing *huntingtin* allele. On the basis of the pedigree alone, the daughter has a 25% change of inheriting the grandfather's disease-producing *huntingtin* allele (**choice B**); however, she would like more information. Because her father (II-1) does not wish to be tested or have any information known about his genetic status with respect to Huntington's, it is unethical to test the daughter for the triplet repeat expansion. The results would necessarily reveal the status of her father also. By doing an indirect genetic test, one can see the daughter has inherited one of her marker alleles (DS2) from the grandfather via her father. This means that she has a 50% chance of developing Huntington's because there is a 50% chance that DS2 is a marker for the disease-producing *huntingtin* allele in the grandfather and a 50% chance it is not (and DS3 is). Notice the result does not reveal additional information about her father (II-1). Before her testing, he had a 50% chance of having the disease-producing *huntingtin* allele. His risk is still 50% with the information from the daughter's test. However, if the father (II-1) does develop Huntington's in the future, that will then mean that the daughter has a 100% chance of having the disease also (**choice D**).

If her marker status had been DS1/DS1, her chances of developing Huntington's would have been near 0 (**choice E**) because she did not inherit these alleles from her grandfather. One came from her grandmother (via her father) and one from her mother. This result still would not reveal additional relevant information about her father (II-1), whose risk would remain 50%.

Index

A

Abetalipoproteinemia, 230
Acetyl CoA carboxylase, 219
Ackee fruit, 243
Acne, isotretinoin therapy for, 150
Acrocentric chromosomes, 349
Active muscle, 165
Acute intermittent porphyria, 272–273
Acute myocardial infarction (AMI), 192
Adeno-associated viruses (AAV), 91–92, 93
Adenosine, 6, 7
Adenosine deaminase (ADA) deficiency, 294
Adenoviruses, as gene delivery vector, 90–91
Adipose tissue
   GLUT 4 in, 170
Adjacent segregation, chromosomal translocation and, 356
   Robertsonian, 358, 359
ADP-ribosylation, 139, 140
Aerobic glycolysis, 171
Agarose gel electrophoresis, of PCR products, 106
Age of onset, disease-causing mutations and, 317
AIDS patients, measuring viral load in, 110
Alanine cycle, 208
Albinism, 267
Alcaptonuria, 267
Alcohol
   consumption of, extreme exercise and, 209
   metabolism of, 209, 209–210
Alcoholism, hypoglycemia and, 208, 208–209
Allele frequency, 334–335
   Hardy-Weinberg principle and, 336
   sex chromosomes and, 336
Alleles, 303
Allele-specific oligonucleotide (ASO) probes, 389–390, 390
Allelic heterogenicity, 267, 295, 314
Allopurinol as enzyme inhibitor, 122
α-tocopherol (vitamin E). See Vitamin E entries
Alternate segregation, chromosomal translocation and, 356
Amino acid activation, 66
   tRNA and, 54, 54–55
Amino acid metabolism, 261
   disorders of, 265–266, 266
Amino acids
   classification of, 115, 116–117
   essential, 119
   glucogenic and ketogenic, 205
   products derived from, 271
   protein turnover and, 118–119
   structure of, 115
   tRNA and, 44, 54, 54–55
Amino groups, removal and excretion of, 261, 262, 263
Aminotransferases (transaminases), 263
Amniocentesis, 396
Anaerobic glycolysis, 171
   in ischemic episodes, 173
Aneuploidy
   autosomal, 350
   nondisjunction as cause of, 352, 353–354
   sex chromosomes, 351
Angelman syndrome, 321, 322
Anticipation, in inheritance, 318–319, 319
Apoproteins, 45, 222
Arsenate, 173
Ascorbate (vitamin C), 147
Aspirin, 193
Atherosclerosis, 227–228, 229
ATM gene, and DNA repair, 25, 27
ATP production
   citric acid cycle, 187, 188, 189
   galactose metabolism, 177
   glycolysis, 175, 176
   pyruvate dehydrogenase, 180, 181
Autosomal aneuploidy, 350
Autosomal dominant diseases, 306
   incomplete penetrance for, 315
Autosomal dominant inheritance, 305, 306
Autosomal Dominant Inheritance
   disease associated with. See Autosomal dominant diseases
Autosomal recessive inheritance, 306, 307
   disease associated with, 307
AZT (zidovudine), 23

B

Bacterial toxins, ADP-ribosylation by, 139, 140
Barbiturates, 273
Barr body, 309
Bases, 5
B-DNA, 9
β-globin, 304
β-islet cells, glucose sensing in, 172, 174–175
β-oxidation
   of fatty acids in mitochondria, 239, 241
   of palmitate, 241

Bile duct occlusion, 277
Bilirubin, 276
  jaundice and, 276–277
  metabolism of, 275
Biochemical reactions, 119
  energy and rate comparisons, 120
  Michaelis-Menten equation and plot, 120–121, 121
  one-carbon units in, 269
Biotin, 146
Biotin deficiency, 207
Bisphosphonates, 149
Blood group glycoproteins, 61
Blotting techniques, 99
  ethidium bromide stain, 100
  Northern blots, 100, 103
  probes for, 100–101, 101
  Southern blots, 101, 101–103, 102
  types of, 99
  Western blots, 100, 104
Body mass index (BMI), 371, 372
Brain, 247
  bilirubin damage, 276
  ketogenolysis in, 247
  metabolic fuel patterns in, 164
Branched-chain ketoacid dehydrogenase deficiency (maple syrup disease), 267, 337
BRCA-1 and BRCA-2 gene, 25, 27

C

Calcium homeostasis, 148–150
Carbamoyl phosphate synthetase, 264
Carbohydrate digestion, 169
Carbon monoxide, 192
γ-Carboxylation, vitamin K-dependent, 153, 154
Cardiac muscle, 164, 166
Cardioprotection, omega-3 fatty acids providing, 217
Carnitine acyltransferases, 241, 244
Carotene (vitamin A). See Vitamin A entries
Catecholamine synthesis, 269
cDNA
  gene cloning applications, 90, 96
  produced from mRNA, 88
cDNA (expression) libraries, 89
  and genomic libraries compared, 89
Cell cycle
  eukaryotic, 4
  eukaryotic chromosome replication during, 18, 19
  phases targeted by chemotherapeutic agents, 4
Centimorgan (cM), 385
CFTR protein, 59
Chaperones, 59
Chargaff's rules, 9
Chemical energy, capturing, 191
Chemotherapeutic agents, 4
Chest pain, ischemic, 192
Chloramphenicol, 58
cholecalciferol. See Vitamin D
Cholesterol
  metabolism of, 230–232
  regulation in hepatocytes, 225–226, 226
  synthesis of, 231, 232
Cholesterol ester transfer protein (CETP), 227
Chorionic villus sampling, 397
Chromatin, 11, 11–12, 12
Chromosomal abnormalities
  inversions, 361, 362
  isochromosome, 363
  numerical, 349–355, 354–355
  ring chromosome, 362
  structural, 355–361
  uniparental disomy, 321
Chromosome banding, 348
Chromosomes, 303
  abnormal. See Chromosomal abnormalities
  nomenclature for, 349
Chronic granulomatous disease (CGD), 212
Chronic myelogenous leukemia, 358
Chylomicrons, 222, 224, 225
Ciprofloxacin, 23
Cisplatin, 9
Cis regulatory element, 75
Citrate shuttle, 218
Citric acid cycle, 187–188, 188, 189
  oxidative phosphorylation and, 194
Cloning DNA
  general strategy for, 84
  medical applications, 89, 91, 95, 96
  restriction fragments. See Restriction fragment cloning
Cobalamin deficiency, 270
Collagen
  characteristics of, 63
  co- and posttranslational modifications of, 63–64
  disorders of biosynthesis of, 65
  synthesis of, 64
Colorectal polyposis, hereditary nonpolyposis, 28
Common Diseases. See Multifactorial diseases
Competitive enzyme inhibitor, 122–123, 123
Consanguinity, 307, 340
  health consequences of, 340–341
Cooperative enzyme kinetics, 123, 124, 173
Cori cycle, 208
Cortisol, 78
Cotranslational modifications, 62
  covalent, 62
  of collagen, 63
Cyanide, 192
Cyanocobalamin (B12), 146
Cyclic AMP (cAMP) second messenger system, 134, 134–136, 135, 136
Cystic fibrosis, 59, 93, 94
Cytogenetics
  advances in, 363–364
  chromosomal abnormalities. See Chromosomal abnormalities
  Chromosomal abnormalities definitions and terminology, 348
  definitions and terminology, 347, 348
  overview of, 347
Cytosine deamination, 25

Index

D

dATP, 108
Daunorubicin, 9
   ddATP, 108
Debranching enzyme, 202, 203
Deletions, chromosomal, 360, 360–361
De Novo pathways
   nucleotide synthesis and, 287, 288
   purine synthesis, 292
   pyrimidine synthesis, 288, 290
Deoxyguanosine monophosphate (dGMP), 7, 8
Deoxythymidine, 6
Diabetes
   genetics of, 375
   hyperlipidemia secondary to, 229
Dicer enzyme, 94, 95
   ketogenesis, 246
Diet, recommended, 164
Dihydroxyacetone phosphate (DHAP), 170–171, 175, 239
1,25-Dihydroxycholecalciferol (calcitrol), 149
Diploid cells, 303, 349
Direct genetic diagnosis, 389–393
   and indirect genetic diagnosis compared, 396
Direct mutation testing, PCR in, 108
   sequencing DNA for, 108–109, 109
Disease
   abnormal G proteins and, 139
   multifactorial. *See* Multifactorial diseases
   risk factors and liability for, 371
   single-gene. *See* Single-gene diseases
Disease-causing mutations
   delayed age of onset of, 318
   penetrance of, 311
DNA
   denaturation and renaturation of, 10
   genetic information flow from, 36, 37
   hydrogen-bonded base pairs in, 8, 9
   organization of, 10–12, 11, 12
   polymorphic markers of, 379, 380. *See also* individual markers, e.g., RFLPs
   structure of, 9
   transcription of, 33–34, 36
DNA chips, in genetic diagnosis, 390
DNA gyrase, 23
DNA libraries
   types of. *See also* cDNA (expression) libraries; Genomic
DNA repair, 25, 26, 27
   diseases associated with, 27–28
   tumor suppressor genes and, 25
DNA replication, 3–4, 4, 17–18, 18, 19
   steps in, 21–24, 24
DNA sequencing, direct, 392
DNA synthesis, 20, 20–21
Double helix, 9
Down syndrome, 350
   maternal age and, 352
Doxorubicin, 9

E

E. coli heat stable toxin (STa), 136
Edward syndrome, 350
effects of, 295
Ehlers-Danlos syndromes, 65
Electron shuttles, in glycolysis, 175
Electron transport chain (ETC), 189, 191
   chemical energy and, 191
   inhibitors of, 192–193
   oxidative phosphorylation and, 189, 190, 191
   tissue hypoxia and, 192
Elongation step, in translation, 56, 57, 66
Embryos, preimplantation diagnosis for, 397
Energy
   metabolic sources of, 120, 159, 160. *See also* Metabolic energy
   of chemical reaction, 119–124, 120–124
Enhancers, 74, 75
Environmental factors, 314
   genetic factors vs., 375–376
Enzyme inhibitors
   classification of, 115–116, 116
   drugs as, 122
Enzyme-linked immunosorbent assay (ELISA), 109
Enzyme(s)
   branching, 201
   debranching, 202, 203
   dicer, 94–95, 95
   for pyrimidine synthesis, 291
   genetic deficiencies in glycogen metabolism, 203–205
   HGPRT, purine catabolism and, 293
   in sphingolipid catabolism, genetic deficiencies, 250–251
   kinetics of, 123–128, 124
   phosphodiesterases, 135
   water-soluble vitamins and, 145–146
Epithelium maintenance, vitamin A for, 150
Erythrocytes
   glycolysis in, 175–176
   role of HMP shunt in, 211
Essential amino acids, 119
Ethidium bromide stain, 100
Euchromatin, 12
Eukaryotic cell
   co-expression of genes in, 80
   DNA packaging in, 11, 12
Eukaryotic cell cycle, 4
Eukaryotic chromosome replication, 18, 18–19, 19
Eukaryotic gene expression, 73–74, 74
Eukaryotic messenger RNA, 42
   pre-mRNA transcripts, alternative splicing of, 41, 43
   production of, 40–42, 41–42
Eukaryotic ribosomes, 41, 44
Eukaryotic RNA polymerases, 35
Euploid cells, 349
Euploidy, 349
Exercise, alcohol consumption and, 209
Expression libraries. *See* cDNA (expression) libraries
Expression vectors, 88, 89
Ex vivo gene therapy, 90, 92, 93, 94

F

Fabry disease, 251
$FADH_2$, 189
Familial cancer
  incomplete penetrance in, 316
Fasting
  ketogenolysis in brain during, 247
  prolonged, 164
Fatty acid(s)
  activation of, 218
  biosynthesis of, 218–220, 219
  nomenclature of, 217
  oxidation of, 241, 242, 243–244
  synthase of, 219–220
  unsaturated, 217
Favism, 212
Five-carbon sugars, 5
Fluorescence in situ hybridization (FISH), 364
Fluoroquinolones, 23
FMR1 gene expression, 103
Folate deficiency, 271
Folate mechanism, 270
Folic acid, 146
Founder effect, 337
Fragile X syndrome, 103, 311
  anticipation for, 53, 319
Frameshift mutation, 304
Friedreich ataxia, 53, 319
Fructose
  deficiency of, 179
  intolerance to, hereditary, 180
  metabolism of, 179
Fructose-1,6-bisphosphatase, 207

G

Gain-of-function mutation, 304
Galactose metabolism, 177, 177–178
Galactosemia, 178
Gametes, 303
Gaucher disease, 251
  PCR and RFLP for, 391
G-banding, 348
Gene expression
  embryonic, regulatory proteins in, 79
  glucose and insulin gene, 171
  in eukaryotic cells, regulation of, 73–80, 74
  profiling of (microarrays), 103
  RNA interference, 94–95, 95
Gene flow, 340
Gene replacement therapy
  challenges to, 94
  delivery vectors, 90–94, 91–94
Gene(s), 304
  delivery vectors for, 90, 91–92
  environment vs., diseases and, 375–376
Genetic analysis techniques
  blotting techniques, 99–104
  mapping and linkage analysis, 382–384, 382–386
  polymerase chain reaction, 104–106

Genetic code, 49, 50, 66
Genetic diagnosis
  applications of, 396–397
  indirect, 392–395
  prenatal, 396–397
Genetic drift, 338–339, 339
Genetic fingerprinting, 107, 107–108
Genetic imprinting, in Prader-Willi syndrome, 80
Genetic mosaicism, 309
  in Turner syndrome, 351
Genetic regulation
  eukaryotic, 73–80, 74
  overview, 73
Genetic testing, RFLPs and, 102, 102–103
Genomic libraries, 88
  and cDNA (expression) libraries compared, 89
Genotype, 304
Genotype frequency, 333, 334
Glucagon
  in gluconeogenesis control, 78
  insulin and, opposing activities of, 138
Glucogenic amino acids, 205
Glucokinase
  GLUT 2 and, 171
  hexokinase and, 173
Gluconeogenesis, 205, 206, 207–209
  control by response elements, 78
Glucose-6-phosphatase (G6PDH) deficiency, 203, 204, 207
α1,6 Glucosidase, 203
Glucose transport, 169–171, 170
  palmitate synthesis from, 219
glucose transport and, 171
GLUT 1, 171
GLUT 2, 170, 171
GLUT 3, 171
GLUT 4, 170, 171
Glutamate dehydrogenase, 263
Glutaminase, 263
Glutamine synthetase, 263
Glyceraldehyde 3-phosphate dehydrogenase, 174
Glycerol 3-phosphate, 220, 221
Glycerophospholipids, 221
Glycogenesis, 199
Glycogen granule, 199
Glycogen metabolism, 200
  genetic deficiencies of enzymes in, 203–205
Glycogenolysis, 199, 201, 201–203, 202
Glycogen phosphorylase, 201–202
Glycogen storage diseases, 203–205
Glycogen synthase/synthesis, 199, 200
Glycolysis, 171, 172, 173–174
  ATP production and, 175
  electron shuttles and, 175
  in erythrocyte, 175–176
  intermediates of, 175
Glycoproteins, 61
Glycosyl α1,4:α1,6 transferase, 201
Glycosylation, 61, 62
Gout, 287, 293, 294

G proteins, 133, 134
   in signal transduction, 139
Gray baby syndrome, 58

H
Haploid cells, 349
Haplotype, 384
Hardy-Weinberg equilibrium, 334–335
   for dominant diseases, 336
   in PKU, 335
   practical application of, 335
HDL (high-density lipoprotein), 225, 226
   atherosclerosis and, 227–228, 228, 229
Heme
   catabolism of, bilirubin and, 276
   synthesis of, 271–272, 272
Hemizygotes, 308
Hemochromatosis, 274, 314
   ASO probes in, 389–390, 390
Hemoglobinopathy, 118
Hemolytic crisis, 276
Hepatic glycogen phosphorylase deficiency, 204
Hepatocytes
   cholesterol regulation in, 226, 227–228
   role of HMP shunt in, 210
Hereditary fructose intolerance, 180
Hereditary nonpolyposis colorectal cancer (HNPCC), 28
Hers disease, 204
Heterogenicity, allelic, 314
Heteroplasmy, 313, 314
Heterozygotes, 310
   manifesting, 310
Hexokinase, 173
Hexose monophosphate (HMP) shunt, 209, 209–210, 210
   role of, 210
HGPRT enzyme
   purine catabolism and, 293
   RFLP analysis and, 395
High altitude, adaptation to, 176
HIV testing, 109, 110
Homeodomain proteins, 80
Homocystinemia, 268
Homocystinuria, 268
Homogentisate oxidase deficiency (alcaptonuria), 267
Homologous chromosomes, 303
Hormones
   and signal transduction, 131
   classes of, 132
   lipid-soluble, 140
   water-soluble. *See* Water-soluble hormones
Human Genome Project, 85–89, 86–87
   major goal of, 88
   polymerase chain reaction and, 104
   uses of, 85
Huntington disease, 53
   anticipation for, 318, 319
   delayed age of onset in, 318
   polymerase chain reaction amplification, 106
Hydrophilic amino acids, 115, 117
Hydrophobic amino acids, 115, 116
Hydroxymethylbilane synthase deficiency, 272–273
Hyperammonemia, 261, 289
Hypercholesterolemia, 232
   treatment of, 231
   type IIa (LDL receptor deficiency), 230
Hyperlipidemias, 228–230
   niacin for, 147
   secondary to diabetes, 229
   types of, 229
Hyperuricemia, 294
Hypoglycemia
   alcoholism and, 208, 208–209, 209

I
I-cell disease, 62
IDL, intermediate-density lipoprotein (VDL remnants), 222, 224, 225
Ig heavy chain locus, 75
Imprinting, 323
Indirect genetic diagnosis, 392–395
   and direct genetic diagnosis compared, 396
   in DNA and RNA synthesis, 23
In-frame mutation, 304
Inheritance
   anticipation in, 318–319, 319
   autosomal dominant, 305, 306
   autosomal recessive, 306, 307
   mitochondrial, 313
   mode of, in pedigree, 313
   multifactorial, 372, 373
   X-linked dominant, 311, 312
   X-linked recessive, 308, 308–310, 309
Initiation step, in translation, 54, 56, 57, 66
Insulin
   glucagon and, opposing activities of, 138
   glucose transport and, 170
   potassium and, 165
   recombinant proteins, 89–90, 248
Insulin receptor, 136–137, 137
Interphase nucleus, 12
Inversions, chromosomal, 361, 362
In vivo gene therapy, 90, 92
Iron
   deficiency in, 273, 274
   metabolism of, 275
   transport and storage of, 271–272
Ischemic chest pain, 192
Ischemic episodes, anaerobic glycolysis in, 173
Isochromosome, 363

J
Jaundice, 276–277

K

Karyotype, 347, 348
  nomenclature symbols for, 349
Karyotyping, spectral, 364
Ketogenesis, 246
Ketogenic amino acids, 205
Ketogenolysis, 245, 246, 247
Ketone body metabolism, 245, 245–248, 247
Ketones, measurement of, 248
Ketosis, 248
Kinetics of enzymes, 120–124, 173
Klein-Waardenburg syndrome, 79
Klinefelter syndrome, 351
Knockdown vs. knockout gene silencing, 95

L

Lactate dehydrogenase, 174
Lactose deficiency, 178
Large segment deletions, 52
LDL (low-density lipoprotein), 225
  atherosclerosis and, 227–228, 228, 229
Lead poisoning, 274
Lecithin-cholesterol acyltransferase (LCAT), 227
Lesch-Nyhan disease, 287, 295
  RFLP analysis for, 308, 395
Levofloxacin, 23
Lineweaver-Burk equation and plot, 121, 122
  enzyme inhibition and, 123
Linkage analysis, 379
  gene mapping and, 382–384, 382–386, 383
Lipid digestion, 218
Lipid mobilization, 239, 240
Lipid-soluble hormones, 140
Lipid-soluble vitamins, 148
Lipoprotein(s)
  lipase of, 225
  metabolism of, 222, 224
Liver
  damage to, bilirubin and, 276
  glycogen phosphorylase in, 202
  glycogen synthase in, 200
  hepatic steatosis, 209, 220
  urea cycle in, 264, 264–265
Locus/loci
  heterogeneity of, 316
  imprinting and, 320, 322
  modifier, 314
LOD (log of the odds) scores, recombination frequencies and, 384–385
Long-chain acyl-CoA dehydrogenase (LCAD), 394
Loss-of-function mutation, 304
Lynch syndrome, 28
Lyposomal enzymes
  and phosphorylation of mannose, 62
Lysosomal α1,4 glucosidase deficiency, 203, 205
Lysosomal proteins, synthesis of, 59
Lysosomes, 62

M

Malaria, 338
Malic enzyme, 218
Manifesting heterozygotes, 310
Mannose phosphorylation, 62
Maple syrup urine disease, 267, 337
Marfan syndrome
  pedigree for, 393
  pleiotropy in, 316
Maternal age, Down syndrome risk and, 352
MCAD (medium chain acyl-CoA dehydrogenase) deficiency, 243
McArdle disease, 204
Meiosis, nondisjunction during, 352, 353–354
Membrane proteins, synthesis of, 59
Menkes disease, 65
Messenger RNA (mRNA)
  base pairing of aminoacrl-tRNA and codon in, 54
  cDNA produced from, 88
  eukaryotic, 40–42, 41
  prokaryotic, 35, 40
Metabolic energy
  sources of, 159, 160
  storage of, 160
Metabolic fuel
  patterns in tissue, 164–166
  regulation of, 160–161, 162, 163
Metacentric chromosomes, 349
Methanol poisoning, 123
Methotrexate, as enzyme inhibitors, 122
Methylmalonyl-CoA mutase deficiency, 267
Microarrays (gene expression profiling), 103
Microdeletions, chromosomal, 361
MicroRNA (miRNA), 94–95, 95
Microsatellite, 104
Microsatellite(s), 381
  instability of, 28
Microsatellite sequences, PCR amplification of, 107–108, 108
Missense mutation, 304
Mitochondria
  electron transport chain and, 191
  fatty acid entry into, 241, 242
Mitochondrial diseases, 194, 313
  pedigree for, 313
Mitochondrial DNA mutations, 194–195
Mitochondrial inheritance, 313
Molecular biology, 3, 3–4, 4
Molecular cytogenetics, advances in, 363–364
Mosaicism, 309
  in Turner syndrome, 351
Moxifloxacin, 23
Multifactorial diseases
  recurrence risks for, assessing, 374
  thresholds in males and females, 373
Multifactorial inheritance, 371, 372
Multifactorial threshold model, 372–373, 373
Muscle
  skeletal. See Skeletal muscle

Mutations, 51–54, 66
  disease-causing. *See* Disease-causing mutations
  effects of, 51
  genetic variation in/among populations and, 337
  in mitochondrial DNA, 194–195
  in SHH gene, 79
  in splice sites, 42, 52
  large segment deletions, 52
  new, 317
  single-gene, 304
  trinucleotide repeat expansion, 53
  types of, 52
Myophosphorylase deficiency, 204
Myotonic dystrophy
  anticipation for, 53, 319
  RFLP diagnosis of, 391, 392

N
NADH, in electron transport chain, 189, 210
NADPH, in HMP shunt, 210, 211
Natural selection, 337
Neural tube defects (NTDs), 375
Neurodegenerative disease, diagnosis of, 389
N-glycosylation, 61
Niacin (B3), 146, 147, 239
Nitrogen balance, 119
Noncompetitive enzyme inhibitor, 122–123, 123
Nonsense mutation, 304
N-terminal hydrophobic signal sequence, 61
Nucleases, 18
Nucleic acids, 7–9, 8
  and nucleotide structure, 5, 5–6, 6
  bases in, 5
Nucleofilament structure, in eukaryotic cell, 11
Nucleosides, 5–6, 6
  nomenclature for, 6
Nucleosomes, 11, 11–12, 12
Nucleotides
  nomenclature for, 6
  structure of, 5, 5–7, 6
  synthesis of, 287, 288
Numerical chromosome abnormalities, 349–355

O
Obesity, threshold for and prevalence of, 372, 373
O-glycosylation, 61
Omega-3 fatty acids, cardioprotective effects of, 217
Oncogenes
  translocations involving, 358
One-carbon units, 269
Ornithine transcarbamoylase, 265
Orotic aciduria, 289
Osteogenesis imperfecta, 65
  locus heterogeneity in, 317
Oxidation
  fatty acid, 240, 242, 243–244
  LDL, vitamin E role in, 229

Oxidative phosphorylation, 189, 190, 191
  citric acid cycle and, 194
Oxidized compounds, 272
Oxygen (O_2)
  in electron transport chain, 189
  reactive species, 193

P
Palindromes, DNA sequences, 85, 86, 96
Palmitate
  synthesis from glucose transport, 219
  β-oxidation of, 240
Pantothenic acid, 147
Paracentric inversion, chromosomal, 361, 362
Parasites
  and G6PDH deficiency, 212
  purine synthesis and, 292
Parkinson's disease, 269
Patau syndrome, 351
Paternity testing, 107–108, 109
Pedigree, 305
  for autosomal dominant inheritance, 306
  for autosomal recessive inheritance, 307
  for consanguinity, 340
  for mitochondrial diseases, 313
  for X-linked dominant inheritance, 311, 312
  for X-linked recessive inheritance, 308, 309
  in Marfan syndrome, 393
  mode of inheritance in, decision tree for, 313
  new mutation in, 317
  nomenclature for, 305
Penetrance
  incomplete, in single-gene diseases, 315, 315–316
  of disease-causing mutations, 311
Peptide bond formation, during translation, 55
Pericentric inversion, chromosomal, 361, 362
Peroxisome(s)
  proliferator-activated receptors (PPARs), 77
Phenotype, 304
Phenylalanine Hydroxylase Deficiency. *See* Phenylketonuria (PKU)
Phenylketonuria (PKU), 267
  Hardy-Weinberg equilibrium in, 335
Philadelphia chromosome, 358
Phosphatases, 133, 133–134
Phosphatidylinositol biphosphate (PIP_2) second messenger system, 134, 135
Phosphodiesterases, 135
Phosphoenolpyruvate carboxykinase (PEPCK), 207
  in gluconeogenesis control, 78
Phosphofructokinases, 173
3-Phosphoglycerate kinase, 174
Pleiotropy, 316
Polymerase chain reaction (PCR), 104, 105
  agarose gel electrophoresis and, 106
  allele-specific oligonucleotide (ASO) probes and, 389–390, 390
  genetic fingerprinting using, 107, 107–108
  in direct mutation testing, 108–109, 109
  in HIV testing, 109
  reverse transcriptase, 110

Polymerases, 18
  eukaryotic, 22
  in DNA and RNA synthesis, 20, 20–21
Polymorphic markers, 379–380, 380
Polymorphism, 303
Polysomes, 58
Pompe disease, 203, 205
Population genetics
  genotype and allele frequencies and, 333–334. *See also* Allele frequency; Genotype frequency
  Hardy-Weinberg equilibrium and, 334–335
  variation in, evolutionary factors responsible for, 337–339
Porphobilinogen deaminase (hydroxymethylbilane synthase) deficiency, 272–273
Porphyria cutanea tarda, 273
Porphyrias, 273–274
Postabsorptive state, metabolic profile for, 161, 163
Posttranslational modifications
  covalent, 62, 62–63
  of collagen, 63–64, 63–65, 64
Prader-Willi syndrome, 321, 322
  genetic imprinting in, 80
Pregnancy loss
  reciprocal translocation and, 357
  trisomy and, 351
Prenatal genetic diagnosis, 396–397
Probability, of events, 335
Proband, 305
Probes, blotting techniques and, 100–101, 101
Prokaryotic chromosome replication, 18, 18–19, 19
Prokaryotic messenger RNA production, 35–36, 36
Prokaryotic ribosomes, 44
Prokaryotic RNA polymerases, 34
Prolonged fast (starvation state), 164
Propionic acid pathway, 244, 245
Propionyl-CoA carboxylase deficiency, 267
Proteasomes, 59
Protein folding, 59
Protein kinases, 132–133, 133
Protein(s)
  genetic information flow from DNA to, 36, 37
  in DNA replication, 23
  pre-mRNA production of, 43
  recombinant, 84, 89–90, 96
  regulatory, in embryonic gene expression, 79
  synthesis of. *See* Translation
  targeting of, 59, 60, 61
  turnover of, 118–119
Proton gradient, 191
Protozoans, 292
Punnett square. *See* Recurrence risk
Purine, 5
Purine(s)
  catabolism of, 293, 293–295
  metabolism of, overview, 287, 288
  synthesis of, 292
Pyridoxine. *See* Vitamin B6 (pyridoxine)
Pyrimidine(s), 5, 6
  catabolism of, 291
  metabolism of, overview, 287, 288
  synthesis of, 288–291, 290
Pyruvate carboxylase, 207
Pyruvate dehydrogenase (PDH), 180–181, 181
Pyruvate kinase, 174
  deficiency in, 176

Q
Quinolones, 23

R
R ate, of chemical reaction, 119
Rate, of chemical reaction, 119–124, 120, 120–124
Rb gene, 25, 27
Reciprocal translocation, 356
  after birth, 357
  consequences of, 356
  pregnancy loss and, 357
Recombinant DNA
  medical applications, 89–96, 91–95
Recombinant plasmid, 86
Recombinant proteins, 84, 89–90, 96
Recombination mapping, 384
Recurrence risk, 304
  for autosomal dominant diseases, 306
  for autosomal recessive diseases, 307
  for X-linked dominant diseases, 311
  for X-linked recessive diseases, 308
Red blood cells, 164
Regulation, 160–161
Response elements, in gluconeogenesis control, 78
Resting muscle, 164, 165
Restriction endonucleases, 85, 85–87, 96
  sites for, 381
Restriction fragment cloning
  restriction endonucleases in, 85, 85–87
  using vectors, 86, 87
Restriction maps, 86
Retinal rod cell, signal transduction in, 151, 152
Retroviruses
  gene therapy, 90–91, 91, 94
  reverse transcription, 5, 23
Reverse transcriptase, 23
Reverse transcriptase PCR (RT-PCR), 110
Reverse transcription, of mRNA, 88
RFLPs (restriction fragment length polymorphisms), 381
  and genetic testing, 102–103, 103
  in analysis of PCR products, 391
  indirect genetic diagnosis using, 393–394, 394
  Southern blots and, 101
  VNTR sequences and, 102
Riboflavin (B2), 147
Ribonucleotide reductase, 291
Ribose 5-phosphate, 287
Ribosomal RNA (rRNA), 43, 44
Ribosomes
  free, translation on, 58–59
  peptide bond formation by, 55

Ring chromosome, 362
RNA
　editing of, 45
　production of, 34
　synthesis of, 20, 20–21
　types of, 34
RNA-induced silencing complex (RISC), 94–95, 95
RNA interference (RNAi), 94–95, 95
RNA polymerases, 34–35, 45
RNA processing, 46
Robertsonian translocation, 358–360
Robertsonian translocations, 349, 358–360, 359
Rough endoplasmic reticulum, 58–59

S

Salvage pathways
　nucleotide synthesis by, 287, 288
　purine excretion and, 293
Scavenger receptors (SR-B1), 227
Scurvy, 66, 147–148
Secretory proteins, synthesis of, 59
Sex chromosomes
　allele frequency and, 336
　aneuploidy of, 351
Shiga toxin, 44
Short tandem repeats, 104
Sickle cell disease, 118
　malaria and, 338
　RFLP diagnosis of, 102–103, 103
Signal transduction
　by water-soluble hormones, 132
　hormones and, 131
　in retinal rod cell, 151, 152
Single-gene diseases
　incomplete penetrance in, 316–317
　variable expression in, 314
Single-gene mutations, 304
Skeletal muscle
　glycogen phosphorylase in, 202
　glycogen synthase in, 200
Small interfering RNA (siRNA), 94–95, 95
SNPs (single nucleotide polymorphisms), 381
Somatic cells, 303
Sonic hedgehog (SHH) gene, mutations in, 80
Spectral karyotyping, 364
Sphingolipid catabolism, 250–251
Sphingolipids, 248
　synthesis of, 248, 249
Spinobulbar muscular atrophy, 53
Splice site mutations, 42, 53
Starvation (prolonged fast) state, 164
　ketogenolysis in brain during, 247
Statins, as enzyme inhibitors, 122
Stress, lipolysis of triglyceride and, 239, 240
STRPs (short tandem repeat polymorphisms), 381
　indirect genetic diagnosis using, 393
Structural chromosome abnormalities, 355–361
Submetacentric chromosomes, 349
Subunit assembly, 58
Supercoiling, DNA, 10

T

Tay-Sachs disease, 250
Telomerase, 22–23
Termination step, in translation, 55, 56, 66
Tetrahydrofolate synthesis, 270
Thiamine (B1), 146
Thiamine deficiency, 182
Thymine dimer repair, 25, 26
Tissue hypoxia, 192
Traits, concordance rates in twin studies, 374
Transaminases, 263
Transcription, 34, 35, 36, 46
　overview of, 33, 34
　posttranscription editing, 45
Transcription factors, in eukaryotic gene expression regulation, 75, 76–77
　general, 76
　properties of, 76
　specific, 77–78
Transfer RNA (tRNA), 44, 45
　and amino acid activation, 53–54, 54
Transgenes. *See also* Gene replacement therapy
Translation
　amino acid activation for, 54, 54–55
　amino acids for, tRNA and, 44, 45
　inhibitors of, 58
　modifications after. *See* Posttranslational modifications
　on free ribosomes, 58–59
　on rough endoplasmic reticulum, 58–59
　overview of, 49
　peptide bond formation during, 55, 55–56
　RNA interference, 94–95, 95
　steps in, 55–57, 56, 67
Translocations, 355
　involving oncogenes, 358
Transport kinetics, 124
Trans regulatory element, 75
Triglyceride(s), 222
　glycerophospholipids and, 221
　insulin and, 165
　synthesis of, 220–221, 221
Trinucleotide repeat expansion, 53
Triple repeat expansions, diseases associated with, 319
Triploidy, 350
Trisomy 21, 350
　maternal age and, 352
Tumor suppressor genes
　and DNA repair, 25
Turner syndrome, 351
Tyrosine kinase, 136–137, 137

U

Ubiquitin, 59
UDP-glucuronyl transferase deficiency, 277
Uncouplers, 193

Uniparental disomy, 321
Unsaturated fatty acids, 217
Upstream promotor elements, 75
Urea cycle, 264, 264–265
   genetic deficiencies of, 265
Uric acid, excessive, 295
Uridine monophosphate (UMP), 7, 8

V

VDL remnants (IDL, intermediate-density lipoprotein), 225
Vectors
   for gene delivery, 90–94, 91–94, 96
   restriction fragment cloning using, 85, 86, 97
Verotoxin, 44
Viral load, measuring in AIDS patients, 110
Viruses, as gene delivery vector, 90–94, 91–94, 96
Vision, vitamin A and, 151, 152
Vitamin A (carotene), 150–151
Vitamin A deficiency, 148, 153
Vitamin A toxicity, 153
Vitamin B6 (pyridoxine), 147
   deficiency, 273, 274
Vitamin B12 (cobalamin) deficiency, 271, 289
Vitamin C deficiency, 155
Vitamin D
   calcium homeostasis and, 149
   deficiency, 148, 150
   synthesis and activation of, 148, 149
   toxicity, 150
Vitamin E deficiency, 148
Vitamin E (α-tocopherol), 148, 156
   role in LDL oxidation, 229
Vitamin K, 149
   anticoagulant therapy and, 156
   carboxylation dependent on, 154
Vitamin K deficiency, 155
   and vitamin C deficiency compared, 154, 155
Vitamins. *See also* individual vitamins
   homocystinemia caused by deficiencies in, 268
   lipid-soluble, 148
   water-soluble, 145–146
VLDL (very low-density lipoprotein), 224, 225
   metabolism of, 224
VNTR (variable number of tandem repeat) sequences, 381
   RFLPs and, 102
von Gierke disease, 204

W

Water-soluble hormones, 132
   cyclic AMP and PIP_2 second messenger systems and, 134, 134–136, 135
   G proteins and, 132–133, 133, 134
   insulin receptor and (tyrosine kinase), 136–137, 137
   protein kinase activation by, 133, 133–134
   signal transduction by, 132
Water-soluble vitamins, 145–146
Watson-Crick DNA, 9
Well-fed (absorptive) state, metabolic profile for, 161, 162

X

X chromosomes, 303, 347
   inactivation of, 309, 310
Xeroderma pigmentosum, 28
X-linked dominant inheritance, 311
   diseases associated with, 312
X-linked recessive inheritance, 308
   disease associated with, 308
   X inactivation in, 309, 310

Y

Y chromosomes, 303

Z

Zellweger syndrome, 77
Zinc-protoporphyrin complex, 274

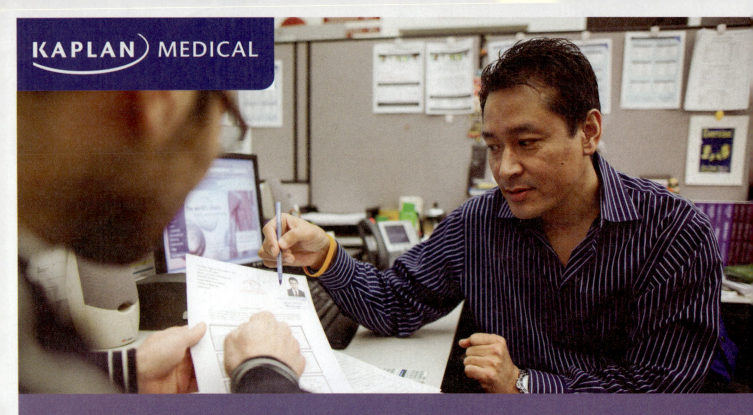